Nursing Ethics Through the
Life Span
second edition

Elsie L. Bandman, RN, EdD, FAAN
Professor of Nursing
Hunter-Bellevue School of Nursing
Hunter College of the City University of New York
New York, New York

Bertram Bandman, PhD
Professor of Philosophy
Brooklyn Campus, Long Island University
Brooklyn, New York

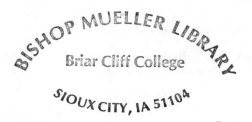
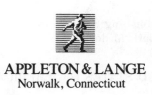
APPLETON & LANGE
Norwalk, Connecticut

0-8385-7052-6

Notice: Our knowledge in clinical sciences is constantly changing. As new information becomes available, changes in treatment and in the use of drugs become necessary. The authors and the publisher of this volume have taken care to make certain that the doses of drugs and schedules of treatment are correct and compatible with the standards generally accepted at the time of publication. The reader is advised to consult carefully the instruction and information material included in the package insert of each drug or therapeutic agent before administration. This advice is especially important when using new or infrequently used drugs.

90 91 92 93 94 / 10 9 8 7 6 5 4 3 2 1
Prentice Hall International (UK) Limited, *London*
Prentice Hall of Australia Pty. Limited, *Sydney*
Prentice Hall Canada, Inc., *Toronto*
Prentice Hall Hispanoamericana, S.A., *Mexico*
Prentice Hall of India Private Limited, *New Delhi*
Prentice Hall of Japan, Inc., *Tokyo*
Simon & Schuster Asia Pte. Ltd., *Singapore*
Editora Prentice Hall do Brasil Ltda., *Rio de Janeiro*
Prentice Hall, Inc., *Englewood Cliffs, New Jersey*

Library of Congress Cataloging-in-Publication Data

Bandman, Elsie L.
  Nursing ethics through the life span/Elsie Bandman, Bertram Bandman.—2nd ed.
     p.   cm.
  Includes bibliographies and index.
  ISBN 0-8385-7052-6
  1. Nursing ethics.   I. Bandman, Bertram.   II. Title.
  [DNLM: 1. Ethics, Nursing. WY 85 B214n]
  RT85.B33 1990
  174'.2—dc20
  DNLM/DLC
  for Library of Congress   89-6522
                                                                   CIP

RT
85
,B33
1990

Acquisitions Editor: Marion K. Welch
Editorial Service: Tage Publishing Service, Inc.
Production Editor: Mary Beth Miller
Designer: Janice Barsevich

PRINTED IN THE UNITED STATES OF AMERICA

*With fond recollections of Albert and Erna Bandmann
and to our daughter, Nancy Bandman, who adds joy and
meaning to life.*

Contents

Preface

We are gratified at the reception of this book's first edition. We have heard suggestions from students and colleagues and have tried to incorporate these into our revision. Between the first edition and this revision several issues, concepts, and topics in health care have had significant impact on nursing. One is the issue of the just allocation of scarce health care resources in the face of an ever increasing world population, especially that of the elderly. The issue is to decide who gets how much of the available goods of health care in a world of finite resources. The marvels of diagnosis, treatment transplants, and such life-supportive procedures as fetal intervention and artificial organs raise critical issues of allocation.

A further development is the current emphasis on virtue ethics, including the ethics of caring. We have tried to explain this development in relation to rights-based ethics. We believe virtues such as wisdom, courage, responsibility, commitment, and caring complement, rather than oppose, values associated with social justice such as respect for rights.

Our aim in this revision of our book is to increase its usefulness to our readers. The students enrolled in our courses for whom this text was required generously shared their opinions regarding the book's content and its format. Nursing colleagues attending national, regional, state, and local meetings graciously and often spontaneously shared their experiences in teaching nursing ethics using this book. Consequently, the revisions reflect these suggestions. The expanding development and use of medical technology was emphasized in the text wherever it became a critical factor as in the reproductive phase of development. The particular moral problems of human immunodeficiency disease syndrome (AIDS) were discussed throughout the book consistent with the disease's presence throughout the life span. The content allocated to discussion of the models of morality was increased from one to two chapters. The chapter on decision making that includes fallacies is completely new. To sharpen the relation between the parts of the book, we have reduced the parts from three to two. These now read: The Moral Foundations of Decision Making in Nursing, and Nursing Ethics Through the Life Span.

We wish to express our thanks to Marion Kalstein-Welch for her unfailing enthusiasm and support for our work.

Elsie L. Bandman
Bertram Bandman
New York City
1989

Preface to the First Edition

This book is about the moral problems of everyday nursing practice. These problems occur throughout the life span of clients. Emphasis is on the nurse's role in moral reasoning and evaluation of these problems, leading to effective and justified decision making.

As clinicians, managers, patient advocates, counselors, and teachers in health care delivery systems, nurses are key figures in developing a moral climate for health consumers and providers alike. This book provides a developmental framework for the application of relevant ethical principles. This framework consists of models of nurse-patient-physician relationship, and of guidelines to decision making and critical reasoning as the foundation of nursing practice. Ethical frameworks and decision making guidelines are essential to the nurse practitioner who cares for clients receiving complex technology, radical surgery, and potent drugs.

Among important values affecting clients and nurses are their rights. Human rights are not artifacts to be left in the reception rooms of clinics and hospitals. Everyday problems show that rights are morally significant to health care participants. Rights in health care are individual passports; permits and licenses to acceptable health care standards which promote maximal self-determination and well-being. To paraphrase John Rawls, as truth is to the realm of facts and descriptions, so rights based on justice are to social institutions. Human ideas and institutions without truth and rights are empty. Applying rights to nursing practice, persons are regarded as centers of self-determination and well-being. Concepts of universality, justice, utility, and altruism, complement rights at the core of client-nurse-physician relationships.

Selection of one principle over another for a given case is less a matter of preference than of careful weighing of relevant diagnostic, prognostic, and treatment data in the context of the client's goals, values, and rational life plans. These considerations merge into the more general concern for the client's well being expressed in shared decision making. This work applies nursing strategies, guidelines, and canons of critical reasoning to the making of ethically justifiable decisions. Due regard is given moral assumptions, inductive and deductive inferences, and exposure of fallacies in argument as keys to sound and justifiable conclusions.

The organization of this book is intended to serve a variety of institutional purposes. First, the book can serve as the basis for a complete course on nursing ethics. Each chapter can be used for one, two, or three classes a week dealing with the topic, themes, and cases of the chapter. The book will cover a whole semester, giving the student a deepening understanding of the moral problems relevant to each developmental epoch of the life span. The role of the nurse is extensively developed.

A second use of the book is as a companion text in the core nursing courses of the integrated curriculum. However the curriculum is formulated, whether from a human-development, adaptation, crisis, systems, research, or health-deviations perspective, this text is useful for developing the ethical aspects of nursing care throughout the life span. Thus, the book can be used profitably throughout the entire curriculum over several years.

A third use of this book is in courses that examine the foundations and trends in nursing from a broad social and historical view. Knowledge of the ethics of nursing fulfills the essential criterion of a professional as one practicing within the framework of an ethical code based on moral principles. This book aims to provide a beacon for future development of the role of the nurse as patient advocate in health care policy formulation.

The fourth use of this book is to provide practitioners with essential knowledge relevant to the ethical problems that arise in everyday practice. Actual cases are presented with discussion aimed at showing the relevance of ethical principles to nursing practice. The roles of nurses are developed in relation to each developmental epoch in the life span.

The book is organized into three major divisions and may be used in any sequence. Part One discusses the moral significance and foundations of nurse-client-physician relationships. Nursing models, roles and professional codes are analyzed and evaluated. Part Two focuses on models of morality, values and priorities, and critical reasoning as worthy guidelines to effective decision making. Resulting principles and guidelines in nursing ethics are then put to work in the third and largest part of the book, the application of nursing ethics throughout the life span. The third part begins with the procreative family and progresses through the life span. Systematic moral-philosophical consideration is given to nursing problems in the procreative family, abortion, infancy, childhood, adolescence, adulthood, the aging, and the dying.

Each chapter presents actual cases which are typical of those encountered in each developmental stage. Analysis of the ethical issues and problems is designed to help connect the underlying ethical principles with nursing practice as a basis for problem resolution. These features point to an enriched role for the place of reason in nursing ethics.

In Part One, Chapter 1, the moral foundations and significance of nursing as a humanistic profession are explored. Chapter 2 examines and analyzes models of patient, nurse, and physician relationships. Chapter 3 evaluates the ethical codes of nursing and medicine. Part Two, Chapter 4, can be used first, since it presents an orientation to the dominant ethical principles and values relevant to health care. This is followed by two chapters on decision making. Chapter 5 deals with nursing strategies and guidelines, and Chapter 6 with critical reasoning. Both chapters bear directly on facilitating shared decisions of the client with the interdisciplinary health care team. Part Three can be used first for provoking student thinking about specific ethical problems relevant to particular developmental epochs from infancy to death. This can be interspersed with examination of Chapter 4, "Models of Morality in Everyday Nursing Practice," and with the chapters on ethical decision making, followed by chapters in Part One. We are suggesting that at most points, the book moves freely from the general to the particular and vice versa. This maximizes its flexibility for use.

In closing, we wish to express our appreciation to Richard Lampert, editor-in-chief, for his interest and helpfulness throughout the development of this work, and to Marion Kalstein, Kathleen Kelly, and Kevin McKenna for its successful completion. Moreover, we appreciate the works and encouragement of colleagues and friends in nursing ethics, most notably Catherine P. Murphy, Philip Pecorino, Arthur Caplan, Anne J. Davis, Mila A. Aroskar, Leah Curtin, Josephine M. Flaherty, James F. Childress, Myra Levine, James L. Muyskens, Andrew Jameton, Rick Moody, Sally Gadow, Stewart Spicker, and Sister Marie Celeste Allen.

Elsie L. Bandman
Bertram Bandman
New York City
1985

PART ONE
Moral Foundations of Decision Making in Nursing

CHAPTER 1

The Moral Significance of Nursing

Study of this chapter enables the learner to:

1. Give reasons for the importance of moral education for nurses.
2. Justify the participation of nurses in moral decisions affecting individuals, groups, families, and health care delivery.
3. Understand definitions of nursing as premises for reasoned arguments and choice in nursing ethics.

INTRODUCTION

The contribution of the art and science of nursing to health care is a proud chapter in the history of humankind. Primary commitment to the health and well-being of the client and family is a characteristic of nursing. Nurses continue to respond to the health needs of people in an evolving scientific and technological society.

The persistent thread that runs throughout nursing history is the continuity of care and nurture of human beings regardless of status or diagnosis.[1] In return, society recognizes the profession's authority and expects members of the profession to act responsibly. Self-regulation is a characteristic of an accountable, therefore mature, profession.[2] The nurse's interaction with the patient is guided by moral principles of "respect for human dignity and the uniqueness of the client."[3] The nurse is expected to meet the patient's health care needs with concerns for the client's safety and best interests uppermost. The nurse's diagnosis of the patient's health needs is based on assessment processes of physical, psychological, and social responses of the client as well as perception of the individual as a whole human being who values life.

WHY NURSING ETHICS?

Through advances in medical technology, the opportunities for intervening in patient destiny by restoring heartbeat, respiration, and other vital functions are many. The future promises even more ways of controlling vital functions and altering body parts. Nurses are part of these interventions. At the primary level of prevention and care, patients and families look to "their" nurses for information, advice, and support when facing difficult decisions of this nature. At the secondary level of curative care, nurses are actively involved in monitoring and sustaining treatment modalities such as life-support systems. At a societal level, nurses are or are expected to be actively involved in policy formulation within the health organization, in professional societies, and in legislative bodies.

Thus, nursing is part of the health care delivery system. More than in any other discipline, the practitioner of nursing is in continuous contact with the patient and the family. This position offers unique privileges and responsibilities. Nurses are privy to the patient's most intimate fears, hopes, and regrets. The family's relationship to the patient becomes vividly clear as the illness strips interactions of veneer and superficiality. The depth of the family's care or lack of concern and respect for the patient is revealed as illness progresses. By word and deed, the nurse manifests to the family a sense of caring and of fundamental human dignity. Thereby, the nurse contributes to a positive change in the immediate family relations with the patient and with other members of the interdisciplinary health team.

Nurses strive to meet universal human needs for care in illness, the promotion of health, and the prevention of disease. Nurses seek to conserve that which is of value to every individual—the optimum functioning of all body systems and of the whole as an integrated unit. Above all, nursing is a human health service that has the quality of mercy and the potential for ennobling both the provider and the recipient. Nursing's practice "is concerned with humans and is humanizing."[4] A central concern of this practice is to enhance the personhood and the humanity of all involved in care.[5]

Indeed, we identify the nursing of the well and the sick with doing good. But why is nursing good? It is good because nursing aims at doing good in common-sense terms. For example, when we say "Nurse Smith is giving nursing care to Mr. Jones," we mean that Nurse Smith is doing good by providing whatever nursing assistance is of value to Mr. Jones in gaining health. In fact, we identify nursing with the good so naturally that it becomes both a contradiction and morally reprehensible to say, "Nurse Smith aims to harm Mr. Jones." If nurses intend to do good, why do we need nursing ethics?

Good intentions are not enough, since knowledge or ignorance of alternatives is also a cause of good or harm. Reasons for choosing one alternative over another, or refusing treatment altogether, need to be critically examined in relation to other possibilities. Moreover, nurses do not wish to impose their treatment choices on other persons whose autonomy is to be supported. The nurse's beliefs concerning the good life may differ from those of the patient. It is precisely this difference that needs to be acknowledged and respected as a mark of personhood and separateness. Knowledge, therefore, of the views that support reasons for one choice over another are indispensable to the nurse in daily practice and in everyday life. Thus, the function of nursing ethics is to guide the activity of nursing on behalf of the good.

WHAT IS ETHICS? WHAT IS NURSING ETHICS?

A preliminary but useful definition of ethics is that it is concerned with doing good and avoiding harm. Nursing decisions affect people. Nurses thereby have the power to do good or harm to their patients. Possibilities of good or harm depend partly on factual knowledge and partly on values. Both must be consciously and critically evaluated for their potential of good or harm to human beings, well or sick.

An example of good is to educate the patient to continue taking medication and to follow the prescribed diet, if doing so is rationally demonstrable. An example of harm is to avoid and thus deny the nursing needs of a difficult patient, such as an AIDS patient or one who does not conform to the nurse's values. Another example of harm is to withhold information and counseling needed so that the patient can make a decision with which the nurse may not agree.

WHAT IS GOOD OR HARM?

The question arises: What is good and what is harmful? Good for whom? Harmful to whom? The nurse, for example, may unavoidably cause pain to a patient in the process of passing tubes, injecting fluids and drugs, and irrigating openings—all of which may be essential to that individual's survival.

Sometimes it is not possible to do good to someone without also doing harm to that person. A nurse who acts to benefit clients by relieving suffering, restoring and promoting health, or preventing diseases is doing good. The good accrues primarily to the patient. The nurse who consciously practices competently, and intelligently, is also doing good and receiving benefit from the professional and financial recognition of self, fellow professionals, workers, clients, and families.

But dilemmas about how to do good and avoid harm arise. A

dilemma is defined as a problem none of whose solutions is satisfactory. For example, a 38-year-old primipara has an amniocentesis that reveals the fetus as having Down's syndrome. The woman wants very much to give birth. Whereas "good" and "harm" are not always so easily defined, we can find a clue to the good in the example of what the pregnant woman wants, namely, to give birth. The dilemma involves her thwarted will: she cannot give birth to a normal child from this pregnancy. In her thwarted will, we find a clue also to the meaning of the harmful and bad. The mother considers the destruction of the fetus as a harmful act that destroys a life. The woman's husband rejects the possibility of a retarded child and feels the marriage will be destroyed as a consequence. This example gives us still another insight into the problem of defining good and bad.

WHAT IS THE GOOD LIFE?

The good life is a lot of things—a sense of physical well-being; health and safety; activities; processes; and goals pursued and achieved; obstacles removed; all without harm to anyone. We have seen that one of the necessary conditions of a good life is health. A means to health is achieved through nursing.

HEALTH AS A GOAL OF THE GOOD LIFE

The practice of nursing is concerned with doing good. One of the goods and one of the highest values of nursing is its concern with the goals of the good life. Health is conducive to and is part of the good life. On this, Aristotle seems to have had a far better argument than Kant, who held that even good health may inspire pride and thus detract from a person's "good will," which, he argued, is the only unconditional good.[6,7] Aristotle had argued that health is a necessary condition of a completely happy life.

Aristotle also held that the good life for humans, which consists in "living well," depends on the full use of one's limbs and one's senses of sight, hearing, smell, taste, and touch.

FIVE KINDS OF ETHICAL ISSUES IN NURSING

We may single out five kinds of ethical issues in nursing. The first of these issues concerns quantity versus quality of life. A parent asks a nurse to "pull the plug" on her 14-year-old boy who has been comatose for 8 months. The question at issue is: What is the morally justifiable position of the nurse? Nurses are in a position to influence questions concerning the quality of life versus the quantity of life. Families ask nurses whether comatose patients with tubes and needles in nearly every bodily orifice are justifiably kept alive.

A second issue concerns freedom versus control and prevention of harm. One example of individual freedom versus control and prevention of harm is that of a frail, elderly patient who wishes not to have a locking waistbelt, but to walk about freely. This freedom is in conflict with the health care team's effort to prevent harm to this patient. Another example is forced feeding of a patient who refuses to eat on grounds of individual rights and freedom. The film *Whose Life Is It Anyway?* further illustrates the issue of freedom versus prevention of harm. Harrison, the paraplegic patient, argues for the right to die and the health professional argues for the conflicting principle of trying to prevent harm to him. A further example is a nurse's freedom to strike for better working conditions and quality care versus the hospital's efforts to prevent harm to patients.

A third issue that critical thinking illuminates is truth-telling versus deception or lying. Reasons for deception and lying are to get one's way, to avoid harm by withholding bad news, or to conceal an abuse pattern, such as alcoholism or narcotic addiction. A further dilemma occurs for a colleague who discovers the abuse and has to decide whether to join in the concealment effort or "blow the whistle" by telling the truth. A third dilemma occurs if the substance abuser threatens to reveal something that is of a vital professional or personal interest to the would-be whistle blower. An implication of these dilemmas is this final dilemma of what to do about a health professional who is a substance abuser and in a position to cause serious harm to patients. Another example of the issue of truth-telling versus deception is the proverbial "sink test" for certain urine specimens. Here a laboratory technician takes a specimen to be analyzed, pours it down the sink, and lies about the findings.

A fourth issue is the desire for knowledge in opposition to religious, political, economic, and ideological interests. Faith healing may be preferred over scientific medicine. Research is poorly rewarded by society as investigation often raises disturbing questions about the status quo. Research about cigarettes or a sugar substitute may provide evidence that conflicts with economic interests. Commercial and military interests in research are supported far more extensively than research related to health care or environmental safety. A recent example of knowledge versus opposing interests, religious in nature, is the decision of some states to teach Creationism in addition or in preference to traditional biological theories of evolution.

A fifth issue is that of conventional, scientifically based therapy versus alternative, nonscientific therapies. A classic case of nursing is that of a nurse who advocated Laetrile as an alternative to chemotherapy for treating a patient with cancer. Further examples of ethical nonscientific alternative therapies include faith healing and Christian science.

Nursing conflicts generally occur within these five kinds of issues, some of which overlap.

METHODS OF MORAL REASONING

Various efforts and approaches have been developed to help resolve these and related ethical issues. To clarify what ethics is, we consider four methods of moral reasoning.

Formal Aspect. One method of reasoning in ethics is formal, which may be expressed through a professional code. According to the *Code for Nurses*, a code of ethics makes explicit the primary goals and values of the profession. When individuals become nurses, they make a moral commitment to uphold the values and special moral obligations expressed in their code.[8]

The *Code For Nurses* states universal moral principles that "prescribe and justify nursing actions. The most fundamental of these principles is respect for persons, autonomy, beneficence (doing good), nonmaleficence (avoiding harm), veracity (truth-telling), confidentiality (respecting privileged information), fidelity (keeping promises) and justice (treating people fairly)."[9]

The formal mode of ethics deduces what decisions to make on the basis of previously agreed upon principles of ethics. An example of the formal approach to ethics is an ethical system derived from religion that has a creed, code and cult that implies moral rules, such as the Ten Commandments.

Benner and Wrubel cite formal beliefs as long-term change agents for health. "For example, most Americans now have the formal belief that cigarette smoking is harmful."[10] This formalized belief becomes a force for change and the basis for rules that prohibit smoking in public places.

The formal method of reasoning in nursing has several advantages and drawbacks. A major advantage is that if one accepts a moral principle, like doing good, and one notices a health professional harming a patient, one knows that person to be wrong. One serious drawback, however, with the formal method of considering nursing ethics is that it is too inflexible to be useful. A second drawback is that there may be conflicting interpretations of a given value, which cannot all be implemented. A third problem with a formal method of moral reasoning is that nurses do not always feel motivated to implement moral principles of care.

Conventional, Empirical, or Sociological Approaches to Ethics. A second approach in moral reasoning is a conventional or sociological method, in which one elicits moral conduct from an empirical study of one's culture or customs. Nurses in the 1920s, for example, stood up when a physician entered a room and "obeyed" medical orders without question.

A strength of the conventional approach to moral reasoning is that "Custom is king."[11] Herodotus's saying supports behavior that is like most other peoples'. Conventional moral principles like "doing good," "avoiding harm," "truth-telling," and "promise-keeping" gain their appeal by being frequently practiced. These principles rule out murder, rape, theft, and abuse as morally impermissible. Conventional ethics provide us with the core of morality.

A disadvantage, however, of conventional reasoning is the possibility of its becoming static and preventing progressive social changes. If nurses obeyed physician's orders in the 1920s, that does not imply that nurses should do so now or at any time in the future. Independent nursing judgment may augment a physician's clinical judgment. Decisions may be made jointly and be better as a result.

Conventional ethics can be helpful for understanding and acting on core problems of ethics. They do not, however, always help one to understand or justify acting on problems that fall outside the core. In the fringes of ethics, one finds puzzles, dilemmas, and controversial questions which cannot be easily decided. The issue of euthanasia presents an example. One would have to look beyond conventional ethics to justify its acceptance.

Philosophical Models of Morality. The difficulties of the formal and conventional methods of reasoning lead one to consider a third approach to morality. This occurs if one identifies ethics with some philosophical model and shows the interplay and dialogue between such models. In this sense, ethics is more like an art than a formal or factual science.

One method of moral reasoning is to argue by analogy. An example of an analogy in ethics is to compare a fetus to a child by calling it an unborn child or to compare a pregnant woman to a landlady.

Another method of moral reasoning is to refute an argument. One example of refutation is showing that a moral principle is inconsistent. Socrates showed this when Cephalus, a contemporary, told Socrates that the key to a good life is always to return what one has borrowed. Socrates then asked, "What if a man lent you a weapon, then went mad and asked for the weapon to be returned?"[12] The clear implication is that one does not return a weapon to a madman, and therefore the principle "Always return what is lent" is refuted.

Philosophical ethics is about the justification of feelings, principles, and methods of moral reasoning. Unexamined values alone are insufficient as grounds for ethical choices for both patients and nurses. Judgments concerning what is the good are so important in their effect on human life that they warrant critical examination.

There are generally 8 to 14 viable philosophical models of morality. Everyone in search of the meaning of good and its relevance to nursing is involved in philosophical discourse and argues for or against one or more of these models of morality. For example, such an argument may occur when trying to answer the question: Should an elderly patient have a locking waistbelt for his or her protection, or should the patient's refusal of a locking waistbelt to prevent falls be supported?

A strength in appealing to philosophical models of morality is that one does not have to agree to unquestioning authority to settle ethical problems. One is quite free to argue against any, or almost all, existing ethical models. The pro-euthanasia nurse may say, "To *me*, killing that poor old suffering patient is morally permissible." A difficulty with appealing to philosophical models of morality is that one is stripped of a centralized bureau of standards, or umpire, to appeal disputable cases.

Intuition in Moral Reasoning. According to a fourth approach to ethics, one may use ethics in its everyday intuitive role. In this sense, ethics may be revealed through a figure in literature, such as Platon Karataef, a wise peasant in Tolstoy's *War and Peace,* or through Huck in Twain's *The Adventures of Huckleberry Finn.* This is the everyday common sense of the person in the street who expresses moral views.

An attempt to provide an ethical justification may make reference to all four methods. A model of morality usually emphasizes one or more, but not all, of these approaches. Thus, ethics has objective aspects, as well as subjective and relativistic ones. A mistake some people make in considering ethics in nursing or any other field is to regard ethics as exclusively formal, scientific, philosophic, or a matter of everyday intuition. Ethics is a composite of all four methods.

THE ROLE OF CARE IN NURSING ETHICS

One example of a model of morality is the caring model, oriented by an older Agapistic or altruistic model developed by medieval Christian philosophers, such as St. Thomas Aquinas (1225?–1275).

Caring is a form of doing good and avoiding harm and so is central both to ethics and to nursing ethics. So powerful a concept is caring in nursing that it is a contradiction to say with approval, "Nurse White didn't care for her patients." To say this is to condemn the nurse. Underlying the model of caring is the concept of caring. The concept of caring is the rubric, the frame within which all nursing that is moral and centered on the well-being of humans occurs.

The models of morality analyzed and applied throughout this book are means, guidelines, beacons, and principles that guide the nurse's conduct toward patients, fellow professionals, families, institutions, and society. Benner and Wrubel aptly illustrate the concept of caring. "I went into the room and he yelled at me, 'Are you listening?' I said yes pretty calmly, and he began crying softly and talking. He knew I was listening." Mary Culname, R.N.[13]

To Benner and Wrubel, caring means that "persons, events, projects, and things matter to people."[14] Caring covers "a range of involvements, from romantic love to parental love to friendship, from caring for one's garden to caring about one's work to caring for and about one's patients."[15]

Here are some examples of sentences using the word *care*. (1) Be careful; (2) Take care; (3) Handle with care; (4) That mother and father care for their children; (5) The members of that couple care for each other; (6) She cares for her roses; (7) He cares for his grandmother; (8) Alan Jones, R.N. cares for Steve Moss, his 92-year-old patient; (9) Ms. Bariel, R.N. cares for that abused child in Room 403; (10) Some countries guarantee a right to health care; (11) Some poor people received a "care" package. One can see from these examples that to care is to give of oneself to an object or persons.

According to Benner and Wrubel, caring is a response to stress.[16] Stress, in turn, is connected to suffering. Caring is a form of coping, helping those in distress. Nursing is an aid in restoring other people's health care interests.[17] Nurses care by relieving stress and distress in their patients. Caring is commitment, manifest in persistent assistance to stress. Care is practiced with a particular patient. This may explain the appeal of the slogan, "Individualize treatment." It may also represent respect for persons as individuals with varying needs, desires, goals, values, and life styles.

Care in the Context of the Feminist Framework

The care framework well-presented by Benner and Wrubel, has its underpinnings in recent feminist writings, such as the work of C. Gilligan[18] and N. Noddings.[19] According to Gilligan, writers like Rawls, Sandel, and Kohlberg who focus on rights, justice, and fairness, along with aggression and assertiveness, appeal to a masculine orientation in ethics. In contrast, virtues such as love, caring, nurturing, and sympathy appeal to a feminine orientation. To Gilligan, women develop an " 'ethic of care' " whose underlying logic is a psychological logic of relationships, which constrasts with the (generally male) formal logic of fairness that informs the justice approach."[20]

To Noddings, caring is reflected in a mother's choosing to save her child over a neighbor's if both are drowning and the mother can only reach one.[21,22] The ethics of caring, rather than the ethics of equality, universality, or impartiality, guides the mother's ethical decision making. To Noddings, "caring lies at the very heart of morality and gives it stability.[23] The ethics of caring is part of the virtue ethics, the appeal to qualities of character, like courage, generosity, commitment, and responsibility.

Three Philosophical Sources of Appeal in the Ethics of Caring

An ethics of caring gains its appeal from several sources. One is the Aristotelian emphasis on the development of natural virtues, such as prudence, wisdom, temperance, and courage. P. Foot, citing John Hersey's *A Single Pebble,* puts it well:

> It was the head tracker's marvelous swift response that captured my admiration at first, his split second solicitousness when he heard a cry of pain, his finding in mid air, as it were, the only way to save the injured boy. But there was more to it than that. His action . . . showed a deep . . . love of life, a compassion, an optimism, which made me feel very good.[24,25]

See Chapter 4 for a further development of Aristotle's happiness-based ethics.

A question for the supporters of the ethics of caring is not only how well this view helps to resolve questions of ethics, such as charges of subjectivity and relativism, but also how well the ethics of caring helps us resolve major ethical issues in nursing. In succeeding chapters, we will consider this question.

Another source of the ethics of caring is found in altruism or love-based ethics, presented by St. Thomas Aquinas, who saw virtues oriented by religion as pivotal to the good life. A third source of the ethics of caring is found in the early Greek hedonists and later in Hume's utilitarianism, which bases ethics on people's wants and likes and the avoidance of people's dislikes and aversions.

CONCLUSION

Throughout the historical evolution of nursing, health has been regarded as a primary value with nursing playing a central role in helping individuals, families, groups, and society to achieve maximum health potential. Nurses accord high value to the concept of total well-being. Nursing practice presupposes the value of care as essential to a conception of the good. However nursing is defined, the central question of nursing ethics remains: What are morally justifiable reasons for my nursing actions? This text will address these and related questions to provide clarification and illumination.

Nursing is a moral activity. Nursing consists in doing good to patients and avoiding harm. A variety of ethical values, some of which conflict with one another, orient nursing and are well-expressed in the *Code for Nurses*. These include beneficence, nonmaleficence, justice, fidelity, veracity, and respect for the patient's autonomy. A pivotal ethical value perceived by nurses is the concept of caring. This concept has been well-identified in the theory and practice of nursing, even though it presents conceptual difficulties in its application.

Discussion Questions

1. Can one be happy without health? Is Aristotle or Kant right about this? Can one be happy if one is poor? Are people who are rich, good looking, smart, healthy, and who have good parents, good children, and good friends happier than those who are poor, ugly, stupid, sick, and who have bad parents, bad children, bad friends, or no friends? Defend your answer.
2. How is nursing an ethical activity?
3. How does technology affect what counts as ethics?
4. In your own view, what are some major benefits and drawbacks with the concept of care?

REFERENCES

1. American Nurses' Association. *Nursing: A social policy.* Kansas City, MO: Author. 1980; 9.
2. Ibid; 7.
3. American Nurses' Association. *Code for nurses with interpretive statements.* Kansas City, MO: Author. 1976; 4.
4. Patridge KB.: Nursing values in a changing society. *Nursing Outlook.* 1978; 26(6): 356.
5. Ibid.
6. Aristotle. *Nicomachean ethics.* Indianapolis: Bobbs-Merrill; 1962:21.
7. *Fundamental principles of the metaphysics of morals.* Abbott TK and Fox M, (Trans.). Indianapolis: Bobbs-Merrill; 1949:11.
8. American Nurses Association. *Code for nurses.*
9. Ibid.

10. Benner P, Wrubel, J.: *The primacy of caring.* Menlo Park, CA: Addison-Wesley; 1989: 166–167.

11. Herodotus "Custom is King" in J. Ladd, Ethical Relativism, Belmont, Calif, Wadsworth, 1973, p. 12.

12. G.M.A. Grube (tr.) Plato's Republic, Indianapolis, Hackett Publishing Company, 1974, pp. 5–6.

13. Benner and Wrubel, The Primacy of Caring, p. 1.

14. Ibid.

15. Ibid.

16. Ibid; xiii.

17. Ibid.

18. Gilligan C. *In a different voice.* Cambridge, MA: Harvard University Press; 1982.

19. Noddings N: *Caring.* Berkeley, CA: University of California Press; 1984.

20. Gilligan C. *In a different voice;* 73.

21. Fried, C. *An Anatomy of Values,* Cambridge, Mass. Harvard University Press, 1971, p. 227.

22 Williams, B., *Moral Luck,* Cambridge, Cambridge University Press, 1981, p. 21.

23. Noddings N. *Doubts about radical proposals on caring.* In: Burbules N, ed. *Philosophy of Education.* Normal, Illinois: Illinois State University, Philosophy of Education Society; 1986: 83.

24. Foot P. *Virtues and vices,* Berkeley, CA: University of California Press; 1978: 4–5.

25. J. Hersey, A Single Pebble. In Foot P. *Virtues and vices.*

CHAPTER 2

Models of the Nurse-Patient-Physician Relationship

Study of this chapter enables the learner to:

1. Evaluate models of physician-patient relationships for their relevance to nursing practice.
2. Analyze Peplau's interpersonal, therapeutic model of the nurse-patient relationship.
3. Utilize the interpersonal model of the nurse-patient relationship as the basis for implementing the nurse's role as patient advocate.
4. Justify the role of the nurse as patient advocate.

INTRODUCTION

Models are idealized patterns, greatly simplified, for looking at complex events in terms of their essential qualities. A model is an abstract representation of a significant portion of reality. Models essentialize the most general aspects of a given phenomenon. They have been called "candidates for reality,"[1] conjectures of what reality is like. A model is an abstract representation of reality, and is not necessarily pictorial or visual.[2] A model both simplifies and highlights "important features of the subject."[3]

Models oriented by values show different perceptions for understanding the health care process. The use of models refutes the conception that health care is value free and helps to identify clashes of values as they occur in practice between health professionals.

MODELS OF NURSE-PATIENT-PHYSICIAN RELATIONSHIPS

Szasz and Hollander

Three models are defined by Szasz and Hollander, as the basis of the physician-patient relationship with recognition that these models of interaction are present in all human relationships including those between physician and nurse.[4]

Activity-Passivity Model. The model of activity-passivity is that mode of interaction in which the physician is active and the patient is passive. This is an entirely appropriate orientation for infants, comatose and anesthetized patients, and patients in situations of emergency. It places the physician in absolute control, supports feelings of physician power, and minimizes identity with the person of the patient.[5] It is authoritarian and paternalistic.

Guidance-Cooperation Model. The guidance-cooperation model is the basis for most medical practice. It consists of a patient with symptoms seeking help from a physician who possesses knowledge relevant to the patient's needs. The physician offers guidance in the form of treatment. In return, the patient is expected to cooperate by obeying the orders received. The presupposition in this model is that the physician knows what is best for the patient, holds the patient's interests foremost, and is free from other priorities. The patient must be equally convinced of these aims.[6] This model is still paternalistic, although to a lesser degree.

Mutual-Participation Model. The third model is one of mutual participation, based on the premise that equality among human beings is of high value.[7] It is the central assumption of the democratic process as well. This kind of interaction presupposes that the participants have nearly equal power, that they need each other, and that the shared activity will be satisfying to both.[8]

This model is characteristic of concepts of self-help considered important in current health care practice. It also recognizes the patient's experience as an important factor in self-care, especially in chronic illness. The role of the physician in this model becomes one of helping patients to help themselves.[9] It is an interdependent, therefore more complex way of relating on the part of all participants. Szasz and Hollander view this model as both necessary and more appropriate for educated and intellectual patients similar to the physician. They see this model as "essentially foreign to medicine"[10] and point out that, as a principle, with improvement of the patient's health status, the physician-patient relationship should change. It is at this point that psychological needs for domination are likely to interfere with the patient's self-determination. The authors view the physician-patient relationship as being like the changing relationship of the parent to the growing child. As the offspring grows in responsibility and maturity, the parent-child relationship becomes increasingly egalitarian.

From a nursing perspective, the mutual-participation model is essential to the self-determination and autonomy of the patient as endorsed by the American Nurses' Association.[11] This model presupposes that human beings have the capacity for growth and change. Nursing that is based on respect for individual differences recognizes and supports the possibility of choice and self-direction as a value of high priority.[12]

Robert Veatch

Within Veatch's four models of physician-patient interaction are the possibilities for either facilitating or inhibiting an ethical relationship.[13]

The Engineering Model. In his engineering model, Veatch denies any possibility of value-free "pure" science or medicine. Choices are made continually among facts, observations, research designs, and statistical levels of significance within a frame of values by supposedly "pure" scientists. An even larger number of choices of value and significance must be made by persons in an applied field such as medicine in which, unlike engineering and plumbing, values cannot be eliminated in favor of technical advice to a human being.

The Priestly Model. In Veatch's priestly model, the physician assumes the posture of a moral expert who presumes to tell the patient what he or she ought to do in the specific situation. This tradition is based on the ethical principle of "Do no harm." It is expressed in the paternalistic practice of withholding bad news from the patient and giving unrealistic reassurance. It takes away the decision from the patient and gives freedom to the physician instead. It does not permit competent persons to refuse blood transfusions on the basis of religious beliefs, for example. Paternalism lessens the patient's dignity by reducing his or her control over body and life. Truth-telling and promise-keeping become arbitrary individual decisions on the basis of "Do no harm." Deception is similarly rationalized.[14]

The Collegial Model. In Veatch's collegial model, the physician and patient are "colleagues pursuing the common goal of eliminating the illness and preserving the health of the patient."[15] Trust and confidence are central. There is equality. Realistically, however, Veatch contends that there is no basis for equality in the physician-patient relationship since social class, economic status, and educational and value differences make the assumption of common interests an illusion.[16]

The Contractual Model. In the contractual model, Veatch defines the participants as interacting with expectations of obligations and benefits for each. Commitment to moral principles is essential. Moreover, the contract recognizes the patient's ultimate control of his or her own destiny. Therefore, there is a "sharing of ethical authority and responsibility" without the moral abdication of either physician or patient.[17]

Veatch sees the advantages of the contractual model as avoiding the moral abdication of the physician in the engineering model and the patient's moral abdication in the priestly model. Nor does the contractual model contain the false equality of the collegial model. The contractual model provides the patient with freedom of choice and control over significant options, with the physician free to decide the details within that reference frame. Furthermore, this model allows either participant to withdraw from the contract if necessary to retain personal moral integrity.[18]

MODELS OF NURSE-PATIENT RELATIONSHIPS

Hildergard E. Peplau's fundamental view of the nurse-patient relationship is one that builds upon the worth and dignity of human beings, the development of trust, problem-solving measures, and collaboration. The nurse may function as a resource person who supplies information relevant to the patient's problem. The nurse may also function in a counseling relationship, while the patient reviews feelings and events connected with illness. He or she may function as a surrogate parent, sibling, or significant other, permitting the patient to explore and examine feelings associated with these relationships. Finally, the nurse may function as an expert who understands the technical matters associated with the patient's illness. Thus, the relationship between nurse and patient is interpersonal, therapeutic, and authoritative to the extent of the nurse's knowledge on technical matters related to the illness. The process is educative and egalitarian, avoiding the nurse's imposition of his or her values on the patient. The aim is for patients to experience their illness as a way of reorienting feelings and strengthening the personality in positive ways.[19]

Nurses help to reduce the threat of illness to individuals by accepting people as they are and helping them through stress. Together, patient and nurse move through stages of patient dependence, independence, and into the stage of interdependence when both are engaged cooperatively in problem-related tasks. At this point, the patient may utilize available services fully in the service of problem resolution and of moving on to new goals and to new relationships.

The nurse must establish the patient relationship as a helping one. As a resource person, the nurse functions as a source of knowledge on health matters related to the patient's needs. The role of teacher combines all the other roles in the service of patient learning and growth. The role of leader can be exercised in the clinical situation as well as at the local, national, and international level. Peplau raises the issue of democratic nursing practice as one in which the patient becomes an active participant in developing the nursing care plan.[20] The nurse as leader does not dictate patient goals or require that the patient give up independence and submit to the domination of the nurse. Basic feelings of respect for the worth of each individual are necessary for a democratic relationship to be operative.

Similarly, the physician's and the nurse's relationship with the patient is affected by the presence or absence of mutual respect, trust, the sharing of authority, and freedom from surrogate miscasting—a physician misperceived as a father or husband figure and a nurse misperceived as wife or mother.

This model of the nurse-patient relationship may, more than any other nursing model, contain the foundation for a democratic, egalitarian relationship of mutual trust and respect between nurse, patient, and physician compatible with the model of nurse as patient advocate. Peplau's model is also compatible with Veatch's contractual model. Peplau insists on the full participation of the patient, with the selection of goals and problem definition solidly in the patient's control. The nurse facilitates, strengthens, and educates the patient's processes of defining the problem, along with analysis, implementation, resolution, and evaluation of the process and goals. Choices and values supported are those of the patient, with the nurse utilizing Peplau's various roles to enhance the patient's sense of worth and autonomy. The composite of the roles, as Peplau defines them, is the basis for a nursing role as patient advocate.

THE ROLE OF THE NURSE AS PATIENT ADVOCATE

The nurse carries out the role of securing the patient's interests, sometimes as the eyes and ears, arms and legs of the patient. The nurse sometimes even singlehandedly embodies the role of caretaker, protector, and advocate, especially since there are occasions when no one else is in a position to fight as hard to help the patient to win the final battle of life over death. In these multiple surrogate roles, the nurse also becomes a therapist and source of personality strength during the patient's health crisis. The nurse identifies himself or herself as the human equal of the patient, as a person with fellow feelings rather than as one who imposes values and preferences paternalistically upon the patient. The surrogate never loses touch with respect for the patient's autonomy as an individual on an open, democratic, and pluralistic basis.

The nurse who understands these multiple roles promotes, protects, and thereby advocates patients' interests and rights in an effort to make them whole and well again. Where that is not possible, the nurse makes patients as comfortable and free of pain and suffering as possible. In any event, the nurse recognizes that his or her first duty is to protect and care for the patient's health and safety. In safeguarding the patient, the nurse supports and thereby advocates the patient's interests in the restoration of the patient's health and well-being.

The role of patient advocate presupposes that, as Minnie Goodnow held at the turn of the century, "the patient comes first,"[21] that the patient defines what nursing is about, that the patient has rights, and that patients' rights depend on significant others who will protect and care for their rights when they themselves are unable to do so. The nurse as patient advocate is thus the touchstone highlighting and guiding all other nursing functions.

THE IMPORTANCE OF ADVOCACY

Why is advocacy so important? Because without the advocacy and effective protection of rights, there are no rights. Rights depend on backup rights, the rights to be effectively protected in claiming one's rights. There are, we contend, no rights without the kinds of backup rights effectively protected by advocates and by a society that recognizes the role of advocates in providing relief and remedies against wrongdoing. For the role of advocates is to safeguard clients against abuse and violation of their rights.

Two arguments have been put forth against the view that to have rights entails advocacy and protection of those rights. One argument is that propounded by supporters of "natural law," who contend that to have a right is to have a right regardless of particular social circumstances in which such rights may not be honored in practice. Thus, slaves in ancient Greece had the right to be free, even though they were unjustly deprived of those rights. Similarly, Jews incarcerated and incinerated in Nazi gas chambers in World War II horror camps, never lost their rights to be free and the right to live in the natural-law view. Their rights were violated. So also is a woman who is raped. Her rights are violated, but not lost.

A second argument against the need for advocacy is one propounded by J.S. Mill. It is that "the rights and interests of every or any person are only secure from being disregarded when the person interested is himself able and habitually disposed to stand up for them."[22] On this view, we lose the rights we cannot effectively claim by ourselves. We must be our own best guardians of the rights we hold. If we do not safeguard our own rights, it is our own fault if we lose them.

Rights are only as strong as the ability, willingness, and resourcefulness of the people of a society jointly to protect and care for all the rights of its members. Mill's argument, while in part true (since each individual cares more for his or her rights and interests than anyone else), is partly false. The rights of anyone or of all depend on the willingness and ability of other relevant persons to bear correlative responsibilities implied by those rights. No one can protect his or her rights alone, unaided by others. This is especially true of sick and frightened patients unsure of what is happening to them and of the source of help. There are therefore no rights without advocacy of those rights by others. Clearly, the nurse is in a strong position to advocate the patient's rights and interests.

The reasons there are no rights without advocacy, then, are that right-holders may not always be in a position to defend their rights, whereas other persons may be in such a position. Secondly, there are no rights without claims effectively made on behalf of such rights, claims sometimes made by other persons on behalf of rightholders. The right to claim is not necessarily vested in a rightholder alone. Others can and have made claims on behalf of those whose rights have been ignored or violated.

A slave, infant, or patient has rights, even if he or she cannot claim them effectively, because even though these persons are helpless to claim such rights, other people as advocates can represent the interests of a slave, child, or patient. The problem of claiming rights can be surmounted, since suitable and effective representation can and does in fact occur. If a child or patient is helpless, a parent or parent surrogate, sponsor, or advocate can step in to protect him or her. Nurses can also—and do indeed quite frequently—protect patients' rights.

THREE MODELS OF PATIENT ADVOCACY

There seem to be three models of patient advocacy. The first, suggested by Abrams, is on the model of "civil disobedience."[23] On this model, a nurse acknowledges patient advocacy that conflicts with established authority and involves risk taking and consequences for noncompliance.

The civil-disobedience model puts the nurse on the defensive, in the position of having to show a hypothetical or shadowy court of rational authority that his or her action is the right one. The burden is on the nurse to make good this claim against the practices of established authorities. This can be hazardous to job security.

A second, related, model of patient advocacy compares the nurse to a guerrilla fighter, one who fights against the health care system.[24] The model of nurse as patient advocate who combats established authority suffers from a similar defect to the model of nurse as civil disobedient. Both models place the enemy, opposition, or problem in the wrong place and upon the wrong set of persons. The problem is not that of the nurse. The problem is that the patient's rights are disregarded by an indifferent system in which no one advocates for the client's rights to participate actively in his or her own health care.

Instead of health-professional conflict, there is or ought to be a natural alliance between nurse, patient, and physician against ill health and disease. In this respect, health professionals derive more role guidance and support from the concept of a health team than from either the civil-disobedience or guerrilla model of client advocacy. To advocate for the client's need is to be part of and on the health team, working with others for the health of the patient. However, the nurse requires the mutual respect of other health professionals to be a member of this team, freeing the nurse from behaving like a civil disobedient or guerrilla fighter.

A nurse as client advocate and a health team member is part of a third model. He or she has professional "standing." The concept of "standing" employs a term from the law given to those whose views are granted a serious hearing and consideration before a decision-making board or tribunal, without necessarily being accepted. Before such a team, group, committee, board, or tribunal, the most rational view prevails, one that can be verified as providing the best alternative for patient care. This model is one that gives standing to a nurse as a patient advocate. The appropriate use of moral and cognitive authority is preferable to a model of a nurse as a civil disobedient or urban guerrilla.

ARGUMENTS FOR AND AGAINST THE NURSE AS PATIENT ADVOCATE

There are three arguments of varying strength directed against the concept of nurse as client advocate, however. The first is that patient advocacy carries no system of institutional supports. The nurse willing to advocate a patient's rights when it matters most, in situations of conflict between nurses and physicians, is at risk of losing his or her job. Portraying a nurse as client advocate flies in the face of institutional political and economic realities, it is held.

A second argument is that at least some physicians regard themselves as the basic protectors of their patients' rights and resent intrusion by other health professionals into their contractual prerogatives with their patients.

A third argument, due partly but not wholly to the two foregoing arguments, is that nurses have too many other roles to spend time and resources as client advocates, and that wrongdoing, by whomever committed, is adequately corrected by persons other than nurses, such as lawyers.

Against the first argument—that patient advocacy lacks institutional supports—the nurse's role of advocacy is to insure the patient's status as an autonomous human being in a milieu dominated by technology. Patients' rights are in need of being protected; nurses have a natural alliance with their patients. Moreover, institutions are vulnerable to lawsuits and sensitive to negative publicity when violations of patients' rights are exposed. Consequently, nurses are natural candidates for advocacy roles in patient care.

A rebuttal against the second argument is that physicians are not always responsible and accountable. The health care system of "checks and balances" calls for resources, skills, and abilities aimed at protecting patients' rights that are not always guaranteed or implemented by physicians. Moreover, nurses, who increasingly show evidence of higher education, quite naturally provide a form of effective advocacy in the delivery of increasingly complex nursing care. Evidence of high-quality nursing judgments in medical centers points to a natural advocacy role for such nurses.

Finally, there is an argument that nurses have too many important technical roles to have the time, skill, and ability to function as advocates. In response, no other group has more continuous contact with patients and families than do nurses. Therefore, nurses often have the most familiarity with patients' and families' ethical choices and are in good position to protect those interests in serious situations.

CONCLUSION

Nurses, having a natural kinship with values of life and death and the quality of life and health care, show increasing awareness of value questions; the protection of patients' rights is a natural outcome. Patient advocacy is integral with the expanding relationships nurses have in the care of their patients. Models of nurse-patient-physician relationships show that patient advocacy by nurses is essential to patients' health care rights.

Discussion Questions

1. Given Szasz's and Hollander's, Veatch's and Peplau's models, what is your conception of an ethically justifiable model of nursing?
2. What are some major advantages and drawbacks of each of the following models: civil disobedience, urban guerrilla, and legal standing?

REFERENCES

1. Hesse M. Models and analogy in science. In: Edwards P (ed.). *The Encyclopedia of Philosophy*. New York: Macmillan; 1967; 5, 358.
2. Black M. *Models and metaphors*. Ithaca, NY: Cornell University Press; 1962: 236.
3. Scheffler I. *Reason and teaching*. Indianapolis: Bobbs-Merrill; 1975: 68.
4. Szasz TS, Hollander MH. *The basic models of the doctor-patient relationship*. A.M.A. Arch Int Med. 1956; 97:585.
5. Ibid.
6. Ibid.
7. Ibid.
8. Ibid.
9. Ibid.
10. Ibid.
11. American Nurses' Association. *Code for nurses with interpretive statements*. Kansas City, MO: 4.
12. American Nurses' Association. *Nursing: A social policy*. Kansas City, MO: 1980, 6.
13. Veatch RM. *Models for ethical medicine in a revolutionary age*. The Hastings Center Report: June, 1972; 3:3.
14. Ibid.
15. Ibid.
16. Ibid.
17. Ibid.
18. Ibid.
19. Peplau HE. *Interpersonal relations in nursing*. New York: Putnam; 1952: 31.
20. Ibid; 49.
21. Goodnow M. In: Carnegie E. *The patient's bill of rights and the nurse*. Nursing Clinics of North America. 1974; 9:557. 1974.
22. Mill JS. *Utilitarianism, liberty, and representative government*. London: Dent. 1948; 208.
23. Abrams N. Moral responsibility in nursing. In: Spicker SF, Gadow S. (eds.). *Nursing Images and Ideals*. New York: Springer; 1980; 153–159.
24. Kosik SH. *Patient advocacy or fighting the system*. Am J Nursing. 1972; 72(4):694.

CHAPTER 3

Moral Implications in Codes of Nursing

Study of this chapter enables the learner to:

1. Examine professional codes for their moral and practical implications.
2. Evaluate the functions of professional codes.
3. Analyze how professional codes affect professional conduct and limit malpractice.
4. Investigate how *The Code for Nurses* provides moral and professional guidelines for defining, justifying, and limiting nursing activities.

INTRODUCTION

Essential characteristics of present-day professions are said to be the development of a code of ethics guiding practice, specialized educational programs, a particular service to society, standards of education and practice, an economic and welfare program, and legal practice acts with licensing and self-government as common elements.[1] Since a code of ethics is a standard incorporated in varying degrees in all practice, education, legislation, licensing, and public participation, codes for nurses and physicians will be analyzed and evaluated in these respects. Professional codes function as a means of self-regulation, serving as guidelines for individual and collective responsibility in response to societal needs for trustworthy, competent, accountable practitioners. Professional codes are regarded as systems of rules and principles by which a profession is expected to regulate its members and demonstrate its responsibility to society.

THE CODE FOR NURSES

The present *Code for Nurses* functions as the basis for professional status in four ways. First, the *Code* shows society that nurses are expected to understand and accept the trust and responsibility invested in them by the public.[2] Second, the *Code* provides guidelines for professional conduct and relationships as the basis for ethical practice.[3] Third, the *Code* defines the nurse's relationship to the client as one of patient advocate, to other health professionals as a colleague, to the nursing profession as a contributor, and to society as a representative of health care for all. Fourth, the *Code* provides the means of self-regulation to the profession.[4]

The *Code for Nurses* is a public statement of belief expressing the moral concerns, the values, and the goals of nursing. The *Code* aims to justify ethical decisions. The *Code* uses both the consequentalist and the absolutist models of morality. The principle of respect for persons is considered the most fundamental value in the *Code*. From the principle of respect comes the principle of autonomy, placing the patient at the center of rational decisions. The principles of beneficence (doing good), nonmaleficence (avoiding harm), veracity (truth-telling), confidentiality (respecting privileged information), fidelity (keeping promises), and justice (treating people fairly)[5] support the value of respect for persons.

In 1988, the American Nurses' Association Committee on Ethics published its responses to nurses seeking ethical guidance regarding specific practice issues.[6] One response was to the issues of withdrawal of food and fluid. Another significant issue was discussed in the statement regarding risk versus responsibility for providing nursing care to patients with serious communicable diseases. These position statements incorporated the values and principles of the *Code* as guidelines to practice.

Specific Provisions of the *Code for Nurses*

1. The nurse provides services with respect for human dignity and the uniqueness of the client unrestricted by considerations of social or economic status, personal attributes, or the nature of health problems.[7]

The nurse begins to fulfill this provision by accepting the client as a stranger who is given interest, respect, and courtesy. Respect for the other is unaffected by socioeconomic status, personal attributes, or the nature of the health problem. The nurse is committed to the principle of the client's right to be "fully involved in the planning and implementation"[8] of his or her own care. Each person has the moral right to decide what will be done to him or to her, together with the right to the information necessary to make those decisions, to understand the consequences, and, on that basis, to accept, terminate, or refuse treatment.

The process of client self-determination may involve the nurse in the roles of resource person and technical expert. The nurse may both supply relevant information and seek the assistance of other professionals in supplementing the patient's or the nurse's own knowledge. The nurse may function as a surrogate authority figure who enables the patient to explore feelings of fear, dependency, suffering, and hopes for total recovery. As counselor and patient advocate, the nurse enlists the client in the process of problem identification, analysis, and resolution of health care needs. The collaboration is directed toward goals of recovery, of optimum function, or of dying peacefully and with dignity.

A nurse who opposes the nature of the health care delivered, such as a decision to abort a fetus or to withhold treatment from a deformed and retarded infant, is justified in refusing and withdrawing from the situation as soon as other arrangements are made that provide nursing care to the patient.[9]

The nursing care provided to the dying is expected to enable the patient to live with all possible physical, mental, and social comfort. It is, above all, the nursing care of the dying that "will determine to a great degree how this final human experience is lived and the peace and dignity with which death is approached."[10] Uses of medical technology such as resuscitation measures and life-support systems pose problems to the dying patient, the patient's family, and health professionals, who must make value-laden decisions. The nurse seeks to protect values of respect for human dignity "while working with the client and others to arrive at the best decisions dictated by the circumstances."[11]

2. The nurse safeguards the client's right to privacy by judiciously protecting information of a confidential nature.[12]

The relationship between nurse and client is expected to be one of trust and mutuality. The client may share intimate, previously hidden facts unrelated to current problems on a confidential basis. However, data relevant to the client's health status needs to be shared with other members of a health care team who have common goals of client welfare. This exception may extend to a court of law, where the nurse may or may not be able to invoke the principle of privileged communication. Otherwise, the nurse is committed to the client's right of privacy on a moral basis that respects human dignity.

Information about the patient's diagnoses, treatment, and care necessary for third-party payment, peer review, and quality assurance procedures are expected to be kept confidential according to written guidelines rigidly enforced.[13] The client's consent must be obtained before the record is used for research or other purposes.[14]

3. The nurse acts to safeguard the client and the public when health care and safety are affected by incompetent, unethical, or illegal practice of any person.[15]

The role of advocate is defined in this provision as one in which "the nurse's primary commitment is to the client's care and safety."[16] As a corollary, the nurse is expected to be alert to practices by any health professional or the system itself that are "unethical," incompetent, illegal, or against the patient's best interests.[17] This requires knowledge of both state practice acts and institutional policies and procedures, as well as a clarification of the term "ethical."

The process of correction begins with the individual who may have caused harm to the patient. If necessary, institutional channels and established procedures are expected to be used for further reporting. Documentation is expected as well.

If the appropriate behavior "is not corrected within the employment setting and continues to jeopardize the client's care and safety . . . the problem should be reported to other appropriate authorities such as the practice committees of the appropriate professional organizations or the legally constituted bodies concerned with licensing. . . ."[18] Although a written grievance must be provided to regulatory bodies, every effort is made to protect the patient advocate.

An effective measure to protect clients and improve practice is the peer review. The method is based on published criteria and the procedures for making recommendations. It is intended as a method for improving health care delivery services and the safety, health, and welfare of clients.[19]

4. The nurse assumes responsibility and accountability for individual nursing judgments and actions.[20]

As an acknowledged professional, the nurse is responsible and accountable for the quality, effectiveness, and efficiency of nursing care provided. Moreover, society expects a profession to be self-regulating. However, safeguards for the patient in the form of professional examination and licensure are operative in most states. These insure minimum competencies. Recently, state regulatory bodies have been created for investigating and prosecuting professional misconduct in addition to supporting the profession's responsibility for setting standards of nursing practice.

Individual nurse responsibility is for the development and implementation of the nursing care plan and for the functions and duties of the role assumed.[21] The areas of nursing responsibility include data collection and assessment, development of the plan and of the goals to be achieved, and the evaluation of the effectiveness of the plan and of the nursing care in reaching set goals.[22]

The nurse is accountable for what is done or not done "to self, to client, to the agency of employment, and to the nursing profession."[23] Accountability includes legal responsibilities. The nurse is responsible for each act or failure to act in a given case. We would add that the nurse is accountable to society for decisions at the policy level affecting the future course of a profession, the institution, or health care delivery.

Evaluation occurs at the subjective individual level and is also done by peers. The process of evaluation by self or by others implies that improvement of practice is continuous. Peer evaluation is intended as a means of self-regulation by the profession itself.[24] Through its *Standards of Nursing Practice,* updated nursing practice laws, and accreditation procedures, the American Nurses' Association demonstrates its accountability to the public.[25]

5. The nurse maintains competence in nursing.[26]

Effective nursing often makes the difference between a client's survival or death, recovery or continued ill health. Therefore, nurses are expected to know what they are doing. Moreover, nurses are expected to maintain competence and remain currently informed of new knowledge. Nursing care is expected to reflect knowledge of new concepts in nursing, new medications, and new techniques.

Present competence measures "include peer review criteria, outcome criteria, and the American Nurses' Association program for certification."[27] Continuing education and advanced formal education are means of keeping current with professional, scientific, and technologic advances. Scientific advances contribute to the rapidly increasing complexity of nursing service and health care delivery. The process of maintaining competence is self-initiated and self-directed with the recognition of the need for appropriate consultation with nurse specialists, educators, administrators, or leaders.

6. The nurse exercises informed judgment and uses individual competence and qualifications as criteria in seeking consultation, accepting responsibilities, and delegating nursing activities to others.[28]

The practice of nursing is dynamic and increasingly complex. In primary care and in the practitioner roles in pediatrics, geriatrics, and family health, for example, new functions are performed by nurses that were formerly those of the physician. The nurse performs a physical examination and history as part of the nursing practitioner's assessment and diagnosis. Consequently, nurses are shifting nursing functions to ancillary personnel. In the process of delegation, the nurse must exercise discretion and judgment in accepting and assigning responsibilities. Consultation is freely used. The primary goal is to insure safe and effective nursing care.

A second goal is to practice within the limits of the legal practice acts for each profession. In some nursing roles, there is a need for collaborative activities to develop joint policy statements with medicine that will define differences in roles and responsibilities. Existing statements of joint policy represent expert judgment and may have standing in courts of law. A third goal is to influence constructive changes in the law.

The delivery of total health services is now beyond the capacity of any single profession. Interdisciplinary team effort in which the members share knowledge, skills, and responsibilities for total patient care nevertheless requires the nurse's recognition of limitations of competence. The nurse needs consultation from appropriate sources. These may include other nurses, physicians, or other health professionals. Distinction in role and functions that are based on education and training call for respect without disparagement of individuals having minor roles.

Personal competence, as well as education and training and policy statements, is assessed before delegating nursing functions to ancillary personnel or accepting medical functions.[29] Any nurse unsure of personnel competence has both the responsibility and, in one view, the right to refuse the assignment in question. This protects both the client and the nurse. The same right and responsibility prevail where functions are delegated that are not nursing responsibilities or that keep the nurse from providing nursing care. Similar precautions are expected to be observed in delegating functions to other members of the team who may be unqualified for the assignment.[30]

7. The nurse participates in activities that contribute to the ongoing development of the profession's body of knowledge.[31]

Systematic investigation is necessary for expanding each profession's body of knowledge. Knowledge, implying truth and beliefs based on adequate evidence, serves as the framework and beacon light of the profession's education and practice.

The American Nurses' Association has developed guidelines for nurses either conducting or involved in research. Research is expected to be conducted by qualified persons or under such persons' supervision. The study design is submitted for approval by an appropriate committee using official or professional guidelines. The purpose, the nature, the goals, and the methodology of the research are evaluated in relation to guidelines for the protection of human subjects.

The subject's right of informed consent, privacy, and dignity are thereby insured. Additionally, the subject has the right to terminate participation at any time. Subjects are protected from undue risks.

These principles are especially important in research consented to by parents or guardians and performed on children, the aged, and the mentally disabled. The nurse who disagrees with the research because of its problematic aspects has the right to refuse to participate or to withdraw on the basis of its adverse effects on patients.[32]

8. The nurse participates in the profession's efforts to implement and improve standards of nursing.[33]

An assumed public concern of professions is that only qualified persons will be admitted to practice. Nursing competence includes a command of skills, academic success, demonstrated responsibility, and a commitment to improve nursing practice for the benefit of others. The selection of students and evaluation of their abilities is an obligation of educators. Helping people involves more than a generous humanitarian impulse. Therefore, the American Nurses' Association has developed standards for practice, education, and service that requires the participation of each nurse for implementation.[34]

9. The nurse participates in the profession's efforts to establish and maintain conditions of employment conducive to high-quality nursing care.[35]

Nurses are now involved in the process of changing the terms and conditions of employment. This provision of the *Code* emphasizes that economic conditions of general welfare are important factors in recruiting and keeping well-qualified nurses functioning at an optimum level.

The most effective method of defining and controlling the quality of nursing care is collective bargaining. The professional state nurses' associations assist and represent nurses in negotiations with employers. One aim is to insure professionally approved standards of practice. Equally important is the support for the rights of nurses to "participate in determining the terms and conditions of employment conducive to high-quality nursing practice."[36] The appropriate channel for nurses to improve conditions of employment ethically and with dignity is through the economic and general welfare programs of the state and national nurses' associations. Increasingly, work contracts have been achieved in previously unorganized health care facilities. Old contracts were renegotiated and revised to the satisfaction of the majority of employed nurses. Some contracts were secured solely through negotiation. Others were secured only after prolonged unsuccessful negotiation and a strike in which arrangements were made to provide care for seriously ill patients in need of nursing care.

The problems of inadequate staffing and salaries will continue to detract from the professional satisfaction of dedicated nurses. An editorial in *The New York Times* discussed the acute shortage of nurses and pointed to the increased opportunities in other fields for men and women who are or could be good nurses.[37] Nevertheless, there are almost two million nurses who might be responsive to improved salaries and conditions of employment in significant ways.

10. The nurse participates in the profession's effort to protect the public from misinformation and misrepresentation and to maintain the integrity of nursing.[38]

This section of the *Code* provides for individual advertising of nursing services through listings and biographies in reputable publications. The nurse may use symbols of licensure such as R.N., earned academic degrees, and symbols of professional recognition such as F.A.A.N. (Fellow of the American Academy of Nursing). No nurse is permitted to endorse, advertise, promote, or sell commercial products, since this may be mistakenly interpreted as an endorsement by the entire profession. In the course of health teaching, several "similar products or services [are expected to] be offered or described so that the client or practitioner can make an informed choice."[39] On the other hand, nurses are expected to advise patients against using products that are dangerous. Violations of these principles by other nurses are expected to be reported to the professional association, as such actions undermine public confidence in nursing.

11. The nurse collaborates with members of the health professions and other citizens in promoting community and national efforts to meet the health needs of the public.[40]

Health care as the right of all citizens is stated in this provision as endorsed by the American Nurses' Association House of Delegates in convention in 1958.[41] Planning for health services to be available and accessible to everyone requires collaboration between consumers and providers of health care at all levels. Nurses have both the right and the responsibility to help achieve quality health care for all by implementing their views through the political process and legislative action. The organization of Nurses for Political Action has been effective in directly communicating the views of nurses on key issues to legislators. The organization has both supported and endorsed political candidates favorably disposed toward nursing interests, health care services, and human welfare.

This provision of the *Code* holds that relationships with other disciplines are expected to be collaborative and supportive. By its very nature, the delivery of complex health care demands an interdisciplinary approach. Likewise, the relationship of nursing and medicine is regarded as interdependent and collaborative "around the need of the client."[42] The changing role of the nurse, particularly primary-care or specialty nurse practitioners, requires colleague relationships with

physicians, with discussion of overlapping, similar, and different functions and areas of practice.[43] An editorial entitled "The Nurses' Discontent" pinpoints the importance of shared responsibility and shared
authority among physicians and nurses delivering comprehensive care
and the demoralization of nurses in the absence of shared decisions.

> Studies suggest that the nurses' discontent runs deeper than money
> or working conditions. They feel that, though they perform crucial
> functions, they are not taken seriously. Hospital rules and traditions
> deny them authority to make even minor decisions. . . . Nurses have
> little say in how hospitals are run. Yet typically, many get to know
> the patients and their problems better than anyone. Some nurses'
> organizations promote the idea of "joint practice," to let nurses par-
> ticipate in decisions about patient care. They have asked that nurses
> be admitted to the groups that set hospital policy. But they have·met
> with stiff resistance from [physicians] and administrators. These
> problems of authority deserve a careful look in considering the short-
> age of nurses.[44]

The challenge to nurses and nursing organizations is clearly set
forth. Nurses serve all of the people. Therefore, nurses have the right
to a voice in all deliberations and decisions affecting the quantity,
quality, and distribution of health care and nursing services.

THE INTERNATIONAL COUNCIL FOR NURSES CODE OF ETHICS

In London in 1899 at a meeting of the International Congress of
Women, a committee was formed as the International Council of
Nurses. In 1905, the American nursing association, the Nurses' Associated Alumnae, with associations from Great Britain and Germany,
became the charter members of the International Council of Nurses.[45]
In 1928, S. Lillian Clayton, president of the American Nurses' Association, identified the principles for which the International Council
stood. These were "self-government of nurses in their associations, and
raising ever higher the standards of education, professional ethics, and
public usefulness of its members."[46] In 1948, the International Council
of Nurses was officially recognized as the voice for all nongovernmen-
tal nursing by the World Health Organization. The Council is the
official representative of all nursing at World Health Organization
meetings.[47]

In 1950, the American Nurses' Association adopted its first complete code of ethics, used as a "model for the *Code for Nurses* adopted
by the Council in 1953."[48] The *Code* was revised in 1973 to its present
form.[49] It is in worldwide use. It is derived from eclectic and conflict-

ing concepts in traditional ethics and emphasizes the nurse's responsibility and accountability.[50]

As a guideline to conduct for nurses all over the world, the *Code* recognizes that nursing practice must reflect and respect cultural and religious differences. As a result, nursing may differ in fundamental respects from one area to another. The *Code* contains the seeds of conflict if the nurse carries the laws and customs of the home area to a different one. Respect for the values of a subculture or minority group is a position that raises the dilemma of whether to respect harmful values or to work for change. For example, an African nurse may be forced to choose between psychotropic drugs and the activities of a local healer for control of the hallucinations and thought disorders of a patient with an acute schizophrenic episode.

The *Code* defines the nurse's relation to people as one in which nursing care is provided in an environment that respects individual values, spiritual beliefs, and customs. Information of a personal nature is to be held in confidence unless the nurse judges it should be shared.[51]

The nurse's responsibility for practice is one of continual learning in order to maintain competence.[52] In specific situations, the nurse sustains the highest possible standards of nursing care and uses judgment in delegating and accepting responsibilities. Personal conduct reflects credit on the profession.[53]

The nurse's relation to society is one of shared responsibility for the initiation and implementation of the health and social needs of the community.[54]

The nurse's relation with co-workers is cooperative. (The physician is not distinguished from other co-workers.) The nurse protects persons receiving care by taking appropriate action when they are endangered.

The nurse's relation to the profession is that of an active role in developing and implementing desirable standards of nursing education and practice, and in contributing to nursing knowledge. Moreover, the nurse is expected to be active in securing fair economic and social working conditions through the professional organization. Women as nurses must still struggle for equality and recognition as persons whose professional lives are separate from their personal lives. The *Code* supports the definition of a professional nurse as a person with rights and responsibilities for self, clients, co-workers, community, and profession and their nursing and health care needs. The World Health Organization recognizes the *Code* for supporting nursing education and practice. It is used as a guide to curricula development, licensing, and legislation in countries involved with shaping their health care systems to serve the people well.

THE AMERICAN MEDICAL ASSOCIATION CODE OF ETHICS

In 1980, the American Medical Association adopted a new, shorter version of its *Principles of Medical Ethics*. This version had been in the process of review since 1977. Previous revisions were in 1903, 1912, 1947, and 1957. The first code for members was adopted in 1847.[55]

Veatch cites two major problems as reasons for the 1980 revision. The first is the Federal Trade Commission's charge of illegal constraints on trade through prohibition of advertising. The new *Code* permits advertising. Similarly, the new *Code* deletes the condemnation of what were called "unscientific cults," such as chiropractic practice.[56] (The 1957 *Code* directed a physician to practice medicine on a scientific basis and to avoid association with anyone violating this principle.)[57] The second set of changes is drastic because they are based on the recognition that the "medical profession is no longer perceived as the sole guardian of the public health, and consequently the traditional paternalism of the profession is in conflict with society."[58] Therefore, the new *Code* is based on concepts of human rights for patients, colleagues, and other health professionals. The responsibility of the physician is to respect those rights and support human dignity, to engage in honest dealings, to maintain patient confidence, and to improve the community.[59] This is the very first time that the physician's responsibility is connected with the rights of patients, with colleagues, and with the rights of other health professionals ("allied professionals" in the 1957 version). The rights of patients to confidentiality are now phrased solely in terms of the constraints of law rather than, in the 1957 paternalistic version, "to protect the welfare of the patient or of the community."[60] The new position strengthens patient confidentiality, but never explicitly defines the physician-patient relationship as a contractual one based on mutual trust or other ethical principles.[61] Confidentiality, for example, could be based on the moral principle of keeping promises.[62] Honesty is another principle in the new *Code* that takes priority over the older paternalistic principle, which allowed deception on grounds of the patient's best interests. Respect for the law and responsibility for changing bad laws as physician responsibilities are made more important in the new *Code*. This can be seen as implying the physician's contract with society for improving it.[63]

The new *Code* ends with a return to earlier principles of physicians' right to choose patients, associates, and environments in which appropriate patient care services are provided. The *Code* committee concluded that these principles were primarily for the protection and benefit of patients. Furthermore, the issue of who is to decide what is in the best interests of patients is still in the firm grasp of the physician group represented by the American Medical Association. Equally clearly, the physicians' freedom to choose whom to serve under what conditions is still in conflict with society's right to draft physicians for service in underserved areas or the armed forces or to restrict them in any way.[64]

On the positive side, the new *Code* abolishes the sexist use of the pronoun "he." More important, it explicates the physician's obligations to society: exposing incompetent or fraudulent colleagues; respecting law and changing it for the benefit of patients; making relevant knowledge available; utilizing the talents of other health professionals; and contributing to improvements in the community.[65] The *Code* committee recognized that "medical ethics are . . . a specific application of the universal norms of moral behavior."[66] Moreover, the *Code* committee acknowledged that "the profession does not exist for itself, it exists for a purpose and increasingly that purpose will be defined by society."[67] In Veatch's view, the new *Code* lays the foundation for a contractual relationship, based on ethically defensible principles, between organized medicine and the society in which it practices. Unfortunately, that time has not yet arrived.

THE FUNCTIONS OF A CODE FOR NURSES

According to *Webster's Collegiate Dictionary,* a code is a "system of principles or rules (moral)."[68] A code, in the case of law, has "statutory force," with enforceable sanctions.[69] Ideally, a professional code regulates the professional conduct of its members by instituting sanctions, directly or indirectly, and thus enforcing its provisions.

The word "professional," used in these discussions of codes, is employed as a persuasive definition. That is, it is used as a value term that exhorts the reader to agree with the writer or speaker. The use of a persuasive definition is in contrast to a lexical or reportive definition that is true or false, such as that of an island as a body of land surrounded by water. The words "professional" and "unprofessional" may also be used persuasively. Ms. Jolene Tuma, R.N., for example, had her license revoked by the Idaho State Board of Nursing in August 1976 on the grounds that her conduct was "unprofessional" for advocating Laetrile and "disrupting" the patient-physician relationship. Ms. Tuma appealed to the *Code for Nurses* to support her view that she was acting professionally.[70]

A professional code may also refer to the shared values and norms to which a profession's majority commits itself. We may recall from Chapter 1 that "moral" means whatever results in good or harm. The principles of the *Code* are designed to bring about good and minimize harm or injury. On this view, there is no way to prevent moral values and principles from consideration in health care matters. Therefore, a professional code may be viewed as a set of moral principles or rules for regulating the professional conduct of its members, preferably with enforceable sanctions, and from which specific directives can be generated for the ongoing governance of its members.

The *Code for Nurses* provides moral guidelines to nursing practice in accordance with consumers' health care interests and rights. The *Code* holds nurses accountable for professionally acceptable standards of nursing care. As the *Code* has evolved, this standard of acceptable nursing care has increasingly placed the client at the center of health care. Meanwhile, both the patient and the nurse are increasingly invested with rights and responsibilities.

According to Veatch, a stark difference between codes before and after World II is the absence of "rights" language in the older versions.[71] The Nazi abuses, Veatch says, gave rise to rules governing experimentation in the Nuremberg Code (1946) and in the Declaration of Helsinki (1964 and 1975).[72] But patients' bills of rights and code reformulation using the language of rights have been a reality only since 1972.[73]

The use of rights language in codes for nurses reflects not only that patients have rights but that nurses also have a role as patient advocates. To carry out their role as client advocates, nurses have special "earned" rights and privileges, which they may invoke even against physicians if those physicians' orders are medically or scientifically contraindicated. The advent of patients' and nurses' rights implies not only a conceptual redrawing of the physician-patient relation, but also a higher set of educational and professional role requirements and responsibilities placed on nurses. One may also find the growth of the nurse's advocacy role occurring as a result of such landmark cases as *Memorial Hospital* vs. *Darling*.[74] Here, the physicians were found negligent along with the nurses in a case involving Dorrence Darling's broken leg, which turned gangrenous and had to be amputated.

By holding nurses and physicians responsible for negligence, the nurses' judgment was identified as a causal factor, one that could have made a difference in the outcome. By holding nurses responsible, the Illinois Supreme Court acknowledged the role and importance of nursing judgment. By doing so, the Court altered the physician's role from the traditional "captain of the ship" to that of a key team member along with other key team members. To hold nurses jointly responsible for negligence against Dorrence Darling, as the Illinois Court did, called for nurses to have greater treatment autonomy and the professional right to advocate clients' rights against physicians if necessary. The nurses in the *Darling* case were cited for not reporting the condition of Darling's leg cast, even if doing so meant reporting a physician's negligence—a kind of reporting that has since come to be known as "whistle-blowing."

One function of the *Code for Nurses*, then, is to upgrade the nursing profession, thus benefitting both patients and nurses, by investing nurses with rights and responsibilities. Rights enable nurses to care more effectively for clients' health care interests and rights—rights which, some nursing scholars believe, cannot be entrusted to physicians alone. But the rights of nurses are not rights *against* patients, for such rights would defeat the point of nursing and nursing advocacy. Rather, nurses' rights are rights to act *on behalf* of their clients, and such rights include nurses' rights against other health professionals, including physicians and other nurses. These rights are invokable if other health professionals fail to promote the rights and interests of patients. On this view, patients' rights come first and justify the earned rights and privileges of other health professionals, on the condition, of course, that professional rights and privileges are consistent with and compatible with patients' rights.

A second function of the *Code* is one consistent with and implied by the first function of upgrading the quality of health care. This function is to set standards to regulate the conduct of nursing practitioners, holding them accountable and morally liable for failure to live up to the standards. For the *Code* functions as an oath or promise made by the profession collectively to the public that these standards will be upheld by the individual nurse.

To regulate the conduct of nurse practitioners, the profession, by logical extension through its *Code for Nurses*, attempts to influence licensure, institutional accreditation, and curricular content.[75] The *Code for Nurses* would otherwise be an exclusively ceremonial statement without influence in the governance of nursing practitioners. Nurses would possibly pay lip service to the *Code*, but it would lack what may be termed "performative" meaning, namely that the *Code* gets things done.[76] The *Code* would have no teeth if it had no "performative force." To have "performative force," the *Code* regulates nursing practitioners by influencing the guidelines for licensure, institutional accreditation, and curricula.

CRITICISMS OF PROFESSIONAL CODES

A criticism of the *Code* and of professional codes generally is that codes reflect vested interests. These interests mask deeper conflicts between the interests of the public and the profession around what Paul Goodman used to call "pork-chop" gains in the form of higher salaries and benefits.

This criticism depends on how the *Code* is formulated, and what functions and interests it can be made to serve. The evidence is that the *Code for Nurses*, while promoting the interests of the nursing profession, is clearly oriented toward serving patients' interests and rights and placing the interests of nurses second to those of patients. This cannot be said of the A.M.A. *Code*, since that code provides for the physician's right to choose whom to serve. The interests of patients and nurses do not collide, but rather dovetail. There are natural points of alliance between patients and nurses, partly due to both being undervalued and underserved.

CONCLUSION

The *Code* provides a floor, a moral basis for justifying nursing action, through its functions of (1) upgrading nursing by investing it with rights and responsibilities for caring for patients; (2) setting accountable moral standards for practitioners; (3) influencing licensure standards; (4) influencing educational and curricular standards of performance and conduct; and (5) appealing through its manifesto-like principles for legal incorporation and public acceptance.

Codes may have important symbolic and regulating functions for professional practices, including nursing. A symbolic function is to remind nurses and other professions of the status and importance of nursing in health care. The *Code for Nurses* carries out this role by stressing the human rights of patients and nurses to self-determination and well-being. The regulating function of the *Code* is to influence standards and practices of nursing.

Discussion Questions

1. How does the *Code for Nurses* influence and guide a nurse's conduct in deciding whether to refuse to help a patient?
2. How does the *American Medical Association Code* compare with the *Nurses Code* regarding the right to refuse to help a patient?
3. Which of the provisions of the *Code* regarding the right to refuse to treat is ethically justifiable in your view, and for what reasons?

REFERENCES

1. Flanagan L. *One strong voice*. Kansas City, MO: American Nurses' Association. 1976: 23.
2. American Nurses' Association. *Code for nurses with interpretive statements*. Kansas City, MO: Author. 1985: 2.

3. Ibid., p. 1.
4. Ibid.
5. Ibid.
6. American Nurses' Association. *Ethics in nursing: Position statements and guidelines.* Kansas City, MO: Author. 1988.
7. American Nurses' Association. *Code for nurses;* 4.
8. Ibid.
9. Ibid.
10. Ibid.
11. Ibid.
12. Ibid.
13. Ibid.
14. Ibid.; 7.
15. Ibid.; 8.
16. Ibid.
17. Ibid.
18. Ibid.; 9.
19. Ibid.
20. Ibid.
21. Ibid.
22. Ibid.; 9–10.
23. Ibid.; 10.
24. Ibid.
25. Ibid.
26. Ibid.; 11.
27. Ibid.
28. Ibid.; 12.
29. Ibid.; 13.
30. Ibid.
31. Ibid.; 14.
32. Ibid.; 15.
33. Ibid.
34. Ibid.; 16.
35. Ibid.
36. Ibid.
37. Editorial: The nurses' discontent, *The New York Times,* August 10, 1981; A14.
38. American Nurses' Association. *Code for nurses;* 10.
39. Ibid.; 18.
40. Ibid.; 19.
41. Flanagan. *One strong voice;* 629.
42. Ibid.; 20.
43. Ibid.
44. The nurses' discontent; A14.
45. Ibid.; 611.
46. Clayton SL. An activity update. In: Flanagan, *One strong voice;* 447.
47. Flanagan. *One strong voice;* 624.
48. Ibid.; 602.

49. Tate BL. *The nurse's dilemma.* Geneva. International Council of Nurses. 1977; vii.
50. Ibid.
51. Ibid.
52. Ibid.
53. Ibid.
54. Ibid.
55. Veatch RM. *Professional ethics: New principles for physicians?* Hastings Center Report. 1980. *10*(3):16.
56. Ibid.
57. American Medical Association. *Principles of medical ethics.* Monroe, WI: Author. 1957.
58. Veatch. *Professional ethics;* 16.
59. American Medical Association. *Principles of medical ethics.*
60. Ibid.
61. Veatch. *Professional ethics;* 16.
62. Ibid.
63. Ibid.
64. Ibid.
65. Ibid.
66. Ibid.; 18.
67. Ibid.
68. *Webster's Collegiate Dictionary.* Springfield, MA: Merriam. 1974; 216.
69. *Black's Law Dictionary,* 14th ed. St. Paul, MN: West. 1969; 323.
70. Tuma J. Professional misconduct. *Nursing Outlook.* 1977. *25*(9):546.
71. Veatch RM. Codes of medical ethics: Ethical analysis. In: Reich W (ed.). *The Encyclopedia of Bioethics.* New York: Macmillan. 1978, *1*: 172.
72. Ibid.
73. Ibid.
74. *Charleston Community Memorial Hospital* v. *Dorrence Kenneth Darling,* 33 Ill 326, 211 (NE 2nd 253 1965).
75. Transcript: *The matter of Ms. Jolene Tuma.* Board of Nursing. Idaho. August 24, 1976; 186–188, 234–235.
76. Austin J.: Performative utterances. In: Austin JL. *Philosophical Papers.* New York: Oxford University Press. 1970; 233–252.

CHAPTER 4

Traditional Models of Morality in Everyday Nursing Practice

Study of this chapter enables the learner to:

1. Identify traditional models of morality used in health care delivery.

2. Apply models appropriately to justify ethical decisions in nursing.

INTRODUCTION

Moral problems arise in nursing whenever and wherever there is the possibility for doing good or harm to someone. All health care policies and practices have consequences—some trivial, some serious, and some life-saving. As significant members of the health care team and as patient advocates, nurses are involved in making these decisions that vitally affect the well-being of patients, families, colleagues, and other members of society.

Nursing decisions and policies, such as those expressed in the *Code for Nurses*,[1] reflect moral values, issues, and problems in everyday practice. Attempts to solve or resolve these issues are expressed through moral views or beliefs. These moral views, which concern predominant ways of looking at values, may be seen as models. A practical model provides an account designed to orient and guide activities.[2] A model of morality characterizes a perspective for viewing moral relationships. These models of morality, which reflect ways of life, overlap.

ALTERNATIVE PHILOSOPHICAL MODELS OF MORALITY

Ethics or morality has both an easy and a difficult aspect. An easy aspect is that an ethical or moral issue arises whenever good or harm results. Almost anything one does in interpersonal relations may cause good or harm. Helping a patient recover health and self-confidence is good. A smile, a frown, a grimace, eye contact or aversion, and a hand extended to another may communicate affection, friendliness, disapproval, rejection, or abuse. Doing good or harm or having them done to us occurs frequently, and these interpersonal actions affect us for better or worse. Deciding what to do for a hope-

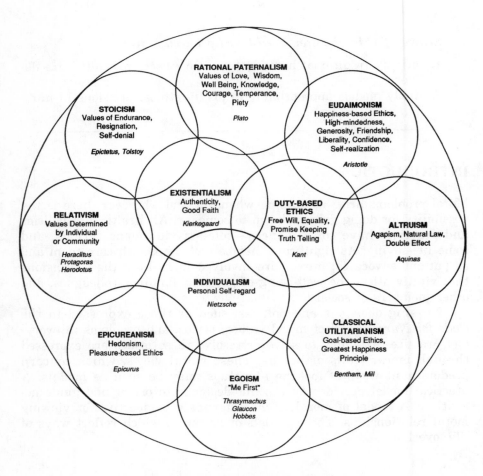

Figure 4–1. Traditional models of morality

lessly defective neonate or an elderly prostatectomy patient whose need for surgery is ignored results in good or harm. The difficult question is how to justify what is said to be good or harmful. Is "pulling the plug" on a 10-year-old comatose patient good or harmful, for example?

As one studies ethics, one finds no single science of moral values. One instead finds alternative models of morality and dialogue between these. Alternative models of morality orient the role of nursing in the care of patients. These models of moral values are like overlapping circles (Figure 4.1). Each model sets out its values along with an attempted justification to some decision-making aspect of nursing. St. Thomas Aquinas, for example, held that human life is a gift that is never to be taken by any human. He used principles of the Christian religion sometimes known as *Agapism* to justify his view on the sacredness of life. The principle that life is a gift is then used to "justify" a nurse's decision to save life at all cost, even the life of a hopeless infant with trisomy 18 (retardation, deafness, and various deformities) or of an irreversibly comatose 10-year-old. There are other models of morality, such as the ethics developed by Nietzsche. His model of morality stresses nobility, courage, stamina, and the role of great leaders in place of equality and democracy. To understand ethics, one cannot take one model of morality for granted as providing the true and final answer.[3] For, the moment one settles on such prized values as democracy and equality, there is an alternative ethical view, such as Nietzsche's that opposes democracy in favor of elitism. There are also related values, such as those of R. Descartes (1596–1650) and Joseph Fletcher, who emphasize the values of consciousness and reasoning.

MORAL ISSUES AND MODELS

Paternalism versus Libertarianism

There are 8 to 14 main models of morality that affect health care decisions. One ethical issue that affects the treatment of patients is that of Paternalism versus Libertarianism. *Paternalism* holds that the state, or one's father, knows best and that each individual is obligated to comply with the authority figure, be it a patient, a nurse, a physician, or the state. Brian Clark's play *Whose Life Is It Anyway?* illustrates the issue between Paternalism and Libertarianism. The physician gives Harrison, the quadriplegic, a tranquilizer against Harrison's objections. The physician also believes Harrison should be kept alive despite Harrison's wishes. *Libertarianism,* on the other hand, holds that individuals have a right to decide what happens in and to their bodies.

A famous ancient Greek philosopher, Plato (428–347 B.C.) is the major philosophical proponent of what might be called *Rational Paternalism*. Plato showed in a dialogue, the *Gorgias,* that the good in a person's own view—what that person desires—is not necessarily good. Plato cites as an example that a person may desire cream puffs at the bakery and confuse such desires with the good. (In modern life, a mother may desire to "pull the plug" on her comatose son, which may not be the wise thing to do.) Another group of philosophers against whom Plato argued in the *Republic* were the *Sophists,* such as Thrasymachus and Glaucon. The Sophists (sometimes known as Egoists, Subjectivists, or Relativists) defended the virtues of selfishness, of looking after oneself first and last, and argued that "might makes right."

Plato, argued against the sophists. Plato believed that looking after oneself first and last or doing whatever one wants if one has the power or can get away with it by stealth, pretension, or lies leads to moral and social destruction. He showed that we live only by living together. We need one another. Plato proposed a social scheme showing how people may live well together. His form of Paternalism is an appeal to knowledge, wisdom, and rationality rather than to force, tyranny, or ignorance. Plato favored a value scheme for individuals and societies in which reason dominates will and will dominates appetite; and he opposed the reverse, with appetite ruling will and reason.[4] Plato's Rational Paternalism rules out the practice of some physicians and other health professionals who place their personal wealth above a patient's health. A Libertarian rejoinder, however, is that life without individual freedom is not worthwhile. A Platonic response is that civilized survival is more valuable than individual liberty or freedom. One issue, then, between Rational Paternalism and Libertarianism, in relation to health care and nursing, is that of freedom versus security and control.

Eudaimonism: Happiness-Based Ethics Through Self-Realization

Aristotle (384–322 B.C.) introduced several major ideas at variance from Plato's. To Aristotle, there is no one method of achieving the good life or in understanding truth or beauty. There are as many methods as there are inquiries, activities, processes, and goals. Plurality replaces unity. There are many goods, such as health, wealth, and victory, not just one.[5]

Experience. Aristotle believed that experience is tangible and concrete; we learn by doing. Contrary to Plato, Aristotle argued that humans rightly prize their senses; sensation is part of human nature.

Self-Realization. The good for humans is happiness. One achieves happiness through individual self-realization. A nurse can make a patient happy by giving the patient hope based on trust. To show how one can realize oneself, Aristotle presents the Doctrine of the Mean. He compares ethical action to aiming at a target. One responds appropriately, not either too strongly or too weakly. To respond appropriately to a patient's health problem—physical, mental or emotional—is to do what is apt, and to avoid extremes that are excessive or insufficient. To Aristotle, for example, being generous is part way between being extravagant and being miserly. Confidence is a mean between arrogance and shame. Courage is a mean between cowardice and foolhardiness.

Stoicism

Epictetus (50–138 A.D.), a major ancient Stoic philosopher, is known for teaching us to recognize the limits of our powers and desires, which may lead us to false hopes and illusions. For Epictetus, modesty, apathy, withdrawal, passivity, resignation, and acceptance of one's lot are appropriate virtues.[6] If one accepts what happens and avoids other desires, then one will have a tranquil life.

In health care, Epictetus's Stoicism has influenced Tolstoy's *Death of Ivan Illich*, Dostoevsky's *House of the Dead*, Freud in his view that life is a struggle to be endured, and Kubler-Ross's work on stages of dying, culminating in the resignation or acceptance of one's death.

The strength of Stoicism is that endurance is a virtue, as is modesty and the recognition of individual human powerlessness in the presence of large cosmic events and forces. In nursing, we are ultimately helpless as we face the forces of life and death. Stoicism helps one accept the inevitable when our interventions fail. A difficulty with Stoicism is that life, ethics, society, and health care institutions call for doers, thinkers, and pioneers. Persistent active interventions in health care make a difference to the survival and longevity of individuals, cultures, and societies.

Natural Law

St. Thomas Aquinas (1224–1274) developed Agapism, love-based ethics, and the concept of natural law. To Aquinas, natural law is higher than any human or civil law. One can appeal to natural law to strike down any law or practice repugnant to natural law, such as abortion, homosexuality, and masturbation.

Aquinas presents four kinds of laws: eternal law, divine law, natural law, and human law. Eternal law is "God's law for the governance of the universe and all its parts. Such laws presumably include the law of gravitation. Divine law directs human beings toward their supernatural ends. Thus, this life is only an initial aspect of one's next and more important life. The most important natural law directs humans to their earthly goals in accordance with eternal and divine law."[7]

According to natural law, the desire for procreation and fruitfulness of the race morally legitimates sexual activity between duly married individuals of the opposite sex. Premarital and extramarital sex and the use of contraceptives are violations of natural law. Sexual activities between members of the same sex are considered immoral. Abortion, euthanasia, usury, war, and murder are also violations of natural law. Finally, "human law governs human beings" within communities, and in accordance with the logically prior types of eternal, divine, and natural law.[8]

A strength of natural law is that it requires legislatures and policy makers to justify laws, policies, and practices. For physicians to require nursing compliance to harmful procedures or medications violates a higher standard. A nurse may appeal to a higher standard the same way one changes a bad law, by appealing to a higher natural law.

There are difficulties, however, with natural law, such as the following: What truth is there in divine, eternal, and natural law? How can such truths be established? How does one justifiably decide what counts as the earmarks of natural law? How do we know that natural law is really what its proponents claim? What shall a nurse do about a terminal patient's wish to be helped to die by having gastric feedings withheld or terminated? Why isn't abortion morally preferable to giving birth to a person with multiple anomalies?

Altruism

Aquinas is justly famous also for his development of Agapistic or altruistic ethics. An important moral point of view that influences and is widely believed to justify moral choices in nursing is a love-based ethics, an ethics based on *agape* or *Agapism*. Love characterizes enduringly positive interpersonal relations, whether it be sexual love, romantic love, parental love, love for one's children, or love of country, customs, culture, and kinships. Love is the tie that binds humans together. Stories, novels, operas, poems, letters, paintings, and sonatas celebrate the force of love in human affairs. People sometimes live for and by one another's love. However, the love people feel for one another knows no greater love than the love of life, which makes all other feelings and love possible. Love is king of the positive emotions, too great and too brilliant to be extinguished or eclipsed even by its rival emotion, hate. Love is the handmaiden of peace, which makes more love possible; but it is opposed by hate, which brings about war and violence.

Perhaps it is no surprise, then, that love is the centerpiece of one of the most influential religions, namely Christianity. A contemporary philosopher, William Frankena, characterizes Agapism as holding that "there is only one basic ethical imperative—to love."[9] There are, according to Matthew 22:37-40, two commandments concerning love.

Thou shalt love the Lord thy God with all thy heart, and with all thy soul, and with all thy mind. This is the first and great commandment, and the second is Thou shalt love thy neighbor as Thyself. On these two commandments hang all the laws and the prophets.[10]

St. Francis of Assisi (1182–1226) extends this love of God and of one's neighbor to the love of all God's living creatures, including birds. This love, and also the test of this love, is that it includes the love of lepers, love of the diseased and dying, love of the poor, love of all living things as God's "creations."[11]

Agapistic or love-based ethics enjoins each person to love others as much as oneself. Such an ethics sometimes calls on people to do extraordinary deeds on behalf of their fellow human beings, which people are not always capable of or interested in doing.

According to Jesus, when someone smites us, we are asked to turn the other cheek. When there is not enough bread and fish, we are taught to share what there is. On this view, we individually gain by giving of ourselves to others. There are two kingdoms: the earth and a higher, eternal kingdom. We live in this kingdom for a short time, but we live in the other one forever.

The ethics of love applied to nursing and health care means that nurses show love, trust, and kindness for their patients. The word "care" is implied by the term "love." Care seems to be a pivotal part of nursing, essential to its calling. An important advantage of a love-based ethics is that love is at or very near the core of all positive emotions, or, to shift the metaphor slightly, love is the fuel and driving force of all worthwhile human feelings.

At least five difficulties exist, however. One is that the force of love seems to derive, as does romantic and sexual love, from desire, and, as such, needs no command or imperative. It is surprising, then, to see love characterized as a commandment in the Scriptures, and to see love characterized by W. Frankena as an imperative. If love, so to speak, flows from the heart, it needs no commandment either from an ancient or recent source.

A second and possibly more insuperable three-part difficulty is that love, as another saying goes, may be blind. It is not always discriminating. One needs a basis for deciding in a pinch to whom to extend love. As one of Bruno Bettelheim's books puts it, *Love Is Not Enough*. There is a need for wisdom, reason, and moral priorities. A second, related part of this difficulty is that there are too many beings to love, and choices need to be made as to who is worthy of love. Third—and this may explain the need to issue a commandment to love—while romantic and sexual love may come "naturally," the love of lepers, the poor, the diseased, and other beings may not be a love that comes so easily. We are limited not only as to who the recipients of love may be, but also as to whom we are capable of and interested in loving. In either case, to borrow an economic metaphor, the demand for love exceeds the supply. There is just not enough to go around.

There is, this rejoinder to the Agapist from the ancient Greek philosopher Aristotle (384–322 B.C.). One cannot be happy, according to Aristotle, without being healthy, reasonably wealthy, and goodlooking. One of two points is that one cannot identify happiness or love exclusively with the otherworldly.[12]

Second, satisfying material conditions of life is necessary for having feelings of love for anyone. The unloved cannot reasonably be expected to love others. A question arises as to whether the religious account of God, the universe, and the role of human beings in the world or the Humanist account of the central role of people in human affairs is a sufficient basis for reducing violence, war, and self-destruction.

Egoism

The difficulties with valuing love of others under all conditions gives rise, in part, to an alternative model of morality, that of self-interest above all. This model is called Egoism. According to Egoism, people are and ought to be oriented by self-love. Self-love is natural. Justice is defined by Thrasymachus as the interests of those who have power. As a model of morality for nursing, Egoist nurses look to patients and institutions solely for the good they can get for themselves.

The basis of modern Egoism is commonly identified with Thomas Hobbes (1599–1679). The main drive in human nature, says Hobbes, is self-preservation. But in a "state of nature," where people are left to themselves, there can be no society at all. In such a state, one in which people act full time on their basic motivations solely to survive, there would be a continuous "war of all against all." There would be no trade and commerce, no growth of knowledge, no arts. Rather, there would be "continual fear of danger and violent death." Human life would be "solitary, poor, nasty, brutish, and short."[13] Hobbes's ingenious solution is to convert this unbearable state of nature into the nature of a state. Such a state is brought about by a *social contract*. This contract provides for individuals to agree to give up their liberty to preserve themselves in a state of nature by any means and to transfer their individual liberty and power to a sovereign whom they agree to obey. The sovereign, in exchange for everyone's obedience, assures everyone's peace and protection. This social contract provides for the exchange of freedom for security. The sovereign keeps individuals obedient by developing a deputized peace force of persons to coerce and control people into continual compliance with civil laws. We are, however, never far from our basic interest in ourselves. Our reason for joining society is self-interest.

The Social Contract

The social contract, begun in ancient Greece by Glaucon, a rival of Socrates, is an important doctrine with implications for social and institutional behavior. The contracts we know are agreements we accept and act by. The Social contract provides that we agree to abide by previous agreements including the law and not to take agreements or "the law into our own hands." On one interpretation of the social contract, the very idea of nurses striking violates this fundamental tenet of the social contract. As the source of all contracts, the social contract requires nurses to accept working conditions in hospitals without resorting to nonpeaceful methods of conflict resolution. A social contract is the agreement to live by agreements, even though those agreements may predate one's own time of life. When innocent Socrates was convicted and sentenced to death, he took the fatal hemlock in preference to escaping from Athens. He thereby showed his acceptance of the social contract. A question arises in nursing as to whether nurses are to abide by bad contracts they had no part in formulating.

Egoism generates the social contract as an alternative to the war of individuals against one another. One agrees to abide by laws and regulations peaceably out of one's own self-interest. The alternative to accepting the social contract is social chaos and fighting at every turn, which is unthinkably harmful to all concerned and is worse than a bad agreement.

The social contract presents a paradox: Agree to agreements that are made without your consent? One agreement is to settle disputes peacefully.

A question arises: Is morality invented or discovered? If morality is discovered, one looks to an external authority to establish it. If morality is invented by people, they decide what is right and wrong. The social contract implies that one invents morality rather than discovers it.

Egoism generates two doctrines: the social contract and the invention of morality. Under Altruism, morality is discovered by some external and superior source of authority. Altruism appeals to natural law. So Egoism and Altruism generate the issue of natural law versus the social contract, the first other than humanly derived, the second derived from within human nature.

A strength of Egoism is that it speaks to people's motivations. Human beings including nurses, physicians, and patients, rewarded by money, power, recognition, status, and prestige, are apt to redouble their efforts. A difficulty with Egoism is, as Plato pointed out, that people live together and need one another. Plato made the point that people need to have their behavior controlled in order to help and not harm themselves and others. For people to do whatever they wish—a belief expressed by the bumper sticker, "If it feels right, do it"—may be inappropriate. One might, for example, fail to respect red and green traffic lights or not answer a patient's call light because one finds that patient a chronic complainer.

Utilitarianism

A modern effort to combine the strengths and also minimize the weaknesses of both Egoism and Altruism is found in Utiliarianism.

Utilitarianism began with David Hume (1711–1776), a great Scottish philosopher. To Hume, ethics depends on what people want and desire. "Reason is and ought to be the slave of the passions."[14] The passions determine what is right and what is wrong. Reason has only two minor roles in deciding what actions to take. Reason can tell us what is true or false and what the facts are; and reason can tell us what means will achieve our ends. But the ends are up to us and depend on our passions.

We act because of our passions. Our passions drive us to prefer pleasure to pain, and we learn to judge these by noticing the uses and consequences of our actions.

Classical Utilitarianism was developed by Jeremy Bentham (1748–1826) and John Stuart Mill (1806–1873). Bentham was the first to develop a "hedonistic calculus." He noted that no matter what moral philosophers and moralists say, we are all governed by two masters: pain and pleasure. The point about ethics is to minimize the first and maximize the second as much as possible. This is now called cost/ benefit analysis, which some people would define as cost/risk/benefit ratio. One may ask about any desire: What does it cost? What is the risk? What is the benefit? To Bentham, the basis for judging any pain and pleasure, the principle of utility, depends on seven criteria. They are "(1) its intensity; (2) its duration; (3) its certainty or uncertainty; (4) its propinquity or remoteness; (5) its fecundity . . . or the chance it has of being followed by 'similar' sensations; (6) its purity" as a pleasure of being followed by more pleasure rather than pain, and "(7) its extent . . . the number of persons to whom it extends or . . . who are affected by it."[15]

An example of Utilitarian ethics applied to everyday nursing is the nurse's decision to give pain medication. This depends on the medication's predicted effect of diminishing or eliminating the intensity of pain considered in relation to its side effects, such as the slowing of respiration. Similarly, a person taking a drink of alcohol does so to get a pleasure of some intensity. Intensity also figures in the most intimate human experience—namely, sexual intimacy leading to and including sexual intercourse. Richard Wasserstrom, a contemporary philosopher, argues that the high degree of intensity in sexual intercourse is a basis for marital exclusivity in our present culture. According to Wasserstrom,

It is obvious that one of the more powerful desires is the desire for sexual gratification. . . . Once we experience sexual intercourse ourselves—and in particular once we experience orgasm, we discover that it is among the most intensive, short term pleasures of the body.[16]

A second criterion, duration, is also of concern to everyone. "How long will this pleasure last?" is a common question. Vacationers and honeymooners alike are known to dread the end of their bliss in some Paradise Island for return to the drudgery and dreariness, drabness, boredom, and monotony of their lives and work. Conversely, how long a patient has to continue a particularly painful treatment again speaks to the relevance of duration in judging pleasures and pains.

Bentham's third criterion, certainty or uncertainty, is an important consideration in health care. Even the most innocuous, routine treatment such as an aspirin tablet or a tonsillectomy has the element of risk in it. For some patients, either of these beneficial therapies ends in death. Considerations of sureness and risk are relevant in evaluating which pleasures and pain to live by. A fourth criterion, propinquity or remoteness, concerns the nearness or distance of an intended pleasure or pain. Patients farthest away from the nursing station are apt to get the least attention. An example of fecundity or fruitfulness that applies to nursing is continuous patient care, preferably by similar personnel, as basic for a patient's healing process.

Purity refers to unmixed feelings. An excess of alcohol may, for example, be followed by a painful sensation. The aim of nursing is one of relieving suffering and promoting health. Nursing is impure when mixed with business dealings with the patient. Finally, extent, to Bentham, concerns the numbers of people affected by a consideration of pain and pleasure. Nurses with six to eight acutely ill patients in their charge will have to distribute their nursing services to a greater extent than if assigned to half that number.

An advantage of Bentham's classical Utilitarianism is that it puts us in touch with feelings of pleasure and pain. A strength of the utility principle is that, in questions of resource allocation, it appeals to the principle of *sufferability,* one that includes the capacity of all sentient beings to suffer. The principle of resource allocation is based on the Utilitarian and also democratic maxim framed by Bentham, "Everybody is to count for one, nobody for more than one."[17] This means that the pleasure-pain calculus considers that "the equal pains or pleasures, satisfactions or dissatisfactions . . . are given the same weight, whether they be Brahmins or Untouchables, Jews or Christians, black or white."[18] The idea that each counts for one is basic to the principle of social equality. In nursing, the equality principle means that nurses are to treat all patients with equal consideration.

A difficulty of Bentham's Utilitarianism is that it leaves too little room for moral values other than pain and pleasure. Other important values are freedom of the will, duty, love, respect for the individual, truthfulness, or even saving an individual's life if doing so collides with the application of the pleasure-pain calculus.

John Stuart Mill attempts to remedy Bentham's difficulties. According to Mill, an action is right if it conforms to "the greatest-happiness principle."[19] Using the utilitarian principle, one appeals to the greatest happiness for the greatest number.[20] This ethics is called "goal based" because it renounces a priori or absolute preconceptions of how best to provide the good that is defined by the greatest-happiness principle. Rather, the Utilitarian ethics follows inductive methods of trial and error, currently called "cost/benefit analysis," with the avowed aim to help the maximum number of persons to flourish. To Mill, "actions are right in proportion as they tend to promote happiness, wrong as they tend to produce the reverse of happiness."[21] To Bentham's criteria, Mill adds quality of pleasure or pain, a quality appropriate for human beings. He adds this further requirement: "Utilitarianism requires" a person "to be strictly impartial as a disinterested and benevolent spectator. . . . In the golden rule of Jesus of Nazareth, we read the complete spirit of the ethics of utility. 'To do as you would be done by' and 'to love your neighbor as yourself' constitutes the ideal perfection of Utilitarian morality."[22]

Mill offers a proof for the principle of utility:

> The only proof capable of being given that an object is visible is that people actually see it. The only proof that a sound is audible is that people hear it. . . . In like manner, I apprehend the sole evidence it is possible to produce that anything is desirable is that people do actually desire it.[23]

In this passage, Mill commits the is-ought fallacy by inferring that what is desired is therefore desirable. That is like saying that, because Hospital X policymakers desire nurses to work a double shift on occasion, such a policy is therefore desirable and ought to be put into practice.

An advantage of Mill's greatest-happiness principle is that it takes the consequences of our actions seriously, a point which no opponent of Utilitarianism can ignore.

Although Mill's Utilitarianism has these strengths, there are several difficulties. Although Mill invokes the ethics of Jesus, Utilitarianism is concerned with aggregate happiness, doing good for the greatest number, which is not equivalent to caring for and loving everyone. A few examples may show the difference between the ethics of Jesus and Mill's Utilitarianism. If a tank with 10 soldiers and an innocent hostage tied visibly to its front is firing at you and 60 friends and neighbors, more lives are to be saved by destroying the tank and all its occupants, including the innocent hostage. Therefore, doing so is not wrong on Utilitarian grounds. But such an action is morally wrong, according to the ethics of Jesus. Similarly, in triage health care problems in which some lives can be saved, Utilitarian ethics emphasizes help to the greatest number. In the face of limited resources, an application of Utilitarianism calls for the subordination of some people, such as the terminally ill, to the care of the majority of persons. However, to pick an analogous problem, if 85 percent of the population of a hypothetical society live well at the expense of 15 percent who live miserably, Utilitarianism seems to have no constraint against such a policy. Some would argue that such a practice is morally wrong. A difficulty of Utilitarianism is that appeal to majority happiness overlooks the value of the individual who, although in a minority, may deserve help. The health care needs of mentally ill, retarded, aged, and other vulnerable patients, for example, may call for taxes the majority opposes.

Utilitarianism has not answered these and other difficulties, as what to do about sacrificing some individuals for the good of the majority. One response is that there are situations in wartime or in disasters in which there is no way other than to consider the well-being and health of the majority while sacrificing individuals. The use of triage—of sorting out the wounded into those who will survive without help, those who will die anyway, and those who can most benefit from help—is an example of the application of Utilitarian principles. A prominent example of concern for the majority's happiness is the military draft, which places a number of persons, usually young men, at risk in defense of the large majority of citizens. Another example of Utilitarian ethics is the distribution of scarce resources in response to majority happiness. Still another example in health care is the risk nurses and physicians take when they are exposed to patients with contagious diseases. An objection to Utilitarianism arises, however: Any such policies, which subordinate certain individuals or groups of individuals, can never be just.

Universal Moral Principles

Utilitarian ethics is opposed by Kantian ethics, the equal and uncompromising application of fixed principles, regardless of changing circumstances. If one chooses not to treat a neonate with trisomy 18, giving the only available respirator to a neonate with only a slight respiratory difficulty instead, one appeals to a Utilitarian principle: Maximize benefit, minimize harm. But if a neonate is a person, not saving is immoral.

Opposed to Utilitarianism is the idea of principled morality or deontological ethics, whose major proponent was the great philosopher

Immanuel Kant (1724–1804). Kant held that an act is good if everyone ought, for rational reasons and in similar circumstances, to act in the same way without exception. The basis for doing this is that it is rational, universal, free and uncoerced.[24] This is called the categorical imperative or universalizability principle, and it tells us to act always on that principle on which everyone in the same situation ought to act. One is to act from the point of view of a rational impartial spectator, which alone is a worthy moral position. Kant cites five examples of categorical imperatives relevant to nursing ethics: (1) Suicide or taking any life is wrong, because if everyone who felt like it committed suicide or killed someone else, the human race would soon be extinct. (2) Keeping promises is right. Breaking them is wrong. Social institutions depend on people, including nurses to fulfill their promises. One may note the relation of promise-making and keeping to the social contract, the rule to abide by rules. (3) Always develop your talents to the utmost of your ability. You owe it to the human race to develop to the optimum. (4) Always help those in need. Everyone at some time or other needs the help of others. (5) Always tell the truth. To be rational and moral requires one to be truthful, regardless of consequences to oneself.

On the basis of the categorical imperative and these examples of always preserving everyone's life, keeping promises, developing one's talents, helping others in distress, and never lying, Kant formulates a substantive principle, which is to act so that one treats oneself or any other person always as an "end" and never as a "means" only.[25] Kant's principle is a welcome antidote to the wanton disregard of patients, family members, and health professionals in relation to hard cases in everyday nursing.

Paul Freund cites an example from World War II showing how the "greatest-happiness" criterion or majority rule prevailed over uncompromising principles. A choice between allocating scarce supplies of penicillin to wounded soldiers in Africa or to soldiers with gonorrhea had to be made. The principled action would have been to give the penicillin to the wounded. But the decision was to give it to those "wounded in the brothels."[26] This decision exposes a moral difficulty of Utilitarianism by appealing to Kantian moral principles, which show no doubt as to who gets scarce penicillin, namely those who are wounded in battle. If, however, one appeals to some version of triage or to the greatest benefit of the greatest number, the appeal to some form of Utilitarianism seems to provide the morally preferable decision. To Ethical Relativists, it depends on one's expected moral values.

However, there is a price one pays in sacrificing moral principles. A war, a sports contest, a business deal may be won; a hospital emergency may be solved, all by ignoring a Kantian moral imperative to keep a promise, tell the truth, or to treat each patient as an end and not as a means only. A price to all concerned is that the moral quality of everyone's life will decline.

There is no room in Kant's categorical imperative for special privileges, irrational acts, or coerced acts. The universalizability principle states the right act regardless of anyone's or everyone's inclination, impulse, convenience, or even of the majority welfare. To act morally is to do what is rational, universal, and desirable for the whole human race, independent of anyone's pleasure, and without regard for the consequences.

There is an important difference between the categorical imperative and the famous Golden Rule, which superficially resembles the categorical imperative. The Golden Rule directs that we treat others as we would like to be treated. The categorical imperative says instead to treat oneself and all others as everyone ought to be treated—freely, rationally, and impartially. If, for example, one enjoys smoking or drinking excessively, then on Golden Rule grounds one may justifiably impose cigarettes and alcohol on others. The categorical imperative rules out such conduct.

There are difficulties, however, with appeal to Kantian principles. One difficulty is that their application is sometimes impractical. Worse, the unswerving application of rigid principles can have disastrous consequences. Moreover, disregarding consequences of actions is a contradiction of what it means to do ethics. Even Kant's principles lead to consequences that are in principle good rather than evil— which explains why people should consider Kant's principles carefully. Even if one acknowledges the essential rationality of Kant's principles, this does not mean one follows every example of his to its inevitable conclusion. To lie to an evildoer such as a Nazi is not necessarily wrong.

CONCLUSION

Philosophical ethics sometimes presents conflicts, dilemmas, problems, tragedies, and stalemates. Philosophical ethics or dialogue between philosophical models or morality also presents reasoned arguments in response to ethical issues in nursing.

To controversy surrounding abortion, the Agapistic responds that abortion is murder. To a Utilitarian, the permissibility of abortion depends on circumstances. Each model presents arguments which the other or others may attempt to refute. How does one judge who is successful? Ethics is not a science, a finished body of true propositions that yields certainty. Nor, however, is ethics purely subjective. For ethics also includes justifying rules that people have for living together.

One can imagine a physician refusing to treat an AIDS patient, leaving it to nurses to treat the patient. One can evaluate nurses and physicians. Jones, an AIDS patient, will suffer avoidable harm, a violation of a fundamental principle both of ethics and of medicine. A moral difference in the two codes of physicians and nurses shows that physicians as a group not only violate a fundamental principle of helping those in need; but that their code sanctions the principle of practicing discriminatory medicine.

Discussion Questions

1. Do nurses act only out of self-interest? Should they? What is self-interest? Does it overlap with interest in others?
2. Can one love others or oneself exclusively?
3. What is the difference between a nurse's motivation and justification for caring for an ICU patient on a double shift?
4. Should nurses receive fees for individual patients, like physicians? Or should physicians receive institutional salaries, like nurses?
5. What is a morally justifiable basis for compensating health professionals on different levels of qualifications, in the giving of primary, secondary and teriary care?
6. Are there true or false statements in ethics? If so, what is an example of a true or false statement in nursing ethics? If not, are there standards for judging right and wrong in nursing ethics?
7. What is the relation of facts and values in nursing ethics?
8. How do facts or clinical assessments of data contribute to moral decision making in nursing?
9. In a case P. Benner cites of an intubated, quadraplegic patient who could not speak, the nurse expert says, "I just knew we could resolve this problem . . . so I intervened in his behalf with his multiple physicians."[27] How could this nurse use clinical data and use a model of morality to make a difference in this patient's life?

REFERENCES

1. American Nurses' Association. *Code for nurses with interpretive statements.* Kansas City, MO: Author. 1976.
2. Scheffler I. Philosophical models of teaching. In: Scheffler I (ed). *Reason and teaching.* Indianapolis: Bobbs-Merrill. 1975; 67.
3. Rachels J. Can ethics provide answers? In: Caplan A and Callahan D (eds). *Ethics for hard times.* New York: Plenum. 1981; 1–30.
4. Plato. Republic. In: Jones WT et al (eds). *Approaches to Ethics.* 3rd ed. New York: McGraw-Hill. 1977; 29–46.
5. Aristotle. *Nichomachean ethics.* Martin Ostwald (tr). Indianapolis: Bobbs-Merrill. 1962; 21–22.

6. Epictetus. The enchiridian. In: Jones WT et al (eds). *Approaches to Ethics.* 3rd ed. New York: McGraw-Hill. 1977; 84.
7. Golding MP. *Philosophy of law.* Englewood Cliffs, NJ: Prentice-Hall. 1981; 31.
8. Ibid.
9. Frankena W. *Ethics.* 2nd ed. Englewood Cliffs, NJ: Prentice-Hall. 1973; 56–59.
10. Ibid; 56.
11. Jones WT et al (eds). *A history of western philosophy.* 2nd ed. New York: Harcourt Brace. 1969. *II*:149–152.
12. Aristotle. *Nichomachean ethics.* Martin Ostwald (tr). Indianapolis: Bobbs-Merrill. 1962; 21–22.
13. Hobbes T. The leviathan. In: Jones WT et al (eds). *Approaches to Ethics.* 3rd ed. New York: McGraw-Hill. 1977; 182.
14. Hume D. A treatise of human nature. In: Johnson OA (ed). *Ethics.* 4th ed. New York: Holt, Rinehart and Winston. 1978; 212.
15. Bentham J. Morals and legislation. In: Jones WT et al (eds). *Approaches to Ethics.* 3rd ed. New York: McGraw-Hill. 1972; 260.
16. Wasserstrom R. Is adultery immoral? In: Arthur J. (ed). *Morality and Moral Controversies,* 2nd edition Englewood Cliffs, NJ: Prentice-Hall. 1986; 19.
17. Hart HLA. Between utility and rights. In: Ryan A (ed). *The Idea of Morality: Essays in Honor of Isaiah Berlin.* New York: Oxford University Press. 1979; 79.
18. Ibid.
19. Mill. *Utilitarianism.* 6.
20. Mill. *Utilitarianism.* 10.
21. Ibid.
22. Ibid; 22.
23. Ibid; 44.
24. Kant I. *Fundamental principles of the metaphysics of morals.* New York: Liberal Arts. 1949; 38.
25. Ibid; 46.
26. Ramsey P. *The patient as person.* New Haven: Yale University Press. 1971; 257–258.
27. Benner P. *From novice to expert.* Menlo Park, CA: Addison-Wesley. 1984; 52–53.

CHAPTER 5

Contemporary Models of Morality in Nursing

Study of this chapter enables the learner to:

1. Clarify values as the basis of moral priorities.
2. Distinguish between alternative models of morality.
3. Justify decisions in nursing ethics in relation to models of morality.

INTRODUCTION

Models of morality intersect with one another in formal, conventional, philosophical, and intuitive ways and within institutions, societies, epochs, and cultures in a dynamism and momentum of their own. Dueling, once regarded as the way men had of settling affairs of honor, is practically extinct. Women were once forbidden to wear trousers, to vote, or to smoke. They may now do much more. Shortly, however, smoking may be banned in public places.

The technology of human reproduction, of transmission, communication, and travel have changed the character of moral problems. Values change with major changes in society.

In this chapter, we consider some major contemporary models of morality that affect nursing ethics. We begin with value clarification, which is useful in identifying one's preferred model of morality.

VALUE CLARIFICATION

Value clarification expresses a person's preferences, likes, and dislikes, such as one's beliefs about the importance of living, dying, God, work, truth, love, family, sex, and pleasure. Value clarification is a process that moves in three stages. It begins with an initial choice of a value from among alternatives. Here one sifts through alternatives and ranks them. In the second stage, one reflects on which of the chosen values are worthwhile to prize. Third, one maps a strategy of action to achieve the values one has chosen and prized. Here one decides to act on one's prized values. Value clarification makes explicit a person's priorities.[1]

A strength of value clarification is that one expresses value preferences and priorities in an honest and straightforward way. Examples are how a nurse feels about the saving of seriously defective neonates, or the value placed on the life of the elderly by society. A drawback of value clarification, however, is that the expression of one's preferences

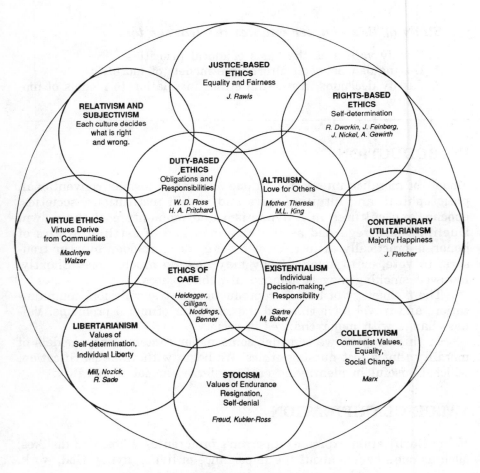

Figure 5–1. Contemporary models of morality.

or priorities does not imply that these preferences are justifiable or that they ought to be preferred. For example, a nurse may prize quiet patients in a quiet ward, but such a value may not be good for the patients. A desire does not imply that the desire ought to be acted on. There is a well-known fallacy in moral reasoning, called the *is-ought fallacy,* which holds that what is does not automatically imply and justify what ought to be. One cannot validly infer that what one desires is therefore desirable. The value of quiet patients may be a clarified value, but it is not thereby shown to be a justifiable value. The harm that a person who drinks and then drives can do shows that chosen or prized values are not justified values. Value clarification calls for further development in the process of justification, which takes us to other important aspects of philosophical ethics.

CONTEMPORARY MODELS OF MORALITY

Individualism versus Collectivism

An example of a contemporary moral issue involving models is that of Individualism versus Collectivism. The first model emphasizes individual liberty, individual self-determination, initiative, self reliance, and self-realization. To an Individualist, social institutions are the sum total of individual efforts and actions. One form Individualism takes is Existentialism, which holds individuals responsible for their actions and inactions equally. If a nurse fails to put the guard rails of a bed up, for example, resulting in an 80-year-old patient's falling out of bed, breaking his hip, getting pneumonia, and dying, the nurse is responsible for killing the patient.

A major Existentialist, Jean Paul Sartre, holds individuals responsible because "we are," he says, "all condemned to be free."[2] To live is, as with Hamlet, to have to decide. One can only be held responsible for one's acts if one is free to choose. To Sartre, to decide is to be free. To choose is to be responsible.

Collectivism, on the other hand, holds society as a whole or a segment of society, such as capitalism, responsible for human problems, including widespread starvation, lack of drinking water, and lack of health care in many parts of the world.

One form of Collectivism originated with Karl Marx (1818–1883). To Marx, individuals are not free, only groups of people with power are free in capitalist societies. Those with power are free to exploit others, turning the majority into wage slaves. This form of Collectivism calls for total social change rather than piecemeal social change proposed by Bentham and by Existentialists.

There are strengths and weaknesses in each of these models. Individualism, expecially Existentialism, emphasizes attractive qualities associated with individual liberty, individual initiative, hard work, and rewards for individual merit. However individuals can amass power and abuse others. Out of such abuse, through exploitation, comes the appeal of Collectivism. This doctrine promises to do for individuals what they cannot possibly do alone, namely, organize to form better rules for achieving social and economic justice. Appeal to collectivities, sometimes identified as corporate bodies, can also provide for more widespread needs and wants than is possible by appeal to Individualism. Collectivities, including corporate organizations, provide security from the basic human wants. They sometimes do so, however, at great cost to individual liberty and to individual self-development.

Contemporary Utilitarianism
Utilitarian ethics is near the forefront of moral reasoning in nursing due, in part, to the rise of science and technology. Questions of how to care for patients with existing shortages, how to decide whom to treat, are questions that are considered as questions of maximizing pleasure and minimizing pain, the Minimax principle. Questions of just allocation of health care resources and nursing services are frequently given a utilitarian approach.

Two forms of contemporary utilitarian ethics are practiced in nursing health care emergencies. One is the use of triage to accommodate questions of scarce health care resources. Using triage, one sorts patients out into those who can essentially recover on their own, those who will die anyway, and those to whom health care can make a difference. Triage is practical in battle, national disasters, and some inner city emergency rooms when the staff is overwhelmed with waiting patients. Conditions of severe understaffing on nursing units with acutely and seriously ill patients sometimes forces nurses to allocate the available time using the principle of triage instead of equal distribution or caring for the most ill.

A second form of contemporary utilitarian ethics, developed by Joseph Fletcher, is called situationalism. In this view, one deals with "here and now" health care problems. According to Fletcher, modern health care is to be restricted to patients who can benefit in relation to quality of life standards, such as neocortical functioning.

Relativism and Subjectivism
Some patients, nurses, and allied health professionals subscribe to Relativism, the view that there is no universal right or wrong but that values are relative to the individual, group, or culture. An example is that in one culture, A, hemodialysis is not given to those who reach the age of 65. In culture B, dialysis is given anyone in need without age or diagnostic restrictions. According to the Relativist model, nei-

ther culture is right or wrong. In some cultures, one cares for AIDS patients; in others not. But on Relativist grounds, there is no right or wrong.

Closely allied to Relativism is Subjectivism. According to this model of morality, there is no right or wrong except what each individual, group, society, or culture thinks is right.

According to the subjectivist view, "beauty is in the eyes of the beholder" and so are truth and goodness. This view is aptly phrased in Shakespeare, as Hamlet remarks that "nothing is good or bad, but thinking makes it so."

An advantage of Relativism and of Subjectivism is that they do not impose an absolute standard of morality to be obeyed without question. A second advantage is that Relativism and Subjectivism foster tolerance of alternative ways of behaving. Closely affiliated with Relativism is Pluralism, which is often an effective antidote to the narrow constraints of an absolute moral standard.

A drawback, however, of Relativism and of Subjectivism is that if nothing is right or wrong, moral education is seriously limited and is reduced to mastery of conventions. One cannot then effectively argue against the lack of health care, the exploitation of nurses, slavery, segregation, racism, sexism, anti-semitism, Naziism, or any other obvious evil. Since there is then no transcultural justification of any moral practice, each culture is the supreme moral lawgiver unto itself. There is then no higher moral court of appeal.

Libertarianism

A morally viable alternative to Relativism is Libertarianism, the view that the most important value is individual liberty. Its progenitor is J.S. Mill, whose classic essay "On Liberty" provided the basis for valuing one's freedom as high as life itself. Robert Nozick, a major proponent of Libertarianism, contends that the best state is a minimal state, one that protects individuals against force and fraud, the "nightwatchman" state.

Nozick's basic tenet is that a state is morally legitimate only if it leaves people alone, unless they harm or deceive others. An individual has a right to keep what he or she earns. The person who climbs the coconut tree and gets the coconut gets to keep it.[3] A nursing or hospital administrator, physician, or surgeon is entitled to charge whatever the traffic will bear. No state is entitled to deprive them of their earnings. For a state to provide more than minimal services of protection against "force and fraud," and then to tax people to pay for public services, such as libraries, museums, schools, hospitals, and welfare,[4] is to coerce people into "forced labor."[4] On Nozick's account, forced labor is a violation of one's right to the free use of one's labor and is immoral. According to Nozick, if one sees a little boy drowning in a puddle of water, one has no moral obligation to try to save the child. It would be nice if one did, but an individual is not morally at fault if he or she ignores the plight of a drowning child. Such a position seems counter-intuitive. A nursing example is that a nurse is not obligated to give mouth to mouth resuscitation to a stranger on the sidewalk in a large city. Nozick reminds us that there are limits to one's obligations. And this nursing example reinforces Nozick's point.[5]

A Libertarian physician, Robert Sade, argues that health care is not a right, but a "purchasable commodity"[6] on the open market. Sade argues that a physician has a right to make a living, like a butcher, baker or candlestick maker.[7]

A strength of Libertarianism is that it stresses the moral value of freedom. Taxation that interferes with people's freedom to keep what they earn is "forced labor" and a loss of liberty.

A difficulty with Libertarianism is that it assumes that the state has nothing to do with helping people achieve economic, social, and political goals beyond the services rendered by a nightwatchman state. Failure to tax a person's earnings for the common good, such as public education, public health measures of disease control, and public hospitals, is irresponsible. People's private earnings are justifiably taxed to provide for the disadvantaged. A person cannot be free if she or he is illiterate, diseased, or hungry. People cannot live free under conditions of ignorance, poverty, and disease.

Justice-Based Rights

To offset the difficulties of Utilitarianism, Relativism, Individualism, Collectivism and Libertarianism, one turns to rights based on justice. R. Rawls attempted to provide an effective synthesis between Utilitarian and absolute ethics. To Rawls, the idea of justice as fairness occupies center state in ethics. Justice is uncompromising. "Justice is the first virtue of social institutions as truth is of systems of thought. A theory however elegant and economical must be rejected or revised if it is untrue; likewise laws and institutions no matter how efficient and well arranged must be reformed or abolished if they are unjust."[8]

We suggest a corollary to Rawls's concept of justice as fairness. Our corollary is that if there are any moral rights at all, there is at least one prior right founded on justice, the equal right of all persons to be free to decide how to live. Such a prior moral right is, moreover, one whose claims are early incontestable and can only be overridden under extraordinary circumstances: (a) favoring the continuation of a person's life and (b) involving the least injustice. The type of exception to be noted is justified only on the grounds that it avoids a greater injustice to everyone's otherwise inviolably equal right to be free to make decisions affecting their lives. For example, a nurse who forcibly prevents a patient from committing suicide for whom there is a viable personal life is morally justified in bringing about this act of minimal injustice.

The equal right to be free to decide how to live, we hold, is based largely on J. Rawls's point that to "respect persons is to recognize that they possess an inviolability founded on justice that even the welfare of society as a whole cannot override."[9] We demur, ever so slightly, however, to Rawls's implication that the "welfare of society as a whole" makes no morally just claim. There is also justice in being on the side of the "welfare of society as a whole."

A conflict between moral rights and claims involving difficult choices calls for a just procedure to avoid a greater injustice, which does not, however, override the claims of justice. That is, justice as "the first virtue of social institutions" cannot be overturned in principle, but always and only by some other just claim. But just claims are never morally overridden by unjust claims, only by those claims that result in helping us avoid a greater injustice. The claims of the majority can never be morally supported at the expense of the minority; nor can a majority morally be put at the service of a minority, such as a society that supports an elite group, such as physicians. An example of a minority being abused by a majority is that the health care needs of a community can be paid for by exploiting nurses as cheap labor. According to Rawls, "the interests requiring the violation of justice have no value."[10] Having no moral merit in the first place, such claims cannot override any moral claims, which collide with the equal right to be free to decide how to live. For example, a hospital administration's demand in contract negotiations for mandatory second shifts by nurses, when needed, conflicts with nurses' just claims to be free to decide when or whether to work a second shift.

We also demur with Rawls that truth is designed for systems of thought exclusively. We hold that truth affects the justice of social institutions. In judging the morality of social institutions, truth and justice are not always separate. For example, if it is true that nurses are underpaid and if it is true that being underpaid is unfair, then it is also true that nurses are treated unfairly.

Rawls identifies rights with justice. To Rawls,

> Justice denies that the loss of freedom for some is made right by a greater good shared by others. . . . Rights secured by justice are not subject to political bargaining or to the calculus of social interests. . . . An injustice is tolerable only when it is necessary to avoid an even greater injustice.[11]

Rawls arrives at the idea of justice as fairness as a central principle through a powerful thought experiment, called "the veil of ignorance."[12] We are all to imagine not knowing our biological, social, economic role, place, or identity in the world. Imagine that we will not know whether we will be born smart or dull; healthy or disabled; white, yellow, or black; rich or poor; male or female; beautiful or ugly.

Under this "veil of ignorance," what rational rules would we agree to live by? Rawls suggests that we would rationally choose to live by two principles. The first is that we would want all people to have equal political liberties, such as the equal right to vote. The second principle in three parts is that social and economic inequalities are justified only if they (1) help "the least advantaged" first; (2) serve "the advantage of all"; and (3) if offices are open to all "on a basis of equality of opportunity."[13]

The Rawlsian conceptual scheme has an important role in health care and nursing in particular, such as fairness and compensation for nurses. Rawls tries to bring together two important values in distributive justice, satisfying large scale for health care needs and for recognizing and rewarding individual merit in providing health care. Rawls's scheme attempts to give appropriate consideration for the advantage of all, including those who are least served, and to recognize merit by rewarding persons on the basis of equality of opportunity.

In health care, appeal to justice as fairness rules out certain profitable practices, such as the exploitation of nurses through unpaid overtime and overcharging the government for patient services not given.

Rawls aims to equalize access to the "primary goods" of life, such as power, money, and good health care. Rawls's work brings home to health care ethicists, including nurses, that there can be no ethics without justice and that justice is to ethics what equal access to health care and to nursing are to a good life for everyone.

One response to Rawls's work is Nozick's, previously discussed, that a society that provides for the "advantage of all" imposes an intolerable burden of taxation in the form of "forced labor."[14] Such a deprivation of a person's liberty can never be just, in Nozick's view.

R. Dworkin presents a different response. Dworkin argues that the function of states is to protect individual rights equally. To Dworkin, individual rights are "political trumps held by individuals,"[15] which no state may take away. However, the emphasis in the concept of rights that Dworkin defends identifies rights with the idea of equality rather than liberty. To Dworkin, individual rights are held equally. In Dworkin's account, people do not have a right to equal shares or equal treatment in the distribution of health care resources, but a right to equal consideration and to treatment as equals. One can recognize that the rights both to liberty and to equality are important to patients and nurses alike.

A further response to Rawls's work, with an important impact on nursing ethics, is the work of Lawrence Kohlberg. He proposes to refute Relativism and Subjectivism by identifying three levels and six stages of moral growth and development. Level 1 is Preconventional. Stage 1 in Level 1 is oriented by fear of punishment and obedience to authority. Stage 2 is instrumental and relativistic. "You scratch my back and I'll scratch yours." The second level is the Conventional Level, with Stages 3 and 4. Stage 3 is marked by "nice-guy, nice-girl" behavior, approved by the peer group. Stage 4 consists in conforming to "law and order." Level 3 consists in Postconventional, autonomous, principled behavior. Here, Stage 5 is a "social contract, constitutional-legal orientation." Finally, Stage 6 consists of a "universal-ethical principled" orientation.[16]

Kohlberg's emphasis is not on conscience, as consciences differ. Kohlberg's appeal is rather to universal principles, like saving life, preventing harm, and truth-telling. Human beings grow morally in these ways and through these six stages, according to Kohlberg.

There are merits in Kohlberg's stages of moral development. One advantage is that Kohlberg provides a good argument against Subjectivism and Relativism. A second strength of Kohlberg's analysis is that it suggests parallels between intellectual and moral development. The brighter one is, the more apt one is to be moral.

There are, however, several difficulties with Kohlberg's analysis. First, an account of how one develops morally, even if true, does not imply or justify how one ought to behave or develop. The is-ought fallacy is committed here. Second, one may arrive at the right moral decision of preventing harm by a conventional or even preconventional, Egoist move. Even Kohlberg's example of stealing a cancer-curing drug for one's wife appeals to self-preservation, a Hobbesian value, at the Preconventional or Egoist stage. Egoism is not always morally wrong. The Egoist action might in some cases be the right thing to do. Third, there are no proofs that the moral hierarchical method, in which one arrives at universal moral principles, is the valid and sound view in all cases. Fourth, if the way one developed morally could not be altered by a moral agent, then one could not be said to have a free will with which to make moral decisions. But if one could do nothing to alter one's moral behavior, there would be no point in telling anyone what optimal, desirable moral development would be. Kohlberg's stages of moral development would be like describing the growth of a tadpole into a frog.

If, however, Kohlberg intended his six stages as a proposal as to how individuals ought to develop morally, in which free will is assumed, then people would have a choice. Where people make choices, good as well as bad may result. If there is a choice as to how to develop morally, then we would have no sure way of knowing how moral development ought necessarily to proceed. Followers of Nietzsche, Thrasymachus, Existentialists, and others who give their moral reasons for denying the moral desirability of the sixth stage have not been shown that their position is morally wrong in all cases. One may prefer truth-telling and doing away with the use of placebos. Yet, there are reasons involving the prevention of harm, that could justify lying and giving placebos, in some instances. To reiterate, Kohlberg has not been able to show that stages of hierarchical moral development from the lowest, Egoism and obedience, to the highest stage of acting on universal principles is the way to become increasingly moral. If Kohlberg were successful, he would show that ethics has a true and valid answer. This, however, has not been shown.

Virtue Ethics in Nursing

Critics of rights in health care point to the high cost of malpractice suits and to the loss of trust and confidence that once pervaded health care delivery systems. These critics call for a moratorium on the language of rights and rules and a revival of concern with traditional virtues that contribute to character and community. Notable among these critics are A. MacIntyre, S. Toulmin, C. Gilligan, N. Nodding, and in nursing, P. Benner and J. Wrubel. MacIntyre emphasizes the cultivation of virtues, such as courage, wisdom, prudence, temperance, honesty, and responsibility.[17] One develops these in families and communities, which are the roots of ethics. Ethics is about character formation, from which laws and rules emerge. But without concrete applications in particular moral concerns, ethics becomes abstract, largely irrelevant, and not significant to the lives of people in communities.

In the same vein, S. Toulmin distinguishes the ethics of intimates from the ethics of strangers.[18] Toulmin draws on Tolstoy's symbols of face-to-face interactions. The people in families, friends, and neighbors with whom one frequently interacts are intimates. With these people one has most of one's daily relationships. The boundaries of ethics are about these interactions. Then there are the distant relations we have with strangers. With strangers there are no deep personal relationships one can or should form beyond politeness.

The ethics of strangers appeals to formalized principles of justice, rights, and rules. Such rights and rules develop adversarial relations that include malpractice suits. We thereby give up the trust we once had in health professionals.

Carol Gilligan takes virtue ethics a step further. She argues that the justice, rights, and rules orientation is designed by and for male domination. An alternative to this view is a feminist ethical orientation concerned with care and nurture.[19]

Nel Noddings focuses on the ethics of care. Noddings argues that if a mother has to decide between saving her drowning child and a neighbor's child, her first concern is and ought to be her own child.[20]

Lastly, Benner and Wrubel apply the ethics of caring, discussed in Chapter 1, to nursing situations. Caring means patients matter as meaningful persons. "Caring . . . fuses thought, feeling, and action.[21] Caring sets up options for dealing with a patient's stressful situations.[22] (See Chapter 1 for an elaboration of this approach to nursing ethics.)[23]

A strength of the ehtics of caring is that it emphasizes features neglected by the rights-based ethics. Justice is not everything. People can only lead a good life if they receive and give care.

A difficulty, however, with the ethics of caring is that it avoids questions like the following: Whom shall one care for? How much shall one care for in relation to intimates? How much care do I have to give? One cannot decide these without considering questions of the just distribution of health care resources. To avoid questions of justice invites ethical Relativism and Subjectivism, where people arbitrarily decide who receives what. The result will be a rationalization of whoever one wishes to care for, leaving others uncared for without ample justification.

VALUES IN CONFLICT

To compound matters even further, people want irreconcilable moral values in health care. They want the prevention of harm,[24] but they also want the minimum of suffering, along with freedom of choice, as illustrated by Jehovah's Witnesses' refusal to accept blood transfusions. People want a long life, pleasure, and affluence. They want both to eat well and to reduce. People want meaningful democratic participation, fair and equal treatment, and speedy and impartial application of justice. They also want their own way, and some people think justice is on their side. They want virtues displayed regularly. They want the good life. One cannot have all these values.

These alternative moral models show that ethics is not a science with verifiable answers. For there is for some issues no rational way to resolve divergencies and conflicts. Nor can one beat someone else's positon down by some definition of what is "ethical" or "unethical," found in a professional code, such as the *Code for Nurses*. Against the idea that there is objectivity in ethics, there are divergencies in moral views, along with tragedy and stalemate. As I. Berlin, a contemporary philosopher, points out, if two patients need one kidney dialysis machine, for the one excluded there is tragedy. For Barney Clark's mechanical-heart operation, there were numerous applicants who have since died. How then are we to decide?

An answer to our dilemma of which ethics to choose, the justice-based or the virtue-based, is to try to combine both. People need both justice and care. But how are we to bring these together?

Paradigm Case Arguments in Health Care

All is not futile. There is a way between the unacceptable alternatives of objectivity and subjectivity in ethics. A promising lead consists of refuting paradigms or standard examples.[25] Paradigms or standard examples are partway between subjectivity and objectivity. In metaphysics, F.H. Bradley once argued that "Time does not exist." Another philosopher, G.E. Moore, then offered this refuting paradigm with the example, "I had breakfast before lunch." A paradigm in ethics is found in the same Moore's classic refutation of Mill, who held that whatever is desired is therefore desirable. Moore cited examples of bad desires to refute Mill's argument.

Four Arguments for Rights

An example of how the paradigm case argument may work in nursing ethics is the view held not so long ago that patients and nurses have no rights. To refute this, appeal is made to standard examples of rights in health care, examples that show how rights function.

Tuskeegee. The ignoble Tuskeegee experiment showed as decisively as any refuting argument can that, if there are any morally justified values at all, they include human rights of patients, subjects, and health professionals to informed consent. From 1932 to 1972 a 40-year experiment was performed to study the difference between those syphilis patients who were treated with penicillin and those who were not.[26] A public health nurse helped persuade over 300 black men with syphilis to forgo the penicillin treatment, even though it had already been tested and was available.[27] According to Elizabeth Carnegie, a nurse, "experiments performed on human subjects by professionals . . . violate" the rights of subjects if done without informed consent.[28]

As this experiment was exposed to public scrutiny, its immorality became obvious. The Tuskeegee experiment was a horrendous evil, a moral outrage, a gross violation of justice.[29] The Tuskeegee example is also a paradigm or standard example against the thesis that the nurse does not need to know anything, that a nurse just takes orders and keeps quiet. The exposure of the Tuskeegee experiment shows that there is no place for ignorant nursing. Nursing based on ignorance is a contradiction. Ignorance includes the moral ignorance of those who unthinkingly cooperate with an evil experiment. A nurse to be effective needs to have a high degree of knowledge, including the knowledge needed to help make justifiable moral decisions, which is possible in clear cases of this kind. As a paradigm case argument or standard example, the exposure of the Tuskeegee experiment is an instance that refutes the contention that patients and subjects have no rights, such as the right to informed consent.

Nazi Experiments. A second argument in favor of informed consent of patients and subjects as a right was the monstrous evil of certain Nazi medical experiments. Dehumanized Nazi experiments "related to sterilization techniques, cold water survival, decompression and heteroplastic transplantation."[30] In addition, the Nazi genocide program, entitled "Euthanasia," which consisted in "techniques of efficient killing," eliminated "thousands of patients with chronic disease or mental illness."[31] According to one writer, a group of Nazi physicians, called "doctors of infamy," under Hitler's chief physician, Karl Brandt, carried out the selection and killing of patients "deemed physically or mentally unfit, with injections of barbiturates, phenol, and in most cases through carbon monoxide gas, the lethal component of exhaust gases from motor vehicles."[32] As a result of Nazi medical atrocities, the Nuremberg Code, an international guideline, emerged after the Nuremberg doctors' trial. Among "its principal points are that informed consent must be obtained from all subjects."[33] Both of these paradigms or standard examples count as refuting arguments against the view that there are no rights for participants in health care, such as patients, subjects, and nurses. The infamous abuses of human rights contributed to what some people call Nuremberg morality; this is made explicit and incorporated in the 1975 Declaration of Helsinki (see Appendix).

The Women's Rights Movement. A third argument in favor of the right to informed consent is the women's rights movement and, in particular, J. Thomson's important article, "In Defense of Abortion." Thomson's argument on abortion, her view of moral rights as a form of self-defense against abuse, contributed strongly to antisexist morality. She emphasized a vital principle in the ethics of health care and in social life that applies to nurses in particular. The principle Thomson enunciated is that to have rights at all is to have rights in and to one's body.[34]

Nurses' Rights. In nursing, Claire Fagin and her teacher Hildegard Peplau refuted the idea that patients and nurses have no rights by arguing that nurses have a right to refuse to administer electroconvulsive therapy (ECT).[35] Another refutation in nursing is the argument against the "master-of-the-ship" doctrine that the physician knows best. In *Charleston Memorial Hospital* vs. *K. Darling,* physicians were held responsible for neglecting the patient. One nurse was also charged with neglecting to report her observations, which could have saved the 18-year-old Darling's leg. After 14 days in a poorly prepared cast, Darling's leg turned gangrenous and had to be amputated.[36] The *Darling* case showed that responsibility is not confined to a physician or the hospital alone. It is also attributed to nurses. With responsibility, training, and ability come decision-making rights or privileges to decide within rules, such as those enjoyed by auto drivers or professional practitioners. One writer calls these "discretionary rights."

Rights as a Form of Moral Standing

Although one may not think too well of some recent abuses or excesses of rights assertions, the paradigm examples cited show the role and justification of human rights. Rights as rallying symbols, cries, and slogans are generated by detecting and exposing violations of justice. To have rights is to have a form of moral standing. When you have rights, like your right to a paycheck, you know where you stand and where others stand. Your right to your paycheck means it is yours and your employers, if they have not paid you, owe it to you. The attempt to take your paycheck away from you is a gross violation of justice.[37] A right is a justified option or permission to do, to have, or to claim that which one regards as one's due.

The Meaning and Importance of Rights

There are five conditions that help define rights. The first is that to have a right is to be free to exercise it or not as one chooses, without being blamed or punished for exercising or not exercising one's right. Thus, my right to vote means I may vote, I have permission to vote, and I may rightfully demand or claim that right; but I am not required to vote, and no penalty or harm should come to me if I choose not to. Similarly, a patient's right to treatment means a patient may demand or claim the right to treatment but is not required to undergo it if he or she so chooses.

A second condition of any right of importance is that others have duties to facilitate one's exercise of rights in appropriate ways. The poll watchers and police have a duty to protect my right to vote if I exercise that right. Similarly, a patient's right to treatment means relevant health professionals have corresponding duties to assure and protect that patient's right.

A third condition of any right is that one's right accords with rationally defensible principles of justice. Such principles generally coincide with equality, impartiality, and fairness. They also reconcile conflicting claims of need and merit in a fair proportion. Rights based on justice rule against legal and institutional rights that have no basis in justice. If Barney Clark, the mechanical-heart recipient, for example, had been the richest person in need of this operation, giving him the first heart for that reason would have been unfair or unjust. This third condition of a positive right importantly includes a right to be cared for or the right to assistance in living.

If there is a conflict between a liberty right and the right to be cared for, one tilts in favor of the right to be care for. People who smoke or patients who test HIV positive cannot be left alone to decide to act on their liberty right to pollute the environment or to have indiscriminate sex. The right to be cared for overrides one's liberty rights where harm to oneself or others results.

A fourth condition is that a right of importance is enforceable. Other relevant persons are both to recognize and effectively protect a person in the exercise of his or her rights. According to L. Becker, a philosopher, enforceability means that "if I have a right to your help . . . and you refuse, some sort of arm twisting is in order."[38] Enforceable rights are specific and special. In nursing, the enforceability provision means that in a hospital that honors a bill of rights, provision is made for mechanisms called "whistle-blowing" for reporting violations of patients' rights. Patient-care and ethics committees may also provide for implementation of human rights in the health care setting.

A fifth and related condition is that if a right is violated, set aside, or overridden in favor of some other right or value, the person whose right was violated or set aside is given compensation. The concept of rights violations implies that something is owed to the victim.[39] Rights thus imply freedom, duties, and justice. These conditions, in turn, imply enforceability and compensations for violations or infringements. These conditions show how seriously a society takes rights and therefore how important such rights are.

R.M. Hare distinguishes three senses of rights. To have a right in a minimal sense means that one is not wrong to do X. To have a right in a second sense means that others are wrong to interfere. A third sense of a right is that others have a positive obligation to assist rightholders to exercise their rights. Hare's distinction helps nurses to assess the strength of patients' and nurses' rights. A patient may have a right in the first sense without having a right in the second or third sense. For example, Jones has a right to play cards but not to keep the lights on after hours. A nurse has right to advocate higher pay, but she may not have a right in the second or third sense.[40] Hare's distinction between these three senses of patients' and nurses' rights helps nurses decide what kinds of rights they and their patient's have.

The Transcendence of Human Rights

Resulting human rights are moral rights of a very important kind, shared equally by all persons. These human rights are the union of two kinds of rights; self-determination or liberty rights and rights to be cared for or well-being rights. To have a full fledged set of human rights, however, is to have both liberty rights and rights to be cared for. One can critically evaluate legal and institutional rights by reference to human rights. The importance of rights is the conceptual link they provide between being a rightholder and being a person. To deny patients and nurses their status as rightholders, with all the conditions implied, in effect denies their status as persons.

Rights and Moral Standing

To have moral standing means that persons are entitled to be recognized and heard, and to have their views considered fairly and equally. Rights to protected freedom and care serve as a basis for claims and actions. To have moral standing is to be respected.[41] It is also to act responsibly by respecting the rights of others, and thus working within the rules for achieving and maintaining everyone's moral standing. A right as a form of standing is a social achievement, not a self-evident characteristic found in human nature; nor is a form of standing an inalienable birthright. There are no rights against wildlife or against events in nature, like snow, rain, typhoons, or lightning. Rights are for people, and accorded by people and the duties rights imply are imposed upon and accepted by people as well.

The Justification of Rights

The justification of rights consists in showing, through standard examples, why a world with rights is morally preferable to one without rights. Rights enable people to do things, like vote, pray, go to school, go to a hospital, receive social security, and do things to enjoy life. Rights are like red and green traffic lights, showing where people stand. A view of rights that regards rights as a form of moral standing, as entrenched and seriously held social values, places rights partway between moral objectivity and subjectivity; as being in some respects objective and in other respects subjective. Rights, after all, result from interests and desires. Yet rights are also a composite of other values, like freedom, love, restraints, duties, and justice. Beyond that, rights break down in the recognition that tragedy and stalemate, too, are aspects of the ethical life of human beings that no formalization or objectivity can overcome.

RIGHTS AND VIRTUES

Can ethics rationally help us to resolve disputes? Are the ethics of rights and virtues incompatible? We think rights and virtues fit together. Rights worth having are a composite of certain virtues, such as respect, dignity, freedom, fairness, and care. But rights based on justice are not the whole of ethics either. There are acts of extra devotion, courage, wisdom, prudence, temperance, generosity, friendship, and trust that are foundational to moral rights. A community or individual who does not have these virtues has no moral rights either. There is no necessary opposition between rights and virtues, providing their structure and functions have been carefully thought through.

To offset relativism in judging nursing acts, there are moral principles, guidelines, composites of the ethics of rights and virtues. These partially overlapping principles include consistency, coherence, truth, respect for rights and for life, liberty, and the pursuit of happiness, autonomy, promise-keeping, loyalty, care, generosity, sympathy, fidelity, freedom, equality, fairness, courage, beneficence, and nonmaleficence. These principles provide parameters and defining characteristics of ethics.

We can apply these principles into reasoned arguments, which appeal to rights and virtues. One might defend the principle that Feminism is good as follows:

> Ideas, individuals and institutions that promote the decent and caring treatment of people are good.
> Feminism promotes treating people decently and with care.
> Therefore, Feminism is good.

One may refer to those moral ideas that merit special attention and recognition as rights. Respect for Feminism merits attention and recognition as a right. Therefore, all feminist principles, like caring, may be identified as rights to be cared for.

CONCLUSION

A world with justice-based rights, despite the drawbacks rights present, is morally preferable to a world without rights or to a world with rights reserved only for owners of power, goods, and people. A world with justice-based rights for all persons, including patients and health professionals, elevates everyone's moral standing. Truths and rights are to ideas and to social institutions what virtues are to individuals. Ideas, institutions, and individuals without truths, rights, and virtues are morally unguided.

Discussion Questions

1. What difference does a just society make in an equitable work load and salary scale for nurses?
2. Why is Gilligan's identification of feminine and masculine virtues, such as caring and justice, appropriate or inappropriate?

3. How would you show that the Rights-based ethics and the Virtue-based ethics are compatible or incompatible, one with the other?

4. On the basis of the models of morality, what justification, if any, is there to the American Medical Association creating sub-professional groups, such as physician assistants or Registered Care Technologists (RCTs) to supplement nurses?

REFERENCES

1. Steele SM. Harmon VM. *Values clarification in nursing.* 2nd ed. New York: Appleton-Century Crofts. 1983; 13–14.
2. Warnock M. *Existentialist ethics.* London: Macmillan. 1967; 39–49.
3. Nozick R. *Anarchy, state and utopia.* New York: Basic Books. 1974.
4. Ibid.
5. Ibid.
6. Sade R. *Medical care as a right: A refutation.* N Engl J Med. 1971: 285–1288.
7. Ibid.
8. Rawls J. *A theory of justice.* Cambridge, MA: Harvard University Press. 1971; 3–4.
9. Ibid; 3.
10. Ibid; 3–4.
11. Ibid; 4.
12. Ibid; 136–142.
13. Ibid; 302.
14. Nozick R. *Anarchy, state and utopia.*
15. Dworkin R. *Taking rights seriously.* Cambridge, MA: Harvard University Press. 1978; xi.
16. Kohlberg L. Stages of moral development as a basis for moral development. In: *Moral Interdisciplinary Approaches.* Paramus, NJ: Newman. 1971; 86–88.
17. McIntyre A. *After virtue.* 2nd ed. Notre Dame. IN: University of Notre Dame Press. 2nd ed. 1984.
18. Toulmin S. *The tyranny of rules.* Hastings Center Report. 1980.
19. Gilligan C. *In a different voice.* Cambridge, MA: Harvard University Press. 1982; 1–3, 20, 171–174.
20. Noddings N. *Caring: A feminine approach to ethics and moral education.* Berkeley: University of California Press. 1984.
21. Benner P and Wrubel J. *The primacy of caring.* Menlo Park, CA: Addison-Wesley. 1989; 1.
22. Ibid; 1.
23. Ibid; 1.
24. Hutt P. *Five moral imperatives of government regulation.* Hastings Center Report. 1980. *10*(1):29–31, 1980.
25. Macklin R. *Return to the best interests of the child.* In: Gaylin W. Macklin R. (eds). *Who speaks for the child.* New York: Plenum. 1982; 294–295.

26. Marshal CL. Marshal CP. Poverty and health: The United States. In: Reich W. (ed). Encyclopedia of Bioethics. New York: Macmillan. 1978, 3:320.
27. Carnegie E. The patient's bill of rights and the nurse. In: Nicholls M. Wessels V. (eds). *Nursing Standards and Nursing Process*. Wakefield, MA: Contemporary Publishing. 1977; 69.
28. Ibid.
29. Cranston M. *What are human rights?* New York: Taplinger. 1973; 68.
30. Vastyan E. Medicine and war. In: *Encyclopedia of Bioethics* 1696.
31. Gruman GJ Death and dying: Euthanasia and sustaining life: Historical perspectives. In: *Encyclopedia of Bioethics. 1:*267.
32. Redlich FC. Medical ethics under national socialism. In: *Encyclopedia of Bioethics. 3:*1016.
33. Ibid; 1018.
34. Thomson J. In defense of abortion. In: Feinberg J. (ed). *The Problem of Abortion*. Belmont, CA: Wadsworth. 1973; 128.
35. Fagin C. *Nurses' rights*. Am J. Nursing. 1975. 75(1):82,.
36. *Charleston Community Memorial Hospital v. Dorrence Kenneth Darling*, 33 Ill. 326, 211 (NE 2nd 253, 1965).
37. Cranston, M. *What are human rights?* New York: Taplinger. 1973; 68.
38. Hare RM. *Moral thinking*. Oxford: Clarendon Press. 1981; 151–152.
39. Becker L. Individual rights. In: Regan T Van DeVeer D (eds). *And Justice for All*. Totowa, NJ: Roman and Littlefield. 1982; 203.
40. Ibid.
41. Singer P. The concept of moral standing. In: Caplan A Callahan D (eds). *Ethics for Hard Times*. New York: Plenum. 1981; 31–36, 40-41.

CHAPTER 6

Ethical Decision Making in Nursing

Study of this chapter enables the learner to:

1. Apply the principles of self-determination, well-being, and equity as an integral part of shared decision making.
2. Identify common fallacies of reasoning used in reaching unsound conclusions.
3. Assess the patient's capacity, voluntariness, and access to essential information as the basis for effective participation in shared decision making.
4. Utilize nursing guidelines and strategies in supporting the client's full participation in shared decisions.

INTRODUCTION

The rapid evolution of health technology in health care has brought about better health, increased quality and length of life, and "new sources of hope for the ill."[1] The "technological revolution"[2] has widened the range of treatment choices within health care. The question has moved from that of acceptance or rejection of a single intervention for a specific condition to the more complex question of which intervention to choose. Since each of these options carries different estimates of success, different side effects, and different degrees of intrusiveness, the implications for the patient's way of life are profound. Mass media provides graphic, intimate details of artificial heart and organ transplants, in vitro fertilization, and fetal surgery to a curious public. The ends and limits of health care are widely debated on television and in the press. Consequently, consumer expectations have changed. Generally, patients expect to maintain control and to be responsible for decisions involving their health consistent with their values, goals, and life styles.

The role of the health care professional is being redefined as well. The authoritarian attitude of care providers is now much less acceptable. Patients and families expect that professionals will share their knowledge with them as the basis for informed consent. Thus, the ideal is rational decision making on the basis of fully shared knowledge, explicit ethical principles, and freely given consent. This chapter will examine the values related to and supportive of this model. Fallacies of argument impede ethical decision making; so common fallacies are discussed. The patient's capacity and competence will be analyzed as necessary conditions for participation as an autonomous person. Lastly, a guideline that incorporates these concepts is offered as an approach to decision making. The term "approach" is selected, since ethics is not a science with true or false answers. Ethical decisions cannot be reached "simply by following handy formulas. No matter how carefully one issue has been resolved, the solution cannot be applied in cookbook fashion to another problem. Rather each issue . . . must be examined in the context of its particular circumstances."[3]

PITFALLS OF REASONING: FALLACIES

Despite the best intentions of participants, road blocks to effective decision making occur through errors and fallacies. Exposing and confronting fallacies in reasoning helps to minimize them. The recognition and correction of fallacies as errors in reasoning facilitates effective and justifiable decision making in nursing.

Fallacies are errors in reasoning. Fallacies are committed innocently out of lack of knowledge of methods of reasoning or are deliberately used to falsify the case or to mislead the listener. Fallacies may be used by anyone. Their use is prominent in advertising, in political rhetoric, and in selling a product or an idea. The health care delivery system and practitioners of all kinds are not immune to the use of fallacies. There are varying numbers of fallacies cited in the literature. Those most applicable to nursing will be discussed here.

The Is-Ought Fallacy

The is-ought fallacy is committed when someone argues that because X *is* the case; therefore, X *ought* to be the case. The letter X stands for some practice, policy, procedure, decision or custom. A frequent fallacy is

> This patient *is* to be resuscitated if cardiac arrest occurs; therefore, all patients *ought* to be resuscitated in arrest.

One can substitute the terms "dialysis," "life support systems," or "artificial feeding" for the term "resuscitated." Another example of this fallacy is

> Nursing *is* the bedside care of sick individuals; therefore, nurses *ought* to be trained at the bedside of sick individuals.

An obvious implication here is that formal college education for nurses is unnecessary or that all nurses should give bedside care to patients. Another example of this fallacy is the statement

> "A nurse *is* required to work a double shift whenever necessary in this hospital; therefore, double shifts *ought* to be required of all nurses during this period of acute shortage."

Still other examples of the is-ought fallacy are such statements as

> "A nurse *is* a low-paid health care provider; therefore, nurses *ought* not to expect high salaries."

> "A nurse *is* subordinate to a physician in rank and education; therefore, a nurse *ought* to obey a physician without question."

Many more examples from nursing are available. The point is that the is-ought fallacy consists of moving from a given present case, practice, policy, decision, or custom (the "is") to a statement of obligation. The fault in reasoning is that if X *is* the case, it does not follow that X *ought* to be the case. Not everyone *ought* to be resuscitated, or kept on life support systems, or be dialyzed, or given organ transplants, or provided with artificial hearts. It is logically fallacious to proceed from the "is" to the "ought;" the "ought" does not necessarily follow.

Appeal to Force
This fallacy consists of making another accept the conclusion of an argument on the basis of force alone. A surgeon presents this argument to a patient regarding elective surgery.

"If you don't get that fibroid tumor removed, you'll die." A physician orders an overdose of morphine that the nurse refuses to give, to which the physician responds "I'll get you fired." A nursing administrator tells a nurse who is a single parent whose two young children are cared for by another parent who must return to her own children, "Either you work the next shift, or you'll be fired." These are appeals to the sole use of force and lack rational support. The nurse in the intensive care unit, however, who says to the patient, "I have to give you this injection (or treatment) to relieve your pain (or ease your breathing, or slow your heartbeat, or clear your passageways)" is appealing to force on a rational basis with supporting evidence for her conclusion.

Abuse of the Person

Another fallacy in argument consists in abuse of the person instead of rational, relevant reasons for a decision. In the fallacy of *personal abuse*, a nurse may criticize a physician for repeated resuscitation of a terminally ill patient on the grounds that the physician "cannot accept defeat" or "is afraid of death."

In *circumstantial abuse*, one person blames another for concluding X on the grounds of membership or inclusion in a group that habitually does something blameworthy, X. For example, Nurse A chides Nurse B for refusing to care for an abortion patient on the grounds that Nurse B is a Catholic. Nurse B being a Catholic may be true, but is irrelevant to Nurse B's opposition to abortion that may include B's longing for a child of her own and rejection of women who terminate their pregnancies. Or the fact that Nurse A and Nurse B graduated from the same baccalaureate program in nursing and A praises the practice of B does not entitle Nurse C to say by way of abuse, "Oh, but you both graduated from Hunter." Nurse C's argument is irrelevant to whether Nurse B is or is not an expert practitioner.

A third version of abuse is known as *tu quoque*, "You're another." Nurse A goes off duty early for class, but Nurse B also goes off duty early to go shopping, and the unit is left dangerously understaffed. The charge by either A or B of "You're another irresponsible nurse" is fallacious since "two wrongs don't make a right."

The fourth version of the abuse fallacy is the *genetic fallacy*. Instead of refuting or accepting evidence on relevant grounds, persons are abused on the grounds of their origins. "The reason you have AIDS is that you come from the slums." Obviously, AIDS is contagious and without social consciousness.

Appeal to Populace

The fallacy in the argument, "Everybody does it," is that since "everybody does it," it must be good. For example, Nurse A says that "Everybody is working three twelve-hour shifts a week; therefore, to do so must be good." Nurse A's argument does not prove that this schedule is good. Nurses may spend days recuperating from this schedule. Popularity does not prove worth.

Appeal to Authority

As might be expected, the appeal to inappropriate authority is a frequent pitfall of reasoning in the health care system. The fallacy consists of persons with appropriate authority presenting themselves as authorities outside or beyond their fields, or areas of expertise. Minimally, to have appropriate authority is to have the required credentials. For example, a physician may decide to resuscitate a young patient with a severe debilitating form of leukemia who specifically refuses resuscitation. The physician argues that he or she knows the value of life far better than the young patient who does not realize how rewarding it is to be alive. The physician is going beyond his or her appropriate authority.

The Slippery-Slope Fallacy

The use of the slippery-slope fallacy in an argument assumes that if one exception to a rule or principle is allowed, then an uncontrollable set of events with unwanted consequences will follow. Thus, if active, voluntary euthanasia is permitted, even under strict controls, then the killing of persons with Alzheimer's disease or other forms of dementia or senility in the elderly will follow. Similarly, if abortion is permitted, then infanticide of the severely handicapped will follow. Likewise, hospital administrators who oppose collective bargaining argue that if nurses are permitted to make salary demands, the cost of hospital care will be unaffordable to the public. Counter arguments can be made to slippery-slope fallacies. Active voluntary euthanasia is practiced in such countries as Holland without any decrease in either the quality of care given to the demented and senile elderly or in the commitment to their survival. Abortion is legally practiced and morally supported as a means of population control in China, for example. The result is a tremendous outpouring of love for the permitted child by the parents and a great deal of effort in areas of child care, health, and education. Universal respect for the elderly Chinese as a source of wisdom and authority continues as it has for centuries.

Slothful Induction

This fallacy is the refusal to allow any evidence that contradicts the conclusion of one's argument as a way of protecting one's conclusions against criticism. For example, a nurse who supports abortion argues for the primacy of the woman's right to her own body. The nurse who opposes abortion argues for the primacy or equal rights of the fetus. Neither looks at the evidence of the tragic national need for sex education and family planning that could decrease the incidence of teenage pregnancy and a woman's forced choice between her own well-being and that of a potential human being she is carrying in her body.

The dogmatic beliefs of a group regarding the supremacy or inferiority of members of a race, tribe, class, or culture without regard for contradictory evidence is a further example of slothful induction. Historically, such slothful believers have raged against evolution, immunization, and the equality of races and sexes. The antidote to the fallacy of slothful induction is to open all arguments to inquiry and to contradictory evidence. A nurse or physician who refuses to question any ethical argument or conclusion because it was put forth by an authority is commiting the fallacy of slothful induction.

The Fallacy of Accident

This fallacy consists of the indiscriminate application of an ethical principle to every situation without regard for "accidental" differences or circumstances. For example, the Kantian imperative of always telling the truth, if applied indiscriminately, can have tragic results. Some individuals are terrified by the thought of cancer and consider it an immediate death sentence that in some cases they prefer to carry out themselves by suicide or by rejecting all treatment. Most patients need support, sympathy, and encouragement during the process of accepting painful truth.

Complex Question

This fallacy consists of asking a question whose answer depends on the affirmative answer to a prior question. The question "Do you want cardiopulmonary resuscitation?" presupposes that you may experience cardiac arrest. The question to patients, "Will you take this surgery (or treatment, or medication) and live or not take it and die?" is an example of the fallacy of bifurcation or *exclusive alternation* or *black-or-white thinking*. Boldly presenting two alternatives does not mean that there are not more alternatives or even that one of the two is not a real alternative.

VALUES SUPPORTIVE OF SHARED HEALTH CARE DECISIONS

In addition to the avoidance of fallacies in decision making, the application of the values and principles of autonomy, well-being, and equity is important. These principles are an integral part of the justifications for decisions reached and for the nurse's role in achieving them.

Values Expressed in Nurse-Patient Relationships

The role of the nurse in shared decision making rests on important premises of this work. The first premise is that every competent adult has the right to decide what will be done with his or her person, that is, to accept, terminate, or refuse treatment. The second premise is that the patient's care, safety, and well-being are the nurse's primary commitment. This view places the patient in the center of professional scrutiny and activity with full patient involvement, understanding, and agreement. The third major premise of this work is that the present and increasing complexity of health care requires an interdisciplinary approach to patient care situations. An important function of the nurse is to promote collaboration on behalf of the patient among professionals involved in that person's care.

Values and Principles Underlying the Decision-Making Process

The Principle of Self-Determination. Patient self-determination is an important value to be respected and enhanced by nurses and other participants in health care decisions. The American Nurses' Association, in its *Code for Nurses,* supports the self-determination of clients as a moral right.[4] Although the doctrine of informed consent has distinct legal implications, "it is essentially an ethical imperative . . . rooted in the fundamental recognition . . . that adults are entitled to accept or reject health care interventions on the basis of their own personal values and in furtherance of their own personal goals."[5]

> The right to control one's body and one's treatment and the emphasis given to self-determination, privacy, freedom, autonomy, the emphasis on not being deceived, and being given complete and truthful information, all point to an important aspect of a rights-based view, namely the role of an individual patient's will in individual decision making.[6]

This statement takes the position that respect for persons necessarily supports "self-determination as a shield . . . valued for the freedom from outside control it is intended to provide. It manifests the wish to be an instrument of one's own and 'not of other men's acts of will' . . . As a sword, self-determination manifests the value that Western culture places on each person to be a creator—'a subject, not an object.' "[7] This position recognizes that persons define their values and assume responsibility for their particular life-style and health practices.

The Principle of Well-Being. Serving the patient's well-being through improving health is another justifying reason or warrant for nursing and all other health care.[8] "The nursing profession exists to give assistance to those persons needing nursing care."[9] The obligation to promote patients' well-being is assumed to be the operational principle of the health care system by consumers and care providers alike. Well-being is further supported by the principle of beneficence, which says that one ought to prevent harm and promote the good.[10] The nurse sees the nursing role as that of friend rather than as servant to the patient.

In practical affairs, conditions such as diabetes, fractures, and infections may be treated in several ways. Most health consumers accept the decision of the professional in the expectation that the patient's well-being is served by the recommendation of the nurse or physician. However, issues such as amniocentesis and termination of aggressive treatment in cancer patients with metastases for whom treatment is ineffective are value choices rather than purely technical or clinical questions.[11] The patient makes this choice on the basis of furthering his or her well-being. A still different way of serving well-being is achieved by supporting the patient's preference for one intervention over another that is recommended. For example, a patient with a slipped disc can be treated medically, orthopedically, or surgically. Previous episodes of prolonged bed rest for this specific patient were so depressing that the patient prefers the greater risk of surgery.[12] A professional baseball pitcher may prefer continuous cortisone for his inflamed elbow rather than move to the outfield.[13]

Evaluating the patient's choices in terms of well-being emphasizes nursing and provider commitment to principles of promoting the good and avoiding harm by limiting the alternatives. Patients cannot demand whatever they wish. The choice is "among medically accepted and available options, all of which. . . have some possibility of promoting the patient's welfare, including always the option of no further medical interventions, even when that would not be viewed as preferable by the health care providers."[14]

Clearly, the definition of well-being is a broader concept than self-determination alone. The concept of well-being takes the patient's best interests into account in relation to the patient's self-determined goals and values. This process requires dialogue between practitioners and patients in which the patients' views, goals, and values are related to the available treatment options. Thus, the principle of self-determination expands to include the contribution of relevant practitioners concerned with the patient's well-being in the process of shared decision making. Self-determination and well-being may therefore be regarded as compatible values. The compatibility of self-determination and well-being takes the form of shared decision making. Shared decision making recognizes the professional's expertise along with patients' evaluations of their options, the consequences of each option, and relevance to their well-being. Shared decision making also permits consideration of the well-being, goals, and values of family members. Constraints arise against permitting a patient to exhaust family resources when little or no patient benefit is likely.

The Principle of Equity. The ideal that people be treated "fairly and equally with all concerned"[15] has implications for the consumer and provider of health care. A traditional approach "is the Aristotelian principle of formal justice that like cases be treated alike."[16] This principle is applicable in the practice of government support of all dialysis treatments for everyone with end-stage renal disease. Arbitrariness is in principle eliminated. The principle of treating like cases alike also implies that differences are treated differently.

To treat patients fairly may be to treat them differently, since their needs differ. There are, however, practical difficulties in applying both parts of this principle. Nursing resources are especially difficult to distribute fairly. Even patients with identical surgery and expected out-comes in the intensive care unit have different physical responses, emotional reactions, and interactional needs. Rarely is the nursing service adequate to meet all the patient care needs defined by responsible nurses. Nevertheless, a major value of nursing practitioners is to promote the well-being of their patients. Nurses do this by respecting their patients' rights and treatment options. In this way, patients are treated fairly as equal participants in making shared health care decisions.

ASSESSMENT OF PATIENT CAPACITY AND COMPETENCE

Fulfilling the principles of autonomy, well-being and equity calls for familiarity with obstacles to reasoning, such as fallacies. To recognize, and thereby avoid, fallacies requires that the patient has the capacity to participate in the decision-making process. The nursing goal is to facilitate the patient's participation in decision making and that requires an accurate assessment of capacity.

Nursing Goals

Fallacies as errors in reasoning may be committed by persons with the capacity to be rational. But some individuals lack both the capacity for rational thinking and for the correction of their fallacies in thinking. These differences need to be clearly differentiated since the goal of the decision-making process is to "advance the ability of patients to maintain control of, and be responsible for, decisions regarding their lives and their health."[17] To be an effective participant in the decision process, three factors are essential.[18] First, the patient possesses the capacity to participate. Second, the decision is voluntary. Third, the patient acquires access to essential information relevant to the health problem and to related life goals, plans, and values.

Patient Capacity

The capacity to participate effectively depends on the "mental, emotional, and legal" ability to do so.[19] The "decision-making capacity is specific to a particular decision and depends . . . on the person's actual functioning in situations in which a decision about health care is to be made."[20] Obviously, infants, young children, comatose persons, and severely mentally disabled persons are incapacitated. They require separate consideration. In borderline cases, careful assessment of the patient's comprehension and reasoning by nurses in contact with the patient in various situations and times of day and night is a major contribution to the evaluation process. Thus, nurses are in the best position to evaluate the effects of psychotropic drugs on the patient. Through observation, nurses can identify gaps in patients' information and supply the missing knowledge. Eventually, the patient's capacity or incapacity to make a decision regarding treatment must be established and resolution secured.

Determination of the patient's capacity to make a decision relates to the individual's abilities, the demands of the decision task, and the probable consequences of the choice. The President's Commission views the capacity to make decisions as requiring:

1. Possession of a set of values and goals;
2. The ability to communicate and to understand information;
3. The ability to reason and to deliberate about one's choice.[21]

A framework of goals and values is necessary for the patient to decide what is good or bad for him or her. The ability to seek, receive, and give information with understanding requires language and conceptual skills sufficient to grasp the task at hand. Life experience is useful for appreciating the significance of alternative medical interventions and life-styles.[22] The capacity to reason and to deliberate enables the patient to evaluate the effect of alternative decisions on his or her goals and plans.[23] This capacity includes the ability to weigh probabilities and possibilities in terms of present and future consequences to the self.

The President's Commission suggests criteria for assessment of the patient's capacity to make a particular decision regarding treatment. These criteria are

1. The ability to understand relevant facts and values;
2. The ability to weigh a decision within a framework of values and goals;
3. The ability to reason and deliberate about this information;
4. The ability to give reasons for the decision, in light of the facts, the alternatives, and the impact of the decision on the patient's own goals and values.[24]

In everyday practice, it is only those patients who disagree with a health professional's recommendation who are scrutinized regarding their decision-making capacity. If the patient agrees with the decision, and the family does too, the patient's capacity remains unquestioned.

Patients' refusal of treatment detrimental to well-being gives grounds for questioning the patient's decision-making capacity. The patient's refusal is the beginning—rather than the end—of dialogue with the patient around the problem situation. If the patient both fully understands the situation and demonstrates sound reasoning ability, the patient's decision to refuse treatment is final and is to be respected.[25]

Patient Incapacity to Make Decisions

The terms *incompetence* and *incapacity* are roughly synonymous, although *competence* is a legal concept determined by a court. Decision-making capacities are an important requirement for exercising self-determination rights. Infants, small children, the comatose, the severely retarded, and seriously disturbed persons are identified as clearly lacking decision-making capacities. One problem, however, is to determine appropriate criteria for deciding hard cases on the border of incapacity. Examples are patients who are mildly retarded, young children and adolescents, and those who become increasingly senile. Especially difficult are patients who refuse treatment that will aid them to achieve autonomy. Macklin supports overriding a psychiatric patient's right to refuse treatment in such cases. A compelling reason for the apparent arbitrariness is that a patient's rational powers and autonomy are increased by treatment when the patient's consenting organ itself, the mind, is affected.[26]

The reason for having a clear boundary is that a competent patient may forgo, refuse, or terminate treatment, whereas incompetent persons' "wishes may be overridden in order to protect their lives and well being."[27] When persons are considered incompetent, other interested persons exercise decision-making capacities on behalf of the incompetent. A father, knowing his 10-year-old has cancer in the leg, may consent to surgical amputation of his son's leg while actively seeking the child's assent to the procedure as life-saving.

A person judged competent (and this is a legal and minimal indicator of capacity) is one who is put in a position to exercise and enjoy self-determination rights.

On this view, as expressed by Kant, "the ability to be self-determining" involves the ability to be self-legislating." To be self-determining means one "is able both to formulate purposes, plans, and policies . . . and to carry out these decisions, plans or policies without undue reliance on the help of others."[28] However, to be a person or moral agent, in this view, implies the ability also "to adopt rules" that a person "holds to be binding on himself" or herself and on "all rational beings."[29] The capacity to be self-determining, on this view, depends on a person having a "rational will."[30]

On the basis of these two views, there are two standards to deal with those who lack a decision-making capacity. These standards are "substitute judgment" and "best interests." The standard of substitute judgment "requires that the surrogate (the person who stands in for the incapacitated person) attempt to replicate faithfully the decision that the incapacitated person would make if he or she were able to make a choice."[31] There are constraints imposed on the surrogate, namely "the same limitations that society legitimately imposes on patients who are capable of deciding for themselves."[32] There are, additionally, "reasonableness" requirements concerning certain risky procedures, for example; a substitute decision maker may not make these decisions on behalf of an incapacitated person.[33] On the other hand, "decision making guided by the best interest standard requires a surrogate to do what, from an objective standpoint, appears to promote a patient's good without reference to the patient's actual or supposed preferences."[34]

The substitute-judgment standard is intended to be faithful to the tradition that honors individual self-determination. The best-interest standard, on the other hand, is intended to carry out the patient's rational interests, those the patient would choose if that person were rational. For example, an incapacitated Jehovah's Witness known to refuse blood transfusions will be treated differently by each standard. If the standard of substitute judgment is used, a Jehovah's Witness may die from lack of blood. With the best-interest standard, the Jehovah's Witness patient may be given a transfusion and saved.

The nurse's role as advocate and watchdog is to protect the patient's best interests and impose rational restraints against legally and morally impermissible health care interventions. But which of these standards to use is sometimes an intractable dilemma. If priority is given to a patient's well-being over self-determination, then the best-interest standard is invoked. In emergency situations, the best-interest standard is usually applied. The further away the health care members are from a patient's circumstances, the more apt these health care members are to invoke the best-interest standard. A difficulty with the best-interest standard, however, is that appeal to this standard may mask an ambiguity—the patient's best interest or the best interests of other people in society. These two standards do not always coincide. Nevertheless, the best-interest standard may present a rational form of the Golden Rule. This cannot always be said of the substitute-judgment standard.

The substitute-judgment and best-interest standards may be regarded as bipolarities. Justifiable health care decision making takes appropriate account of both. One guideline for ethical decision making is to respect and develop the grounds for self-determination wherever possible. This value is at the core and foreground of personhood, and one's best interests are at the periphery and background, marking the boundary between a person's life and death. Well-being depends on self-determination and the fulfillment of one's best interests. When these conflict, as they do for Jehovah's Witnesses, the best-interest standard prevails.

Two concentric circles may portray the relation between self-determination and one's best interests, with rational self-determination at the core of a person's being. This value is sometimes called *independence* or *autonomy*. When independence fails or is inoperative, as it is in infancy and in a comatose state, the best-interest standard comes into play.

Patient Voluntariness

The second necessary condition for informed consent is that the patient's final choice is voluntary, free from coercion and manipulation. The principle of voluntariness is both a legal and a moral imperative that respects the self-determination of the patient.

Serious illness is coercive of patient and health professional alike, since there are often no options or unsatisfactory options available. The limits are real and beyond human control. Thus, voluntariness is often partial in specific cases. Limited voluntariness in patients who are acutely or seriously ill and dependent on professional expertise for guidance is clearly evident. These patients are particularly susceptible to subtle, or even overt, manipulations of their wills and, consequently, compromise of their voluntariness. A great deal of routine nursing and health care falls into the category of forced treatment, since it is given without the informed consent of patients. Patients are expected to turn, cough, breathe deeply, get out of bed, and urinate, for example, on the nurse's command. Routine laboratory and diagnostic tests are usually ordered and performed without the patient's consent on the assumption that the patient's admission to a hospital is in itself a consenting act.

Forced treatments include interventions given without patients' consent or even against their objections. Mandatory vaccination, chlorinating the public's drinking water, and sedating violent mental patients are examples of forced treatment performed to serve the public good. The use of force is not necessarily wrong as these examples show.

A coerced decision results when a patient is threatened with undesirable consequences unless he or she agrees to the intervention. Psychiatric patients may be threatened with discharge unless they agree to electroconvulsive therapy as the "only hope for lifting depression after drugs fail." Patients who refuse treatment such as getting out of bed when the nurse is ready to do it may receive threats of the nurse's being too busy or unavailable later on. The greater the disparity in power and status between the patient, the nurse, and the physician, the greater the potential for the abuse or neglect of voluntariness among "captive" patient populations such as those in nursing homes and mental institutions. Sometimes the family coerces a patient to accept an unwanted intervention with little hope of benefit. Conversely, the family may either directly or subtly manipulate a patient into refusing expensive treatment with potential benefit.

Manipulation of the patient to secure agreement to an intervention is easily accomplished with clients who completely trust and depend upon their physicians and nurses for decisions. Such patients regard themselves as ignorant. They grant health professionals expertise and adherence to the moral principle of serving the patient's well-being. Therefore, it is easy "to package and present the facts in a way that leaves the patient no real choice. Such conduct, capitalizing on disparities in knowledge, position, and influence, is manipulative in character and impairs the voluntariness of the patient's choice."[35]

There are many forms of manipulation. Information can be withheld or distorted. The patient is not informed of alternatives. Risks or possible complications of the recommended treatment are overlooked or minimized. The manner of presenting information strongly influences the patient's perception and response to it. The facial expression, the tone of voice, the relative physical position of the informant and the informed (the informer standing and looking down at the patient), and other aspects of a presentation selectively slant the message toward a particular direction. Information can be presented in so general and positive a way that risks or alternatives are minimized "without altering the content. And it can be framed in a way that affects the listener—for example, 'this procedure succeeds most of the time' versus 'this procedure has a 40 percent failure rate.' "[36]

Patients' Access to Essential Information

A third aspect of patient participation in health care decisions is open, continuous communication between professionals and patient related to "the facts, values, doubts, and alternatives on which decisions must ultimately be based."[37] The objective is to establish a dialogue so as to enhance the self-determination and well-being of the patient.[38] A recitation of facts and risks couched in technical jargon followed by the signing of a standardized consent form may satisfy legal requirements but hardly fulfills the ethical imperative of respecting a person's self-determination.

The President's Commission views the core substantive issues to be discussed by patient and professional as

1. The patient's current medical status, including its likely course if no improvement is pursued;
2. The intervention(s) that might improve the prognosis, including a description of the procedures involved, a characterization of

the likelihood and effect of associated risks and benefits, and
the likely course with and without therapy;

3. A professional opinion, usually, as to the best alternative.[39]

The patient's current medical status is recognized as the physician's responsibility in the American Hospital Association's statement
of *A Patient's Bill of Rights,* adopted in 1973. The statement affirms
the patient's right to know his or her diagnosis, treatment, and prognosis.

The privilege of a medical diagnosis is reserved by law for licensed
physicians. Some states, of which New York is one, use the word
"diagnosing" in the nurse practice act. A nursing diagnosis is distinguished from a medical diagnosis as "that identification of and discrimination between physical and psychosocial signs and symptoms
essential to effective execution and management of the nursing regimen."[40] Thus, the nurse's role consists of supporting the patient's right
to know his or her medical status, and clearly identifying and sharing
the patient's psychosocial response to that knowledge so that nursing
care restorative of well-being can be provided.

Those medical and nursing interventions that a nurse performs
are appropriately discussed with a patient as part of health teaching
and health counseling. These functions are explicitly stated in the
New York State Nurse Practice Act (as one example of laws in states
that use this concept), which defines professional nursing as "diagnosing and treating human responses to actual or potential health problems, through such services as case finding, health teaching, health
counseling, and provision of care supportive to or restorative of life
and well-being. . . ."[41] In the opinion of Jane Greenlaw, R.N., J.D.:

> As long as you make it clear that you're giving your opinion as a
> nurse, and speaking only from your own experience and knowledge,
> you can feel free to answer questions about the patient's course of
> treatment. You can relate your experience in caring for other pa
> tients undergoing the same treatment and answer questions about
> alternative treatments.[42]

On this view, the nurse can discuss medications, temperatures,
blood pressures, wound care, and any other nursing or medical interventions that the nurse performs "supportive to or restorative of life
and well-being."[43] The nurse can facilitate the patient's discussion of
values and goals in relation to the nursing care plan and goals.

Holder and Lewis, a lawyer and philosopher, view "the negotiations necessary to obtain the patient's informed consent as the responsibility of the person who will perform the procedure. . . . The
physician may delegate the discussion to another but retains the legal
responsibility to make sure the patient understands."[44] The nurse's

legal responsibility for a preoperative consent form consists of witnessing the patient's signature as the act of that person. The nurse's moral responsibility is to support the patient's right to understand the purposes and significance of the proposed intervention. If the patient's knowledge is seriously deficient, the nurse's duty is to inform the responsible person so that the proposed surgery or diagnostic procedure is performed on the basis of a fully informed consent in relation to the patient's own values and goals.

Ironically, minor surgery, for which written consent is routinely secured, may be far less risky than many drugs that nurses give without question to themselves or to patients. In interventions of this kind, nurses have an unusual opportunity to teach the patient regarding drugs and their effects. Drugs are both lifesaving and life-threatening, as when unexpected reactions and interactions occur. This is health teaching directed towards the patient's understanding of the specific intervention used, the benefits, the side effects, and risks. This function supports the patient's self-determination and well-being.

A third substantive issue is the professional's opinion of the best choice. In cases of surgery or a serious diagnosis, the professional is usually but not always the physician. The only justification for any intervention is the benefit to the patient. "The decision . . . has two components: whether to treat and how to treat." The decision belongs to the patient. In studies conducted by the President's Commission, the findings showed that little or no discussion of treatment options occurred between physicians and patients in hospital settings. Physicians generally made the decisions and proceeded to treat without patient participation.[45]

Most treatment refusals studied were related to lack of information regarding the purpose, nature, and risks of diagnostic and therapeutic measures ordered. "Conflicting information given to patients by different health care professionals"[46] was another source of treatment refusal. This is a predictable occurrence in hospitals where patient care is provided by many different people and communication among these people is not direct. The result is that patients are insecure about who is in charge, who has the qualifications, and who is to be trusted. In situations where the authority structure is clear, where professional roles of nurses and physicians are clarified, and where the lines of communication are open and direct, the nurse and physician can relate to the patient as colleagues equally concerned with the patient's participation in shared decisions. Professional collaboration is essential for enhancing patients' participation in decisions and for coordinating activities toward this goal. The element of uncertainty can never be eliminated in patient discussions. Instead, it is given its due in relation to the probabilities of success based on empirical data.

Patients who are acutely ill, distressed, and in pain are constrained in their ability to understand, accept, and use the information communicated to them. The physicians and nurses are usually strangers. The language may be technical. The hospital setting may be frightening. If all the health professionals involved with each patient are clear about what is to be communicated regarding the physician's treatment recommendation, the discussion can proceed and enlarge as the patient's state of readiness and receptivity improve. Time is required.

Written and audiovisual materials discussing specific interventions are useful in non-emergency situations. Some physicians require patients to write their own consent forms for elective surgery as a test of their understanding and as the basis for further patient participation in the decision process. The inclusion of families can be significant in the patient's understanding of the physician's or nurse's treatment recommendation.

GUIDELINES FOR SHARED DECISION MAKING

Strategies to Maximize Participation

The aim of the nursing strategies used in this context is to facilitate relationships between patients, nurses, physicians, professionals, and families "characterized by mutual participation and respect and by shared decision making."[47]

An important nursing function is to coordinate the medical, technical, and nursing activities on behalf of the patient's well-being into a meaningful process that the patient and family can utilize in the shared decision process. This function is stated in nursing laws and codes as patient education, health teaching, and health counseling.[48] The process of communicating essential information to the patient may be carried out independently as part of the nursing care. The patient's response is shared with other health professionals and family as discussion and deliberation around the patient's well-being ebbs and flows when needs and concerns change. In everyday practice situations, nurses "typically have a central role in the process of providing patients with information."[49] Nurses are increasingly viewed by the public and by themselves as patient advocates. In this role, nurses help patients gain better health and more control of their participation in health care.

Nurses also facilitate patients' informed participation by functioning as interdisciplinary team members working with others to solve patients' problems. The client benefits from the improved communication and easier access among professionals whose focus as a team is on the whole patient rather than on a limited aspect. A team that functions effectively can better manage interdependent problems and integrate services.[50]

Questions of what person or persons or discipline will serve as primary communicator arises when people from many disciplines work with each patient. A related question is how to communicate consistent messages to the patient and family. A further question relates to the communication of the team concept to the patient and to the family.[51] One measure of effective communication is the consistency of messages from health professionals to client, and the accuracy of the client's information.[52] This is in contrast to settings where there is little communication among professionals. This results in the patient's receiving separate, different, and sometimes conflicting messages from individual professionals.

Formal interdisciplinary team meetings are the ideal. Meetings are held regularly with a focus on client problems and management issues. Problems are usually aired and settled by the group, which uses negotiation and conflict resolution processes. Meetings enable nurses to communicate patient concerns in a systematic fashion to an interdisciplinary group in which the problem can be analyzed and the nurse's perceptions, inferences, hypotheses, and recommendations confirmed or disconfirmed by a group whose focus is the patient's well-being. The nurse is recognized as a colleague in a vital professional role. The principle of feedback is utilized in all interactions. The nurse's contribution to patient care is formalized, recognized, and placed in the context of total care to the patient and family.

CONCLUSION

Choice is an important value for every person. Nursing strategies for facilitating patients' choices enhance the values of personhood, especially at critical times in a person's life, when he or she is ill, incapacitated, dying, or vulnerable due to age, mental disability, or socioeconomic status. A nurse often knows what to do and how to do it, and who can best do that which is needed for maximizing the patient's well-being. At times, the nurses' priority on behalf of the patient's best interests may conflict with the patient's choices. This may present an ethical problem without a true or final answer. In ethics, one cannot ask for more. As Aristotle long ago pointed out, one cannot expect the same precision in ethics as in mathematics or science.

Discussion Questions

1. How do science and technology promote effective decision making in nursing?
2. How do fallacies interfere with competent decision making by nurses?

REFERENCES

1. President's Commission for the Study of Ethical Problems in Medicine and Biomedical and Behavioral Research. *Making health care decisions.* Washington DC: U.S. Government Printing Office. 1982; 33.
2. Ibid.
3. President's Commission for the Study of Ethical Problems in Medicine and Biomedical and Behavioral Research. *Summing up.* Washington DC: U.S. Government Printing Office. 1983; 72.
4. American Nurses' Association. *Code for nurses with interpretive statements.* Kansas City, MO: Author. 1985; 4.
5. Ibid.
6. President's Commission. *Making health care decisions.* 2.
7. Bandman B and E. The nurse's role in an interest-based view of patients' rights. In: Spicker SF, Gadow S (eds). *Nursing Images and Ideals.* New York: Springer. 1980; 129.
8. President's Commission. *Making health care decisions.* 45–6.
9. American Nurses' Association. *Code for nurses.* 15.
10. Frankena WK. *Ethics.* 2nd ed. Englewood Cliffs, NJ: Prentice-Hall. 1973; 47.
11. President's Commission. *Making health care decisions.* 42.
12. Ibid.; 43.
13. Ibid.
14. Ibid.; 44.
15. *Webster's New Collegiate Dictionary.* Springfield, MA: Merriam. 1974; 386.
16. President's Commission. *Summing up.* 70.
17. President's Commission. *Making health care decisions.* 16.
18. Ibid.; 55.
19. Ibid.
20. Ibid.
21. Ibid.; 57.
22. Ibid.; 58.
23. Ibid.; 59.
24. Ibid.; 60.
25. Ibid.; 62.
26. Macklin R. *Man, mind, and morality: The ethics of behavior control.* Englewood Cliffs, NJ: Prentice-Hall. 1982. 90, 91–95.
27. President's Commission for the Study of Ethical Problems in Medicine and Biomedical and Behavioral Research. *Deciding to forego life-sustaining treatment.* Washington DC: U.S. Government Printing Office. 1983; 124.
28. Houlgate LD. *The child and the state: A normative theory of juvenile rights.* Baltimore: The Johns Hopkins University Press. 1980; 50.
29. Ibid.
30. Ibid.
31. President's Commission. *Making health care decisions.* 178.
32. Ibid.
33. Ibid.
34. Ibid.; 179.
35. Ibid.; 66.

36. Ibid.
37. Ibid.; 69.
38. Ibid.
39. Ibid.; 74.
40. Nurse Practice Act, Title VIII, Article 139, New York State Education Law, 1972.
41. Ibid.
42. Greenlaw JL. *When patients' questions put you on the spot.* 1983. RN *46*(3):79.
43. Nurse Practice Act. New York State Education Law. 1972.
44. Holder AR, Lewis JW. *Informed consent and the nurse.* Nursing Law and Ethics. 1981. *2*(2):1.
45. President's Commission. *Making health care decisions.* 76.
46. Ibid.
47. Ibid.; 36.
48. Nurse Practice Act. New York State Education Law.
49. President's Commission. *Making health care decisions.* 147–48.
50. Bradley JC, Edinberg MA. *Communication in the nursing context.* New York: Appleton-Century-Crofts. 1982; 278.
51. Ibid.; 278–279.
52. Ibid.; 279.

PART TWO

Nursing Ethics Through the Life Span

CHAPTER 7

Nursing Ethics in the Procreative Family

Study of this chapter enables the learner to:

1. Understand the functions, values, and dynamics of traditional and nontraditional families.
2. Distinguish between ownership, partnership, and club membership models of family relations.
3. Facilitate the family's participation in shared decision making in the clinical and ethical aspects of family planning, sterilization, and artificial and in vitro fertilization and implantation.
4. Develop the role of the nurse in genetic counseling based on facilitating the family's evaluation of its goals, values, and rational life plans.

INTRODUCTION

A new family that brings out the best in each member is usually and desirably motivated by love, including sexual love. The morally idealized family of a young male and a young female coming together out of love, care, and respect for each other is aptly dramatized through the visual, literary, and musical arts, in love stories such as *Romeo and Juliet,* in operas such as *La Bohème,* and films such as *The Sound of Music.* Love as a mode of family interaction may also be depicted in sculpture, as in *The Family of Man,* in which a man and a woman with a child between them embrace. Touching, reaching out, kissing, and embracing are expressions of love that bring people, usually of the opposite sex, to want to share the rest of their lives in fun, joy, and happiness. For love is the essential ingredient that binds new two-person families together. This love of two people is ordinarily and desirably transmitted to offspring.

The family is commonly regarded as the source, development, and justification of almost all values. To a recently born child, the family is the substance and boundary of its universe. The family gives stability and sustenance to a child's first experiences, once aptly termed by William James as "a booming, buzzing confusion." The family thus converts the child's initial confusion into an orderly ongoing system. The family is the young child's universe. The child's value relations depend on the love and quality of care of its parents and significant others who share in the parenting.

The first role of the nurse is to strengthen the positive love and to affirm and sustain creative family-life values. The nurse's second task is to help the troubled family achieve the strength and stability of a family that supports each member's worth in the process of growth and development.

FAMILY FUNCTIONS AND VALUES

The American family is changing its values, leadership, size, membership, roles, and functions. Despite change, it remains the basic social unit, the source of human capacities for relatedness and caring for another. Today's family systems are experiencing value conflicts as new life-styles are considered and tested. New configurations emerge as single parents, stepparents, parent and live-in friend, surrogate parents, and lesbian or male homosexual parents form a family in conjunction with one or more children.

Burgess's widely quoted definition of the family reflects its changing character. He defines the family as

> . . . a group united by marriage, blood, or adoption, residing in a single household, communicating with each other in their respective roles, and maintaining a common culture. . . . The family is in transition from a traditional family system controlled by mores, public opinion, and law to a companionship family system based on mutual affection, intimate communication, and mutual acceptance of division of labor and procedures of decision-making.[1]

Mutuality of interests, values, and goals is seen as the basis for becoming partners in a relationship. Increasingly, the goal of individuals starting families is that of happiness and self-actualization through affectionate ties with others. The pursuit of individual goals within a family can sometimes conflict with family Utilitarian goals of the greatest good for the greatest number, which sacrifice the interest of the minority to those of the majority. Kant's ethics of duty can be a powerful force in parental behavior and decision making through the use of a principle that calls for right action without exception.

Some of the functions of the family flow out of its definition. Burgess et al. see the family as most valued because it provides emotional support through reciprocal expressions of love and caring acts. Our culture places a high value on the factor of love and choice of mate. Burgess sees the family's second function to be its commitment to the provision of an environment in which its members share experiences, activities, and companionship. The third function Burgess defines as the care and rearing of children. Lastly, the family is one of society's primary agencies for transmitting the culture from one generation to the next.[2] As the primary unit of society, the family is the center of authority and decisions regarding the procreation of children, the provision of comprehensive care regarding their health and education, and all of the necessary supports to life and well-being.

THREE MODELS OF FAMILY AND MARRIAGE

Ownership Model

One model of marriage and family, regarded as the traditional model by some, is the model of ownership. Here, one member, usually but not always the male spouse, has the unshakable conviction that he is the boss, one who owns every member of the family in a master-slave, dominance-submission relationship. The model of owning something finds natural appeal within human nature in the conviction learned early in life that if one owns anything, one owns one's body.[3] Moreover, in the early, formative years of an infant's life, parents may act wisely by following the Ownership Model, which implies close responsibility and care. One does, after all, speak of "Mrs. Jones's children" in a way that clearly communicates a possessive relationship. To own something is to protect and cherish it. For that reason, the association of ownership with one's body and one's life provides a naturally persuasive case for a woman's rights regarding abortion.

In a family oriented to the Ownership Model, we find a morally "strong role differentiation," to adapt a concept from a recent work by A. Goldman. Such moral role differentiation entitles one person to have special powers, privileges, and exceptions from the moral rules that apply to other family members.[4] The family sovereign may, for example, be given the best food at the table, the best chair in the home, and the most attention, and may never be expected to help with the dishes, the lawn mower, or the vacuum cleaner. The family sovereign may also go anywhere, such as to having the neighborhood bar or to a distant city or country, and may do anything, including having extramarital sexual relations. Other family members must obey the sovereign. The Ownership Model invests authority and the source of all family duties in a single individual and requires unquestioning obedience to the will of the master.

One may distinguish two kinds of ownership. In the benign ownership view, the master rules, with most decisions beneficial to the master as well as to other family members who obey. In this view, the family sovereign makes reasonably good decisions most of the time, is efficient, consistent, and accountable for the general well-being of all family members. But such a sovereign nevertheless exercises sole decision making with unquestioning authority. If that sovereign is incapacitated unexpectedly, absent, or dead, one effect of such a sudden change is to turn a family from order into chaos. For in this kind of family pattern, other family members are unprepared to step in and make everyday family decisions.

A second version of the Ownership Model is a malignant sovereign who shows no responsibility for the good of other members of the family. Such a family sovereign is likely to squander family resources at the local bar or on frequent and expensive outings and to act impulsively and without regard to obligations to other family members. Such a sovereign is truly a tyrant.

In a recent article, M. Robbins and T. Schacht discuss the role of the nurse in family hierarchies. Although "we cannot observe hierarchies directly," they write, "we can infer them from our observations of the sequence and direction of behavior. For instance, who talks first? Last? Longest? Who talks to whom? When? Where? About what? If one family member consistently approaches the staff about the patient's health care, may we hypothesize that he or she holds an upper position in the family and has the task of being an "expert" on the patient's status?"[5]

Although Robbins and Schacht are concerned that a "nurse's attempt to communicate with family members may meet with resistance if the communication inadvertently violates the family communication hierarchy,"[6] our concern is with the nurse's value role in relation to the values of the family. We think, additionally, that a value-oriented nurse may, for example, question the practices of any fixed hierarchical pattern, one implied by the Ownership Model and may participate in the patient treatment plan.

The Ownership Model may also provide a perspective for perceiving nurse-patient-family relationships. The nurse or other health care team members may view patients as subordinate within the health care hierarchy. Nurses and physicians may regard themselves as sovereign beings who in effect "own" their patients, which means that their patients in effect have no right to question them.

Partnership Model

A second model, one more compatible with rights talk and its principles of justice and fairness in a family, is a Partnership Model. According to the Partnership Model, everyone in the family feels that he or she has an investment in achieving wise, benevolent, just, fair, and compassionate decision making. The slogan "all for one and one for all" prompts the members of this family model to cohere. They each stand to gain by committing themselves to the good of the family. All are beneficiaries, and all share the burdens as nearly equally as possible. In a family oriented to a Partnership Model, there is a weak or even no moral role differentiation between family members, due to their different social roles. On this view, the husband who in the Ownership Model never wipes the dishes, does laundry and cleaning, or cares for the children, may well be expected to do so on the basis of a fair and equitable distribution of family chores.

A Partnership Model entails a rights-based view, one with a full complement of rights to make decisions and rights to be cared for. These are rights accorded to each family member or held in trust.[7] In a Partnership-oriented family, the rights of family members are approximately equal.

Two types of Partnership Models may be distinguished. In one kind of partnership, there is a senior partner and a junior partner or several junior partners. Even George Orwell's *Animal Farm* sardonically points out that "some animals are more equal than others." So, too, in some families in which partnership is the practice, there nevertheless is a recognition that one member is the senior partner. Perhaps this seniority is due to age, experience with life problems, an edge in wisdom, financial or physical power within a family, charm, or charisma. But the consequence of such a "senior partnership" may be slippage back to the Ownership Model.

For this seniority version of the Partnership Model, a problem arises that is similar to the use of the "team" analogy in health care. On a sports team, there is generally a captain and even a coach, who gives the orders which other team members follow. In a sense, a political democracy is a partnership. However, anyone versed in *realpolitik* is aware that despite James Madison's noble sentiments to the effect that the people in a democracy are the governors and rulers, in practice, only one person or at most a small number of persons make all the important decisions. Thus, the seniority version of the Partnership Model dominates families and nurse-client-physician-family relations.

A second version of the Partnership Model is that of virtual equality of all family members in decision making. This may be more of an ideal type, one with fewer examples than the seniority version. If rights are taken seriously in nurse-family relationships, then the principle "each member counts equally" is respected. The value placed on partnership in the family may be extended to perceiving the nurse as a partner in the therapeutic process. J. Quint Benoliel writes that

> . . . a nurse-family relationship that promotes partnership as the central means for seeking solutions and resolutions is an essential component of delivery of nursing care in such a manner that the integrity of each person is preserved.[8]

An advantage of the Partnership Model is that shared decision making, whenever feasible, distributes burdens and benefits, liberties and duties on a roughly equal basis. This agrees with Rawls' justice-based model. A Partnership Model provides for open and for self-correcting decision-making procedures in a family. This is in contrast to a single decision maker in the Ownership Model. John Stuart Mill's eloquent reason for freedom of expression readily applies to the Partnership Model of family life. Mill gives the reason for providing the freedom to dissent as an opportunity to substitute truth for error.[9] To paraphrase Mill, a single decision maker under an Ownership Model is robbed of the chance to correct mistakes that comes with the alternative decision makers found in the Partnership Model. Benoliel puts the case for nurse-family partnership well. She writes, "Partnerships with families require an openness to the possibility that there are many different ways of sharing power within groups."[10] A Partnership Model also develops strong bonds and existentially felt commitments to the good of the family.

A drawback of this model, however, is that a Partnership Model-oriented family, sensing few or no bonds or commitments outside the family, may develop insularity and aloofness to persons outside the family. The slogan "One for all and all for one" may exclude others and also result in pitting a family against society. The close-knit family is akin to a close-knit profession whose members may show indifference and callousness to those outside the profession. Likewise, the close-knit family may regard others with suspicion, alienation, and hostility and erect "high fences" or barriers to keep the family in and strangers out.

A result of such family insulation is the development of a dubious notion that the ethics of intimates in the family is all there is and that there are no ethics that applies to strangers.[11] A related difficulty is that a family with strong partnership involvements may suffocate individuals and prevent them from developing separately. Partnerships have their price, and one of the most costly may be the chains all of the members unwittingly wear.

Some further issues arise for nursing in the relationship with families—issues such as the following: Can the nurse be regarded as a full partner and not as an intruder if the nurse voices views that are unpopular to a family? If the nurse's religious, political, and philosophic views affect his or her beliefs on abortion, sterilization, mental illness, euthanasia, and experimentation, and these are in collision with the views held by a family, what significance is to be placed on the nurse's values and what on the family's values?

Club Membership Model

In response to the difficulties of both Ownership and Partnership models, a third model is the Club Membership Model. On this view, the relation of family members is like that of members in a club, who can come and go as they please, use the facilities and locker rooms, play the sports they like, take a shower, and leave when they wish. The members have only to abide by rules involving relations to other members, the use of the facilities, prompt payment of dues, and respect for the property and propriety of fellow members.

In a Club Membership Model, where each person does "his or her own thing," there is weak moral role differentiation among the members, with scope for relativism and moral anarchy. The Club Membership Model endorses liberty or self-determination rights but few subsistence rights to be cared for. Special privileges and powers conferred by the club override moral considerations to outsiders. The Club Membership Model of a family is one of loose affiliation of its members. Alliances between members may be formed, but without deep and abiding alliances to the club. Moreover, the Club Membership Model tolerates indifference to the lives and quality of lives of its members as well as to persons outside the family.

The Club Membership Model is like a professional association, a social institution, or a miniature society. Citizenship is in a society, writ small, but a society nonetheless. Here, personal bonds are loose, with scope for individual self-development and a minimum of Paternalism. The Club Membership Model is also like some family communes, in which the affiliation is loose, roles diffuse, boundaries highly permeable, and the membership continually changing. In this respect, Club Membership is at the other end of the spectrum of behavior controls exerted by the Ownership Model. The Club Membership Model also has advantages and drawbacks. To its credit, it emphasizes individual liberties and noninterference. But to its discredit, there are too few rules to guide its members to care for one another.

Relations Among These Models

Only in the Partnership Model are family members liable to develop autonomous relationships of mutual respect and self-respect. For these reasons, although all three models provide points to consider, one that is maximally rights-based and one that therefore seems morally preferable to the others is the Partnership Model. This model provides a full complement of decision-making rights and rights to be cared for. What counts most in this model is the members' caring for themselves and one another. However, the defects that such a model provides, such as neglect of outsiders and suffocating relations within the partnership, call for appropriate consideration of each of the other models as well.

FAMILY DYNAMICS AND VALUES

Whatever its composition, the family is an interacting, interdependent unit operating by rules and expectations, values, and relations of intimacy. Relations are permeated by feelings of affiliation, loyalty, caring, and pride or conflicting feelings of hate, shame, and rejection. Family experiences are the source of adolescent and adult values, which are usually modified or extended but sometimes rejected in adult life. The most basic values, such as respect for human worth, honesty, and truth-telling, have their roots in family experiences. Stephen Toulmin, a philosopher, distinguishes the ethics of intimates from the ethics of strangers.[13] He argues that the ethics of strangers does not take adequate account of individual circumstances and needs. To strike a balance, Toulmin suggests that we look to Leo Tolstoy, the 19th-century Russian author of *War and Peace, The Death of Ivan Ilich*, and *Anna Karenina*. Tolstoy held that morality was only possible among intimate relations, as in families, between parents and children, lovers, and neighbors. As Tolstoy saw it, ethics is for those people within a person's walking distance. The moral universe stops when one takes a train, for the people one sees there are casual and commercial contacts, not close relations. Moral relations become less significant as one relates to acquaintances and strangers.

Abuse
Although love and consideration among family members is the desirable feeling, other feelings, such as indifference, hostility, impatience, and verbal and physical abuse, do occur. Awareness of abuse may help expose, confront, and minimize abuse and contribute to its replacement by positive love-generating feelings. Family members reflect social, psychological, and economic realities, which may reveal conflicts between spouses early in marriage. Some couples are known to feel disenchantment soon in their relationship and see faults in the other person that grow to intolerable proportions. Such disenchantment may well lead to abuse and even a habitual pattern of abuse between husband and wife, lovers, partners, or companions. Such couples live

together but they cannot stand each other. At worst, they abuse each other. Abuse is also evident in developing family relationships and may become the basic pattern of interaction between husband and wife.

Patterns of abuse make the nursing of such family members difficult. In the Ownership Model, there may be less overt abuse, since the issue of who rules the family is settled. But in either the Partnership or Club Membership model, there may be enough role ambiguity for one- or two-way abuse patterns to set in and become the dominant motif of family interaction.

Identifying abuse and knowing what counts as abuse is important in deciding what to do about it as distinct from some lesser wrong. For abuse is a serious harm or offense. The occurrence of abuse justifies interference with the abuser's right to freedom. Abuse may be direct or indirect, active or passive, intentional or unintentional. Abuse involves violation of another's rights.

The nurse's role is to support a victim of violence by letting her know what social, legal, and nursing services and remedies are available. By keeping careful records, nursing agencies can join other social agencies in advocating the victim's interests and preventing recurrence of physical abuse. The nurse's role in developing awareness, recognition, exposure, and confrontation of abuse is designed to minimize and to eliminate it. For abuse, the serious violation of a person's human rights, is the antithesis of decent human behavior. Nurses as nurturers have both a right and a duty to safeguard people, especially the powerless, against abuse.

The concept of abuse also provides a paradigm case argument against the notion that everything is either subjective or relative. To say, for example, that in some families, communities, or countries, it is all right to beat wives and children, is to deny that it may be justifiably judged by others who are more enlightened as abuse. Abuse is morally wrong.

Divorce

Although divorce is a legal event, the process of separation is fraught with moral problems for both spouses and children. Their lives, once intimate and cohesive, are separated, disorganized, and rearranged in new and unfamiliar patterns. Divorce is an increasing phenomenon in American life involving at least one child in most cases.

Divorce does not end the feelings and ties of spouses with children. It simply puts distance between them and enables them to use the children as pawns to continue the conflict if they so choose. Divorce is the end of a marriage, which by its nature places every family member at risk. The process of family rearrangement is slow, involving the ethical, emotional, psychological, physical, social, and economic dimensions of family life over a period of years. The impact of divorce is heavy on each member, but perhaps heaviest on young children whose foundation of security is in the feelings of "omnipotence" and "omniscience" of the parents.[12] The predictability of their world is shattered, and each child carries a load of self-blame and guilt. Children worry about what they did wrong and what they can do to reunite their parents. The child is deeply attached to both parents, and when one parent ostensibly abandons the child, the fear of abandonment by the other parent is usually strong. The family system, however disrupted by marital discord, represents survival to the children affected. Older children of school age and adolescents may be more verbal in expressing their rage and frustration at what they perceive as parental failure, but even they often regress, fail in schoolwork, and engage in antisocial activities in the effort to reunite their parents around their problems.

Levels of vulnerability differ among children, yet all can benefit by adherence to ethical principles governing relations. The process of separation and divorce need not be made any more traumatic than necessary by respecting the rights of every family member to a truthful explanation of reasons for the divorce. Children are powerless, and their rights particularly need to be respected. Children are entitled to the truth in terms they can understand. The difference between truth-telling and deception is vital to the development of the child's autonomy, integral to Kant's ethics. If the parents are divorcing because of one partner's alcoholism, crime, mental illness, or desertion, the children need to know this so that they will not fill in the vacuum with self-destructive mythology. If the parents are separating because one prefers another, or because of incompatibility, this too needs to be said without blame. In this way, the child is not forced to choose between "the good parent" and "the bad parent." The parents must exert themselves to the utmost to avoid adversarial, visitation, and custodial battles involving children. This causes considerable conflict and ambivalence, with possibly permanent damaging effects. Each parent's right to continue relationships with a child needs to be respected and facilitated by the other parent. Parents need to consider the ethical principles of rights and fairness in their relations to each other so that one parent, usually the mother, does not carry an undue share of the physical, psychological, and financial burden of child care. If both parents adhere to Kantian ethical principles of placing their parental duty to their children above considerations of individual comfort and convenience, it is quite possible for parents to unite around such issues as truth-telling and promise-keeping with their children. If the ethical principle of love as concern for the welfare of each family member is paramount, even though parents are divorced, it is possible to change the effects of divorce from crisis proportions to an event with "potential for growth and enhanced maturity"[13] of all concerned. The nurse can facilitate that process through exercise of her role as moral agent reinforcing ethical principles of duty, rights, and fairness.

THE NURSE'S ROLE IN FAMILY ETHICAL ISSUES

What can the nurse do to help a troubled family or parent to decide what ought to be done, in the light of their own value preferences and life situation, about a health problem? The nurse can use a problem-solving method, beginning with an assessment of the facts and a clear definition of the problem by the nurse and parents together. A next step may be for the parents to identify their ethical principles and value choice in relation to the problem and the alternatives. The nurse can facilitate the process by raising questions to clarify understanding of all the options.

Family decisions are of several kinds. Decisions can be made unilaterally by one parent who assumes the authority for the whole family, as in the Ownership Model. Or decisions can be made by majority vote or by consensus, in which discussion continues until there is commitment to the decision, as in the Partnership Model. In some families, there is an absence of deliberation and decision processes so that external events and forces shape the decision, as in the Club Membership Model. The authoritarian family values the duty and responsibility of one or both parents as the main factor in decisions. The family seeking consensus of its members values sharing responsibility and commitment to group decisions.

The nurse can serve as a catalytic agent to the family, identifying the need for decision in the problematic situation by means this family considers right for them. He or she can encourage open discussion of the problem with respect for the rights of all concerned.

Family Planning and Sterilization

For some couples, the number of children conceived and brought to term presents no problems. Such parents regard "life as a gift" to be respected and preserved and the use of contraceptives unnatural. For them, abortion is both tragic and unthinkable. To other couples, the omission of contraceptives with consequences of an unwanted pregnancy are tragic and unthinkable. Other couples decide that for personal and social reasons of overpopulation, they will not have any children. Such individuals may be sterilized.

Those who morally oppose contraception must contend with the inescapable fact of individual, family, and group inability to meet the nutritional, health, housing, clothing, and educational needs of its members.

One argument holds that to bear a child who must then suffer poverty, hunger, disease, and neglect of their human capacities, because there are more mouths to feed than there is food, is cruel and unjust. A new trend of voluntary sterilization is emerging in the United States, with an estimated three million American couples using either vasectomy or tubal ligation. Voluntary efforts here and abroad are insufficient, however. Policy proposals recommend that American aid to emerging countries should be tied to population control. The counterargument is that food and aid should be given solely on the basis of human need. Thus, the ethical controversy continues regarding individual liberty to produce as many children as desired and the duty of parents, and ultimately society, to provide children with the necessities of life, including health care.

Critics of population control say that separating nurture from procreation creates a dualism that downgrades the body as an inseparable element in all human events. A counterargument is that nurture is a significant human commitment to the welfare of another. In contrast, procreation is biological and without commitment to the care of the life generated. Thus, the supporters of family planning say that nurture is ultimatedly the more significant act.

ETHICAL ISSUES IN REPRODUCTIVE TECHNOLOGY

Artificial Insemination

The ethical arguments for and against artificial insemination are related to the differing definitions of the meaning of marriage, parenthood, and the family system and to the rightness or wrongness of reproductive interventions. The Roman Catholic position views artificial inseminations by either donor or husband for reasons of sterility or of fallopian tube closure as morally wrong. A recent Vatican speaker said ". . . artificial procreation is an act of production rather than communion between two people. [It] reduces human beings to objects and degrades their being, value, and dignity. Married couples have no right to children, only the right to perform the procreative act."[14]

The ethical arguments in favor of artificial insemination are based on a definition of marriage of mutuality and happiness. In Joseph Fletcher's conception, "marriage is not a physical monopoly."[15] Agreement to an anonymous donor by husband and wife is necessary for informed consent to the donation. Donation of sperm by the husband to the wife is free of problems to supporters of artificial insemination. The issues become more involved, however, when an anonymous ovum is needed to implant in the wife's uterus, or a uterus is needed in which to implant the wife's ovum to carry the fetus to term for a couple unable to have its own child. Granted, these are futuristic events, but they have a high probability of actuality in the near future.

The argument supporting artificial insemination by donor or by husband is that the human acts of sexual intimacy and procreation are different and separate. The main argument is that parenthood is not primarily a matter of biology but instead a broadly human function of commitment to the care and rearing of a child.

In Vitro Fertilization and Implantation

Similar ethical arguments are used either to justify or denounce in vitro fertilization of the mother's ovum by the father's sperm in a glass dish in the laboratory, followed by implantation of the embryo in the mother's body. Critics of the act say it is unnatural and undermines the marriage covenant of sexual love for procreation. It treats the procreative dimension of sexuality "as a mere biological function and defines parenthood in terms of nurturing life, not generating life."[16] Utilitarian advocates of the procedure point to the happiness achieved by the couple finally able to bear their own child. Others point to the great benefits to genetics and obstetrics coming from this research, which will be of benefit to future generations.

In vitro fertilization experimentation raises ethical issues in policy formation. Should this costly research, which ultimately benefits a few, be financed by scarce public funds needed for the benefit of the many? Is a child conceived in this manner subject to public curiosity, stigma, and rejection as a subhuman being?

Fetal Therapy

The pregnant woman undergoes life-style changes, risks, and discomforts for the sake of her fetus. With technological advances in perinatal medicine and surgery, the fetus is accessible to *in utero* diagnostic procedures and treatment. "The pregnant woman and her fetus are increasingly viewed as two treatable patients."[17] Caesarean delivery and intrauterine transfusions are effective, standard treatments for fetal distress. "Shunt diversions for hydrocephalus or obstructive uropathy are . . . research procedures."[18] These decisions, to treat or not to treat, involve the woman's autonomy and her rights to her own body. The moral conflict is "between the pregnant woman's own health, interests, and desires and her perception of the best interests of her fetus."[19] This poses moral conflicts for the procreative family that must choose to either risk the mother's or the fetus's health. It poses conflicts for the health providers as well. Informing the parents regarding the range of possible outcomes, including the birth of a defective infant despite treatment, is the basis for fully informed consent or fully informed rejection of the treatment.

Surrogate Motherhood

Individual cases of surrogate motherhood in which the genetic father and the artificially inseminated mother have waged bitter, prolonged lawsuits for possession of the contracted infant were national news sensations. In the Baby M example, the surrogate mother, Mary Beth Whitehead, carried the pregnancy to full term on the basis of a financial contract with the genetic father and his wife, then refused to give up the newborn. In still another example, the infant born to the surrogate mother supposedly fathered through artificial insemination, turned out to be grossly deformed and retarded. The identity of the father of this newborn became a legal and moral issue. Neither the contracting sperm-donating male or the surrogate mother desired the defective newborn. A legal suit settled the identity of the father on the basis of scientific evidence as the husband of the surrogate mother. He too rejected the infant.

These two cases illustrate the possible harms to the infant, to the surrogate mother, her spouse and family, and to the genetic father, his spouse and family by the exercise of the liberty rights of the participating adults. Does the love-based model of ethics provide the surrogate mother justification to keep or to regain her infant and to break her promises to the contracting couple? There are several important ethical issues in surrogate motherhood. One is the woman's right to her own body to reproduce a baby for another person. Opposed to this is the idea that the product of a pregnancy, a healthy infant, is not for sale. A group of surrogate mothers demanded the return of their babies and the outlawing of the practice they called "an institutionalized form of slavery."[20]

The New York Task Force on Life and the Law sought legislation to forbid surrogate parenting that makes money from human reproduction, as did the New Jersey Supreme Court.[21] The New York State Task Force condemned the characterization of pregnancy as a service like any other in the marketplace. They rejected a price tag on pregnancy for all women. They gave as their reason that the purchase of another human being is in violation of the "inherent dignity and equality of all persons."[22]

The counterarguments are that the decision shows a lack of compassion for childless couples who want to use the technology to hire a surrogate mother. Theirs is a human need for which they are willing to pay. Some surrogate mothers desire the income and feel compensated for their labor. These are private affairs involving informed consenting adults who can change the conditions of the contract at any time including after the birth of the infant.[23]

Surrogate motherhood evokes conflicts of altruism, justice, rights, duty, subjectivism, and egoism among the participants. Each position has merits, but a decision was reached in the case of Baby M—to award the child to the contracting couple with visitation rights permitted the surrogate mother—that was supposedly in the best interest of the child. Meanwhile the legal battle for custody continues.

The Nurse's Role

The nurse's role is to identify her or his own attitude clearly so as to differentiate those values from the values of the prospective parents and the pregnant woman. This may require consultation and deliberation with colleagues until the nurse is clear on basic ethical values. If the nurse disapproves of artificial insemination, in vitro fertilization and implantation, or surrogate motherhood, then the nurse had best withdraw from participation, since such decisions and technology are legal and clearly the right of consenting adults implementing the principle of moral autonomy.

Genetics

With advances in the science and technology of genetics, scientists can now detect defective genes causing "Huntington's disease, cystic fibrosis, Tay-Sachs disease, two types of muscular dystrophy, and retinoblastoma."[24] Genetic markers have also been identified that in some families "signal susceptibility to Alzheimer's disease and manic depression . . . [and] genetic predispositions to more common disorders including atherosclerosis, arthritis and diabetes. . . ."[25] Genetic marker tests search for a known sequence of genes inherited by families with a genetic defect. The marker appears with the faulty gene. This technique is creating an explosion in genetic findings.[26]

The success of genetic testing in identifying defective genes creates ethical conflicts and dilemmas for individuals, families, institutions, health professionals, and society. An example of the ethical issues is the case of a young Ashkenazi Jewish couple of Orthodox beliefs who marry with the intent of having children. The nephew of one of the spouses is born with Tay-Sachs disease, an inherited disease characterized by mental and physical retardation, blindness, convulsions, and death within the early years of life. It is 100 times more prevalent in Jewish children and especially in Ashkenazi Jews. There is a genetic test for the presence of an essential enzyme. If the mother is pregnant, amniocentesis will reveal the presence of the required enzyme. If the enzyme is absent, the child will be born with Tay-Sachs disease.[27] The alternative is abortion, an unacceptable practice to this religious group.

Prospective parents from vulnerable groups may experience considerable difficulty in even considering themselves as other than young, healthy parents competent to deliver a perfectly normal child. Yet some people, such as the couple in the example given, have a high familial probability of carrying the gene for disease. Genetic screening is a simple, effective way of determining their transmission status regarding Tay-Sachs disease. Genes are the way we project ourselves into the future through our children and their children. The ethical issue is the parents' liberty right to produce children without regard for genetic consequences. The counterargument to reproductive freedom is the parents' duties to the potentially afflicted child, other family members, and to society for the emotional, social, and financial cost of treatment and care.

As tragic as the circumstances surrounding the Tay-Sachs child are to the parents, perhaps the traits for sickle-cell anemia present more difficult decisions. There may be

> . . . no evidence to show that health disabilities are associated with carrying a sickle cell gene, except under extraordinary environmental conditions. The gene for hemoglobin S, even when present in a double dose. . . is remarkable for its variability of expression, and decisions about eugenic interventions to reduce its frequency are fraught with difficulty.[28]

This poses ethical problems for the black or Mediterranean couple regarding screening of a prospective spouse so as to avoid transmitting a double dose of a disease that may be benign, debilitating, or lethal. It also involves the issue of truth-telling to a prospective mate if one has the trait, with the possibility of ending the relationship. There is also the question of the availability of health and life insurance or job security if the truth is told. For a short time, New York State required non-Caucasian, non-Indian, non-Oriental individuals to take a blood test for the sickle-cell trait before issue of a marriage license. This caused public outrage on the basis of its discriminatory effect on blacks. The effect was to stigmatize them, causing peril to their employment, health insurance, and loss of privacy. This law was repealed as ineffective in reducing the frequency of persons in the sickle-cell gene pool.[29]

The case of retinoblastoma is even more complex and requires policy decisions. Retinoblastoma is a malignant glioma of the retina of the eye occurring in young children and showing a hereditary pattern.[30]

> It used to occur in no more than 1 in 30,000 people. It now occurs in England in as many as 1 in every 18,000 births. This exponential increase took place roughly between 1930 and 1960 and [is] almost entirely the result of physicians' being able to detect the tumor, treat it, and allow the individuals to survive and go on to reproduce. . . .
> Between 60 to 90 percent of the individuals actually manifest the tumor, . . . get it in both eyes and would be blinded or die except for new developments in surgery and radiation therapy. Now 70 percent are saved from blindness and at least four out of five survive.[31]

Thus, the disease is costly to treat, requiring highly specialized eye surgery and treatment, is genetically transmitted, and leads to blindness in some cases. Since this is a dominant gene, it will be passed on by the survivors to ever-increasing numbers of offspring, who will in turn require costly treatment and care. The ethical issue then becomes the right of individuals at risk to pass on retinoblastoma to half their offspring, who must then be treated at public expense, versus the right of the state to refuse treatment on the basis of scarce resources and priorities of prevention. Private insurance carriers may also refuse the risk because of its unfairness to other policyholders who bear the burden of cost.

The argument then extends to preferential treatment of retinoblastoma cases, who tend to have above average intelligence. In reality, most states practice preferential treatment. Patients receiving kidney dialysis three times weekly, for example, cost the state very much more than a chronically mentally ill or retarded person living in either a custodial public institution or substandard community facility.

Genetic Screening: Mandatory versus Voluntary

Individuals and society have choices regarding genetic screening. For example, individuals whose parent or grandparent had Huntington's disease, a degenerative brain ailment that appears around the age of 40, have a 50 percent chance of developing it. There are an estimated 200,000 such persons at risk.[32] The director of the Huntington's predictive testing project at Johns Hopkins Medical School says that "nearly two thirds of young adults at risk of inheriting the gene say they would like to know if they have it . . . and many couples are testing fetuses early in pregnancy and aborting those that test positive."[33] Some individuals at risk prefer not to know while others have committed suicide after learning that they have the gene.[34] The individual at risk faces further moral conflicts. Should that person tell the potential marriage partner of the risk of both developing and transmitting the disease of Huntington's, or of Sickle cell anemia, or of Tay-Sachs? What is the duty of the nurse or physician to inform the potential spouse if the person at risk does not do so? Can the spouse and the children receive compensation from health providers for not forewarning them of the harm of genetic disease? Does the individual with the defective gene have the duty to inform close relatives as well?

Experts predict that employers and insurers will soon require genetic information, unless states restrict testing of employees as some states now do in the case of AIDS. The possibilities for discriminating against known individuals carrying a defective gene are enormous. The problems will multiply as genetic screening identifies persons with predispositions for atherosclerosis, arthritis, diabetes, Alzheimer's disease, manic depressive illness and other common ailments. Will the pregnant woman then have a conflict of aborting a fetus who has the potential for heart disease in 50 years?

Mandatory testing, whether done in the premarital, prenatal, or postnatal period, has potential for moral dilemmas and tragic consequences. Mandatory prenatal screening presents women with terrible burdens and tragic choices if the fetus carries a defective gene. Prenatal screening is not morally neutral since the customary intent is to abort a defective fetus. The alternative, that of bearing the child with a known prognosis of disability, suffering, and death from Tay-Sachs, Sickle cell anemia, Huntington's disease, cystic fibrosis, or muscular dystrophy, for example, is equally tragic and possibly more threatening to the survival of the family.

Another response to known heriditary defects, one that violates individual's liberty rights, is compulsory sterilization. Sixteen states still have compulsory sterilization laws.[35] Historically,

> ... by 1931, thirty states had passed compulsory sterilization measures, some of which applied to a very wide range of "hereditary defectives" including "sexual perverts," "drug fiends," "drunkards," and "diseased and degenerate persons.[36]

The parallels to Hitler's program of purifying the race by the elimination of non-Aryans is inescapable. Such a view mistakenly emphasizes biological fitness and denies the negative and positive contributions of the environment to individual worth and capacity.

A third option for the state requiring mandatory genetic screening is illustrated by the case of retinoblastoma, a tumor that leads to blindness or death if untreated. Since retinoblastoma is generally associated with intelligence quotients of 116 to 128 and each case costs an average of $100,000, conservatively, to treat, we have here a classic case of tradeoffs between costs, benefits, and risks, sometimes called cost/benefit analysis. A question is whether society can afford to finance each case of retinoblastoma. A converse issue is that, given their relatively high intelligence levels, society cannot afford to deny treatment to such persons in view of their social, economic, and cultural contributions. A related question, aptly put by Marc Lappe, is: "What are our obligations to those children who are at risk for genetic disease and what are their parents' duties to society?"[37] What if a genetic disease was correlated with lower than average intelligence levels; would society still have an obligation to care for this population? Lappe asks what obligations a society has to the least well off. He also asks, "How do these obligations change when there are scarce medical resources to be distributed?"[38] Are individuals measured by their contribution to the social good? What role do parents have in bearing the cost of treating genetic diseases? Should affected individuals or their families pay for their own treatment? If society as a whole pays, does society have a right to constrain individuals from procreating "by withholding marriage licenses entirely from individuals with a heritable form of retinoblastoma?"[39]

These questions present moral and political issues for the relation of individuals and society, including issues of support and control. To give society a role in deciding who procreates may set a dangerous precedent in imposing restrictions that may not be rational or free from encouragement of selective breeding, a practice once championed by the Nazis. An immediate practical difficulty of any program of selective breeding involving either negative or positive eugenics is that restricting human variety lessens the chances for good as well as bad species modifications. We are left with moral dilemmas that have no satisfactory answers. Each answer implies some serious negative consequences.

These questions involve the issue of Libertarianism in opposition to Legal Paternalism and Legal Moralism. Libertarianism holds that a society is made up of individuals whose most important value is freedom from interference. According to Legal Paternalism, there are some common interests in society that call for justified interferences with individual liberties. These include a lifeguard at public beaches, safe drinking water (presently available to only a small fraction of the earth's population), requirements to wear seat belts in autos and helmets on motorcycles, rules providing for safe production and use of foods and drugs, and rules restricting the underaged from voting and drinking. According to a third position, Legal Moralism, society is viewed as a "seamless web," with individuals regarded as parts of larger wholes. Each individual's place depends on compliance with the requirements of a centralized decision-making group. On this view, the antithesis of Libertarianism, individuals have no private lives free of moral correction. Every social virtue becomes a law, and every sin becomes a crime. Free will is at a minimum. Such a society is somewhat like the order found in the Ownership Model of family ethics.

THE NURSE'S ROLE IN GENETIC COUNSELING

We apply these positions, then, to the role of the nurse in genetic counseling. In this connection, Marc Lappe argues against any restrictions "constraining individuals from procreation." He opposes "intrusion into the privacy of reproductive decision making by the state, which. . . constitutes a greater harm than leaving such decisions to the couples at risk."[40] The nurse, on Lappe's view, does not constrain a retinoblastoma couple against procreation but leaves the decision to them. Lappe prefers "voluntary genetic counseling," which he regards "as superior to compulsory counseling in both outcome and compliance."[41] He is concerned about some state restraints. Blindness is a major health problem in the state; the costs of surgical care are escalating.[42] Lappe proposes a principle consistent with our moral traditions.

> First, recognize that virtually every prospective parent who puts a child at risk for retinoblastoma will have had the same tumor and will have experienced the pain, suffering and other burdens of that condition. [Lappe assigns] primacy to this unique experiential basis for judging over and against rules imposed by society from outside the family.[43]

Families at risk decide, even though Lappe concedes that "society" rather than the average individual family "has the financial resources to cope with the surgical cost of treatment."[44] At any rate, Lappe sides

> . . . with Montaigne who said "I have never seen a father who failed to claim his son, however mangy or hunchbacked he was. Not that [the father] does not perceive his son's defects. . . but the fact remains, the boy is his.". . . love and parental bond establish the grounding for a procreative decision, one which works to the best interests of the child.[45]

Lappe concludes that

> . . . the right to decide [therefore] must be vested exclusively with parents that are involved. We would be best investing the moral authority for making this decision not with the state but with these individuals who primarily bear the burdens of perpetuating their own genes. [Lappe sees the alternatives as] placing the state over the individual [which denies] the deepest feelings that parents have for their children.[46]

Lappe's message is to trust the parent who has had similar experiences. There is something inherently good and wise in parents. With a little care, one hears the refrain "Parents know best" in the form of genetic and moral counseling.

One may note the love-based ethics that provides an important moral premise for Lappe. The bond of love between parent and child suggests an innate wisdom and goodness, which parents, following Montaigne's reasoning, show in their decisions. Leave procreative decisions to parents, therefore. Lappe's advice to nurses may be regarded as a form of love-based ethics. His hypothetical advice to nurses is that in their genetic counseling they leave the option rights concerning procreation basically to prospective parents rather than to the state in either a Legal Paternalist or Legal Moralist form. This view is also identified as a moral-sentiment view, expressed alternatively by Jean Jacques Rousseau (1712–1778) and Leo Tolstoy (1828–1910), both of whom valued the moral sentiments that are found among ordinary people, including peasants, who are viewed as "noble savages." This innate moral folk wisdom is the love parents have for their children. It reveals wise and untutored forms of public and private decency.

But is this view of the goodness and wisdom of parents borne out by evidence? One has only to look at public institutions, such as those for the retarded and abandoned, rejected or abused children, to learn of all the despised and rejected physical, emotional, and mental "hunchbacks" unwanted by parents. The parent does not always know best. Persons in authority, such as physicians, judges, nurses, and other representatives of society have a role in sustaining good family relations even on the basis of paternalistic inteference.

CONCLUSION

A family can be positive if it enables individuals in the family to flourish separately and together. If the relationships are destructive or unwise, intervention by nurses and other relevant persons is appropriate. The nurse can help by supporting positive human relationships. One reason for nursing intervention is that in relations between spouses or parents and children, the stronger does not always know best.

Discussion Questions

1. How would you compare four moral views such as Paternalism, Libertarianism, Agapism and Utilitarianism taken on counseling the family with a sickle-cell trait?
2. Discuss the use of reproductive technology from the view point of Agapism, Utilitarianism, and Kantian ethics?
3. In the three-way relation between the state, the individual at risk or who has a costly hereditary disease, or the procreative couple who bears the major responsibility for providing for treatment? Who, if any has rights to treatment?

REFERENCES

1. Burgess EW, Locke HJ, Thomas MM. *The Family*. 4th ed. New York: Van Nostrand Reinhold. 1971; 1.
2. Ibid.; 2.

3. Thomson J. In defense of abortion. *Philosophy and Public Affairs*. 1971. *1*(1): 47–66.
4. Goldman A. *The moral foundations of professional ethics*. Totowa, NJ: Littlefield, Adams. 1980; 2–8, 20–22, 34–37, 49, 58–61, 65–69, 88–91, 109, 113, 273, 277–278, 281, 282.
5. Robbins M, Schacht T: Family hierarchies. Am J Nursing. 1982. *82*(2): 285.
6. Ibid.
7. Feinberg J. The child's right to an open future. In: Aiken W, LaFollette H. (eds). *Whose Child?* Totowa, NJ: Littlefield, Adams. 1980; 125–153.
8. Benoliel JQ. The nurse-family relationship. 121.
9. Mill JS. *Utilitarianism, liberty and representative government*. London: Dent. 1948; 79.
10. Benoliel: The nurse-family relationship. 121.
11. Toulmin S. *The tyranny of principles*. The Hastings Center Report. 1981. *11*(6): 31–39.
12. Feldman J. Divorce and the children. In: Getty C, Humphreys W. (eds). *Understanding the Family: Stress and Change in the American Family*. New York: Appleton-Century-Crofts. 1981; 336.
13. Ibid.; 333.
14. Berger J. Vatican official assails method of fertilization. *The New York Times*, October 8, 1987; B6.
15. McCormick RA. Reproductive technologies: Ethical issues. In: Reich WT (ed). *Encyclopedia of Bioethics*. 1978. New York: Free Press. Vol. 4; 1456.
16. Ibid.; 1463.
17. Lenon JL. The fetus as a patient: Emerging rights as a person? *AM J Law Med*. 1983. 9:1–29.
18. Committee on Bioethics, American Academy of Pediatrics. Fetal therapy: Ethical considerations. *Pediatrics*. 1988. *81*(6):898–9.
19. Ibid.
20. Schneider K. Mothers urge ban on surrogacy as form of slavery. *The New York Times*, September 1, 1986; A13.
21. Editorial. *The New York Times*, June 4, 1988; 26.
22. Ibid.
23. D'Amato A. Letter to the editor. *The New York Times*, February 18, 1988; A26.
24. Blakeslee S. Genetic discoveries raise painful questions. *The New York Times*, April 21, 1987; C1.
25. Ibid.
26. Ibid.
27. *Taber's Cyclopedic Medical Dictionary*. 1981. 14th ed. Philadelphia: FA Davis. 1427.
28. Lappe M. Genetics and our obligations to the future. In: Bandman EL, Bandman B. (eds). *Bioethics and human rights: A reader for health professionals*. Lanham, Md.: University Press of America, 1986; 86.
29. Ibid.
30. *Taber's Cyclopedic Medical Dictionary*, 1246.
31. Burgess EW, Locke, HJ, Thomas MM. *The family*, 4th ed. 2.
32. Blakesle S. Genetic discoveries raise painful questions.

33. Ibid.
34. Ibid.
35. Lappe M. Genetics and our obligations to the future. 91.
36. Ludmerer KM. Eugenics: History. In: Reich WT (ed). *Encyclopedia of Bioethics*. 1978. New York: Free Press. Vol. 1; 459.
37. Lappe M. Genetics and our obligations to the future. 89.
38. Ibid.
39. Ibid.; 91.
40. Ibid.
41. Ibid.; 92.
42. Ibid.
43. Ibid.; 92.
44. Ibid.
45. Ibid.; 93.
46. Ibid.

CHAPTER 8

Nursing Ethics and the Problem of Abortion

Study of this chapter enables the learner to:

1. Appreciate the moral significance of a couple's decision regarding procreative choice.
2. Understand the Supreme Court and legislative decisions regarding abortion.
3. Identify the uses of reproductive technology in relation to abortion.
4. Utilize the ethical arguments in opposition to and in support of abortion as the basis for forming an individual position regarding this problem.
5. Participate in policy formulation regarding abortion on the basis of ethical reasoning and arguments.

INTRODUCTION

The procreative family has a most important decision to make. To paraphrase a Shakespearean question in *Hamlet* "To be or not to be?" The family asks: To begin or not to begin a new life? Several moral arguments provide justifying reasons in deciding whether or not to initiate or to continue a new life—a decision surrounded by enormous responsibility. The power of life and death is in the hands of those who decide. For this reason all problems in bioethics, in Willard Gaylin's view, keep coming back to abortion. Moral principles are designed to answer whether to end a life or not. As we shall see, these principles, while helpful, do not always work. For this reason, abortion continues to be a problem.

LEGAL STATUS OF ABORTION

On January 22, 1973, in the landmark cases of *Roe* v. *Wade* (410 U.S. 113) and *Doe* v. *Bolton* (410 U.S. 179), the Supreme Court established the right of every woman to have an abortion legally. *Roe* v. *Wade* struck down the Texas statute restricting abortion to instances necessary to save a woman's life. The *Doe* v. *Bolton* case struck down a Georgia statute permitting abortions only if necessary to the woman's health, to prevent the birth of a malformed child, or to terminate pregnancy from rape. The Court's decision invalidated similar laws in other states that restricted abortion.

In the report of the majority opinion, the Supreme Court noted that there is no history in this country of ever prosecuting women for abortions, even for those performed after the fetus entered the "quickening period" (first felt movements of the fetus occurring from the 18th to the 20th week of pregnancy).[1] Moreover, the justices said that, since the adoption of the Constitution and through the 19th century, abortion was in less disfavor than it now is. The Court offered three reasons for the change from the historical right of a woman to terminate pregnancy to the criminal abortion laws in existence in some states. Primarily, the laws were meant to discourage illict sex on Legal Moralist grounds. Secondly, the laws were meant to prohibit abortion as highly dangerous to women who died in large numbers from fatal infections. In regard to this argument, the justices admitted that early abortion mortality rates are now even lower than the rates for normal childbirth. The third reason given is the state's supposed interest in protecting the unborn life, based on the argument that life begins at conception.[2] Historically, however, most laws against abortion were meant to protect women from a very risky procedure.

In the decision favoring abortion, the Court recognized the right of personal privacy in the Constitution, with roots in the First, Fourth, Fifth, Ninth, and Fourteenth Amendments, as well as in the Bill of Rights. The majority of justices said that only fundamental personal rights extending to marriage, procreation, contraception, child rearing, and education can be included in the right to personal privacy.[3] On the basis of these amendments, a woman's absolute, unrestricted right to terminate pregnancy was argued. The Court, however, could not agree to the woman's absolute right to privacy without the state asserting its interests in safeguarding health through maintaining standards of medical practice and "in protecting potential life."[4] The Court refused to accept the fetus as a person because of substantial disagreement on the concept of personhood and the omission of the unborn from consideration in the Fourteenth Amendment. "The unborn have never been recognized in the law as persons in the whole sense."[5]

Without resolving the question of when life begins—whether at birth, at conception, at quickening, or at viability—the Court recognized states' interests in the woman's health and the potential human life approaching term as compelling. The Court summarized its decision in the following provisions:

1. Any state criminal abortion laws such as the Texas type, which "excepts from criminality only a lifesaving procedure on behalf of the mother, without regard to pregnancy state and without recognition of the other interests involved,"[6] violate the due process clause of the Fourteenth Amendment.
   a. The abortion decision in the first trimester is between the woman and her physician.
   b. The state may regulate the abortion procedure to protect the mother's health after the first trimester.
   c. Following the stage of viability (a fetus usually 28 weeks or older, capable of living outside the uterus), a state may regulate, or even prohibit, abortion except where medically necessary to preserve the life or health of the mother.
2. Only licensed physicians are permitted to perform abortions.

Common sense might consider this decision from the highest court of the land to be authoritative and final. Not so. The controversy over abortion continues, and two more Supreme Court decisions affect the implementation of the *Roe* v. *Wade* (1973) decision.

On June 20, 1977, in two cases *(Beal* v. *Doe,* U.S.L.W. 4781 and *Maher* v. *Roe,* 45 U.S.L.W 4787) involving Pennsylvania and Connecticut, the Supreme Court ruled that states are not required to spend Medicaid funds for elective, nontherapeutic abortion. Congress then promptly banned the use of federal funds for abortions, with some exceptions. Thus, quite effectively, the Supreme Court's 1973 decision permitting abortion was seriously restricted by withholding funds for abortions from poor women, the recipients of Medicaid funds for health care, as unnecessary medical service. Thus, one social class, the poor, is singled out for the restriction of the fundamental right to abortion because of the inability to pay. Moreover, the justices' majority opinion argued for the states' "valid and important interest in emergency normal childbirth."[7] On the grounds of the state's significant interest in a woman's pregnancy, the state funds childbirth but need not fund elective abortions. The Court said that while the state may not prevent abortions, it need not help poor women obtain them as a remedy for social and economic ills.[8] The Court left the federal government and the states free to provide or to withhold funding for abortions. Critics of the decision called it a political response to antiabortion groups. Public opinion polls of random and of religious groups show a large majority of those polled in favor of legal abortion and freedom of choice.[9] Even on this point, we do well to remind ourselves of the "is-ought" fallacy, which may be committed if one argues that what people favor therefore justifies a moral policy.

REPRODUCTIVE TECHNOLOGY AND ABORTION

Prenatal Tests of Fetal Health
The possibilities for choosing abortion to end an unwanted pregnancy are growing explosively as a consequence of three new prenatal tests of fetal health.[10]

Chorionic Villus Sampling. This test may be used as early as the ninth week of pregnancy. Cells are taken from the villi, the gestational sac that surrounds the fetus in early pregnancy. In a few days, the results "disclose birth defects like Down's syndrome, Tay-Sachs, or other inherited disorders."[11] The experts believe that its time advantages will result in this test replacing most amniocentesis procedures.

Alpha-fetoprotein Screening. The second test, alpha-fetoprotein screening, is a blood test, which in California physicians are required by law to offer their patients. It is given at 16 weeks of pregnancy to women of all ages. The test measures levels of alpha-fetoprotein that the fetus excretes into the amniotic sac and the mother's bloodstream. The test is used to detect neural tube defects. If the neural tube fails to close at the top, the baby is born anencephalic and dies at birth or soon after.[12] If the neural tube is open at the spine and the spinal cord is exposed, the infant has spina bifida and probably hydrocephalus and mental retardation.[13] The test also detects risk of Down's syndrome.[14] Neural tube defects occur in about 1 in every 1,000 births to women without family histories of birth defects. This test is the only way to find such affected fetuses.[15]

Amniocentesis. The third test is amniocentesis in which cells obtained from the amniotic fluid surrounding the fetus are grown. This procedure can only be done at about the fourth month of pregnancy and the result takes two weeks to develop. At four and a half months of pregnancy, abortion is physically and emotionally more difficult for the woman. This test detects such genetic defects as Down's syndrome and Tay-Sachs disease.

The Benefits, Harms, and Risks of These Tests
The benefits of the alpha-fetoprotein screening test is that younger women below age 35 are normally not offered amniocentesis. Yet,

since younger women are the majority of the pregnant population, they bear 80 percent of the babies with Down's syndrome. With this test, these women are informed of the increased risk of carrying a fetus with Down's syndrome or with neural tube defects and then offered amniocentesis.[16] Another benefit of this test is that women over 35 with normal levels of alpha-fetoprotein are at low risk of having a fetus with Down's syndrome and on this basis can choose to reject amniocentesis.[17]

The harms and risks of amniocentesis and the chronic villus sampling tests lie in the one-half to one and a half percent of miscarriages induced by the test.[18] The variation is reportedly due to the skill and expertise of the obstetrician performing the test.[19] The harm of the alpha-fetoprotein test lies in the suggestiveness of the results and the need for follow-up tests hazardous to the fetus.

Although these tests offer clear benefits of choice to the pregnant woman based on hitherto unavailable information, they also present difficult decisions about which prenatal tests to accept and how to act on their results. Because the tests are so often a prelude to abortion,[20] they add to the growing clamor of public opinion around the legalization and public support of abortion. These tests offer the pregnant woman data regarding the health of the fetus as the basis for exercising her right to abortion.

Fetal Reduction

Some infertile women have resorted to either the use of fertility drugs or to *in vitro* fertilization and implantation. Consequently, some women have had multiple pregnancies of as many as eight fetuses with little chance of survival of any. One approach to this problem is selective abortion of the most accessible fetuses seen through the sonogram by injection with a lethal dose of potassium in the first trimester of pregnancy.[21] Most pregnancy reductions leave the woman with twins as a margin of safety or, in some cases, with the healthiest single fetus. Some of the decisions to reduce the number of pregnancies were made for the woman's convenience. Other abortions were made solely to ensure the survival of at least one or two of the multiple fetuses.

Arguments for and against this experimental procedure ranged from support for a woman's absolute right to her body to a total rejection of abortion in any form. Richard McCormick argued that the procedure could be justified when all the fetuses would otherwise die. "It is against the abortion position of the Catholic Church, (but) . . . I just don't think that the abortion position of the Church was formulated and designed with any circumstances like these in mind."[22] John Fletcher, another ethicist, said that the reduction did the "least harm for the most potential good."[23]

The Use of Embryonic Tissue

Another moral dilemma has arisen from the growing clinical need for human fetal tissue. Fetal grafts from the human embryo are considered to be a major advance in treating degenerative disorders such as Parkinson's disease, radiation disorders, juvenile diabetes, and repair of damaged hearts.[24] Fetal tissue reportedly integrates and survives longer in the host and resists rejection better than adult tissue grafts.[25] Research using embryonic cardiac cells for cardiac repairs is more feasible than total heart transplants according to this author. A moral dilemma arises from the massive need for human embryonic cells, the current inability to grow them without using fetuses for "personal or commercial exploitation."[26] An aging society with increasing degenerative diseases and growing demand for their treatment by the best means available will "further polarize attitudes toward abortion."[27]

ETHICAL ISSUES IN ABORTION

Even if there were a clamor for legalization of abortion, questions continue to rise as to whether abortion is morally permissible.

Positions on abortion are largely justified by opinions held on the status of the product of pregnancy. At one end of the spectrum, the Catholic church, through its Popes Pius XII and now John Paul II, views life as sacred and to be preserved from the moment of its conception. All abortions, even for therapeutic reasons, are illicit.[28] This view holds that a human being emerges at conception through the parental combination of genetic packages with all of the potentialities of a person in the zygote. Counterarguments to this most basic position point to the fact that a

> zygote is not irreversibly an individual until around the end of the second or the beginning of the third week of life. During this time it may split, forming identical twins (or triplets, etc.) . . . there is evidence that twinned individuals may recombine, forming again a single genotype.[29]

This weakens the argument that a human exists from the moment of conception.

An argument favoring abortion is that, since the embryo lacks electrical activity in the brain, it is simply living tissue, which may be eliminated like other unwanted tissue, such as the appendix or tonsils. The counterargument of those opposing abortions is that reflexes are present in the embryo and, although lacking in brain activity, "its potentialities for full human life and personhood set it apart as quite

different from a being whose permanently nonfunctioning brain sig-
nals that he is dead."[30] The counterargument is that, as Dedek and the
Supreme Court decision point out, the fetus is a potential person and
not actual, "just as the acorn is potential but far from the reality of an
oak tree. Acorns are not oak trees"[31] after all. Thus, the counterargument against abortion rests on the potential personhood of the fetus,
who has the same right to life as any other person.

Judith Thomson, a philosopher, who defends abortion under certain circumstances, confronts the premise of the fetus as a human
being from the moment of conception. She acknowledges that human
development is continuous and to draw a line of personhood at any
point, whether at conception, quickening, viability, "understanding,"
"reasoning," or "life projects," is to make an arbitrary choice. The same
kind of thing might be said about the relation of the acorn to the oak
tree, but, she argues, "it does not follow that acorns are oak trees."[32]
Arguments of this sort are notorious examples of the slippery-slope
fallacy.

For the sake of developing both sides of the argument, Thomson
grants that if the fetus is a person from the moment of conception,
then, like every other person, it has a right to life. Likewise, the
mother is a person and has a right to her life and to decisions determining what is allowed to happen in and to her body. At this point,
the antiabortionists believe that a person's right to life, in this case
the fetus's, outweighs "the mother's right to decide what happens in
and to her body. . . . So the fetus may not be killed; an abortion may
not be performed."[33]

Thomson responds to this point with her well-known analogy of
waking up back-to-back with a famous unconscious violinist. The violinist has a lethal kidney ailment and is plugged into your compatible
circulatory system. To unplug him would be to kill him. The hospital
director soothingly tells you, "But it's only for nine months." But do
you have to agree to it? Thomson asks. And what if it were nine years
or your lifetime? The hospital director says, "Too bad. Everyone has a
right to life, and this violinist is a person. His right to life outweighs
your right to your own body. Therefore, you cannot be unplugged from
him ever."

This is an outrageous argument, in Thomson's view. It is especially outrageous in instances of pregnancy through rape or when the
mother's life is in danger because of pregnancy. If, on this view, the
mother and the fetus have an equal right to life, why not flip a coin,
or grant that the mother's right to life plus her right to what happens
in and to her body outweighs the fetus's right to life?

The antiabortionist view is that performing an abortion is direct
killing, whereas not doing anything is only letting the mother die and
not killing an innocent person, namely the fetus. The direct killing of

an innocent person, such as the fetus, is regarded as murder and therefore not permitted as preferable to letting either the mother or the fetus, or both, die. Thomson responds that it cannot be murder for the mother to save her life by performing an abortion. No woman need sit by passively waiting for her death. Using the violinist analogy, she has only to unplug herself. Thomson believes that to refuse an abortion to such a mother "is to refuse to grant to the mother the very status of person which is so firmly insisted on for the fetus."[34]

Thomson sees this situation as analogous to that of a mother trapped in a very tiny house with a rapidly growing child; she will be crushed to death by the lack of space. Thomson argues that third parties, such as health providers, may refuse to choose between the mother's life and the fetus's life, but the mother, who is the person housing the child, has the right of self-defense against threats to her life. She owns the house.

Thomson likens the houseowner analogy to that of two people freezing to death, with one the owner of a coat that will save his life. The coat owner has the right to the coat. So does the pregnant woman own her body, which houses the fetus. Therefore, the health provider can refuse to act in not performing an abortion, but someone needs to protect the rights of individuals both to their own bodies and to their own coats.

Thomson then considers the case for abortion when the mother's life is not at stake. She sees the antiabortionist argument here as resting on the fetus's claim to a right to life. This view regards the right to life as unproblematic. Thomson says that life is not unproblematic. In her view, the right to life includes the right to the "bare minimum . . . for continued life."[35] But what if the bare minimum is something to which the person has no right, such as continuous free food, clothing, shelter, health service, and loving care?

Thomson raises the counterargument to this position, which is that even if no one has a right to be given anything, there is a right not to be killed by anyone, by unplugging, shooting, or knifing. But to refrain from unplugging the violinist is to allow him to continue the use of your kidney. Although he has no right to the original use of your kidneys, the antiabortionist arguments says that the violinist has the right against you "not now to intervene and deprive him of the use of your kidneys."[36] The right to life in Thomson's view does not guarantee the use of another's body even if such use is lifesaving, contrary to the antiabortion position. Thomson uses the example of a gift box of chocolates to two brothers to illustrate her case. If the gift was to both jointly and the older brother eats the whole box without giving any to his brother, he is unjust, for the younger brother was given half. Contrariwise, unplugging the violinist is not unjust, since you gave neither him nor anyone else the right to the use of your kidneys.

Unplugging him would surely kill him, but not unjustly and without violation of his right to life, since the use of another's body is not guaranteed in the right to life.

Thomson then responds to the charge of abortion as unjust killing. Certainly the rape victim has not given the fetus "a right to the use of her body for food and shelter."[37] But isn't there some sense in which a woman engaging in intercourse who then becomes pregnant is at least partly responsible for the life within, even if she did not invite it in? (It is a statistical fact that not all contraceptives are 100 percent effective.) Does the woman's partial responsibility then give the fetus the right to the woman's body, and can the woman now kill it even to save her own life? Thomson points to the argument that a fetus's right to life as an independent person is fallacious since, in fact, the fetus is dependent on the mother and the mother has a special kind of responsibility for its well-being. Nurses know the significance of the mother's nutrition, health habits, and life-style in supporting the fetus's proper growth and development. Thomson uses other analogies to support her arguments in defense of abortion. If, for example, I open the window of my home and a burglar climbs in, it would be incorrect to say, "Ah, but you opened the window and now he's in, and therefore you're partly responsible and must let him stay."[38] Or, for example,

> People seeds drift about in the air like pollen, and if you open your windows, one may drift in and take root in your carpets or upholstery. You don't want children, so you fix your windows with fine mesh screens, the very best you can buy. As can happen, . . . one of the screens is defective; and a seed drifts in and takes root. Does the person plant who now develops have a right to the use of your house?[39]

The required move might be to seal your windows and doors and to live with bare floors and without furniture. Surely a person plant who enters your house does not have a right to a place in the house, any more than a burglar has who came into your house without permission. A woman could have a hysterectomy to avoid unwanted pregnancies, but like the person who keeps the person plants out of her home, a woman who wishes to avoid rape would never leave home without an army. Since this is virtually impossible for most persons, abortions of unwanted pregnancies are justified.

Some difficulties arise for several aspects of Thomson's argument. One is that to have a right in and to one's body, compared to owning a house, is not absolute. There are exceptions to one's rights in and to one's body. If one has a contagious disease, such as typhoid or smallpox, one cannot go anywhere one pleases. Nor can one use one's body to swim in the community drinking water supply. The "landlord" analogy, to use a metaphor of Stephen Toulmin's about certain abortion arguments,[40] implies that a pregnant woman has the right to decide whether to evict her tenant, and it presupposes that a woman owns her offspring. Some writers even go so far as to assert that a "pregnant woman makes a baby, presumably like a carpenter, sculptor, or architect."[41] Viewing a pregnant woman as a landlady, factory owner, or sculptor begs the question at issue and gives the case away to those who argue that a pregnant woman may do with her body as she pleases. A criticism of the property or artifact metaphor is that a life growing within another person is not quite like somebody's property or factory or simply clay in someone's hands, contrary to the claim of those who write that a mother makes a baby.

A mother does not make a baby, since there are factors outside a mother's power to control affecting the development of the fetus. A mother's contribution to the fetus's physical development is largely involuntary, unlike a carpenter's, sculptor's, or architect's, whose will and design has more to do with shaping the outcome. The mother cannot decide the sex, size, color, or genetics of her offspring, for example. Opposed to the landlady, factory-owner, or sculptor metaphor of a mother-fetus relationship is the comparison of a pregnant woman to a passive receptacle, such as a flower or oven, who does not create the life within her. On this view, God alone makes or creates a baby. The mother is only the one who will help it grow, like a plant growing with the help of water and sunlight. A woman's role is to receive male sperm, which then develops inside her womb. On another view, there are scientific accounts of fetal development which do not invoke God. But "the gift of life," to use St. Thomas Aquinas's metaphor, is not any human being's to take or to destroy under any circumstances. According to Aquinas, "Life is God's gift to man and is subject to His power who kills and who makes to live."[42]

The woman-as-flower analogy also has difficulties. How could one test the assertion that God makes a baby, for example? What kind of gift is life that it cannot be refused or destroyed by anyone else? Is life necessarily or always a gift, even for an infant or older person with multiple physical or mental deformities such as spina bifida, myelomeningocele, or cancer? Another view denies the essentially passive role of women in pregnancy and child rearing. A woman, on this view, has a role and a stake in the outcome. She is no mere receptacle to be filled at will by a male who owns and controls her nature and destiny. To compel a woman to bring to term an unwanted pregnancy is regarded by one writer as "forced labor."[43]

But whether a given practice counts as "forced labor" may be philosophically debatable. For example, Robert Nozick argues that taxation beyond that which is necessary for a minimal state—one that protects individuals against one another—is "forced labor."[44] Ingenious as is Nozick's idea of forced labor, there is room for debate. His argument does not present us with a fixed truth. For example, taxation for libraries, museums, parks, colleges, or public preservation of the wilderness, as Joel Feinberg previously pointed out,[45] hardly constitutes "forced labor."

We can distinguish two senses of forced labor. We are all forced to work to make a living. A woman who wants a child exerts labor and force to bring a fetus through the birth canal. A second sense of forced labor, akin to slave labor that is morally impermissible, imposes the duty to bring a fetus to term. In this negative sense of forced labor, if there are any *a priori* truths in morals, they include the statement that "forced labor," slave labor, is morally wrong. But this principle conflicts with another principle that murder is wrong. Abortion in certain circumstances is murder and is therefore wrong.

The use of the property and the flower metaphors attempts to answer the question, "When does life begin and end?" This question presupposes an answer to the metaphysical question, "Is a pregnant woman one being or two?"[46] To individuate the fetus very early in pregnancy or at the moment of conception is to regard a pregnant woman as two persons, each with equal rights. A conflict then develops between the rights of each, calling for a settlement by a third party such as the church or state. To individuate later in the pregnancy or near the time a woman gives birth is to regard a pregnant woman as one person and, therefore, as the only rightholder. Against this one pregnant person, a growing fetus may be conceived of as an intrusive invader if that fetus is unwanted. The mother decides whom to let into her house or body, as one chooses whom to invite to one's party. On this view, the decision is hers to make. She owns her body and everything in it. The force of the ownership model, is again an intuitively powerful source of appeal when it comes to a woman claiming her rights; for if she owns anything, it is her body.

In opposition, Brody argues that humanity begins with a fetus. A human fetus has the same moral status as a mother, and therefore the same right to live. This means abortion is not morally justifiable, even in cases that threaten a mother's life. By analogy, a bigger, stronger person has no right to kill a weaker one. To Brody, Thomson's self-defense argument does not work, because the fetus is not the mother's pursuer.[47] Instead, the fetus is a miniature human in the sense that it has an essential property of being human, namely a brain,[48] which it develops sometime between the second and twelfth week after conception.[49]

There are strengths and difficulties in Brody's argument. One strength is that his argument refutes Thomson's self-defense argument. Another strength is his appeal to the obvious resemblances between a fetus and an infant human being. A third strength is the respect Brody engenders for the living and the moral wrongness of killing.

A difficulty with Brody's argument, however, is that he is nowhere able to equate human life as a set of conscious acts with the undeveloped fetuses' states of mind. This discrepancy between ordinary humans and fetuses undermines his claim that fetuses are human.

The philosophical point is that, while each side has its devotees and battalions, neither side has as yet delivered a decisive refutation of the other. There is not sufficient evidence to show that either God or a mother makes a baby. Neither the receptacle nor property metaphors will do in answering the objections raised by the other side. An acorn may not be an oak tree, and a fetus may not be a person, but without acorns and fetuses it is unlikely that there will be oak trees or persons. Appeal to the principle of potentiality cannot be lightly dismissed.

Nor, however, can one dismiss the woman's role in our culture in caring for and carrying the burden of bringing up her offspring long after its birth. She ought therefore to have a large decision-making role in deciding whether to foster or terminate the life inside her. For if the mother cannot sustain the life once born and promote the child's actualization of its potential for full personhood, then she might do better to terminate such a being earlier in its development rather than later.

A recent variation on the pro-choice argument claims that in our culture only a woman and not the male parent, physician, nurse, or any other person has a right to decide whether to abort. The decision is the woman's, the argument goes, not because of her right to her body, but rather, according to a view recently put forward by Allison Jaggar, on the basis of two other principles.[50] The first principle is that the right to life means "the right to a full human life." Jaggar contends that a newborn has the right to a full human life, and if the woman is unable or unwilling to provide such a life, she has a right to terminate her pregnancy. The right to life of a fetus is not merely a right to be born. A person's right to life is a right to the means necessary to a full life, such as adequate nutrition, shelter, clothing, education, health care, love, and affection. A newborn being's right to a full life and to all the means necessary to achieve it leads to Jaggar's second principle, "decisions should be made . . . only by those importantly affected by them."[51] Since in our culture the main onus and responsibility of parenting rests on a woman, she, being most importantly affected, is the one to decide. "This principle provides the fundamental justification for democracy."[52] A woman's role in giving birth terminates approximately 20 or more years after birth, after a mother has provided the major conditions for the child's being on the way to achieving the right to a life of fulfillment and decency.

To Jaggar's argument we would add this further post-Malthusian point. (Thomas Malthus [1766–1834] argued that, while the earth's food supply goes up in an arithmetical progression, the population moves up in a geometric progression.) Abortion is regrettable and may well be a serious trauma to a woman. To abort goes against the drive to support life. Contraception is preferable to abortion in controlling population growth. However, abortion is morally more desirable than serious overpopulation, in which each individual cannot be given an opportunity and the conditions for "a decent and fulfilling human life." A family that has more members than it can amply provide for has to give each individual fewer resources, including love. A consequence of placing no restrictions on reproduction is to have too many people struggling over meager resources, with a consequent increase in violence.

THE NURSE'S ROLE IN ABORTION

Jane Smith is a 17-year-old freshman student at a large state university. She is a graduate of a small-town high school in a rural county, sexually inexperienced and socially naive. She becomes pregnant and is rejected by her lover as "irresponsible and dumb." She does not inform her parents, who are against premarital sex and abortion. She cannot provide for a baby, has never worked, and is without skills. She comes to the college health service for advice. What kinds of moral justification could you provide for and against abortion?

In response to the unhappy situation just depicted, the first step might be for the nurse to help the young woman give careful consideration to the alternatives of aborting or continuing the pregnancy. What are the main arguments relevant to the issue of abortion on a personal and on a social policy scale? What are the arguments for and against abortion useful to the nurse as a counselor?

The nurse primary-care practitioner cited in our case study has at least three positions he or she may take regarding the college student's request for advice regarding an unwanted pregnancy. The nurse should have reflected earlier on the ethical issues so that he or she has thoughtful, deliberate ethical justifications and not scattered reasons for counsel to the troubled young student. If the nurse assumes that human life begins at conception and that this person has a right to live that overrides the unwed mother's right to rid herself of an unwanted pregnancy, the nurse concludes that abortion is wrong. The nurse's conviction that abortion is morally wrong does not, however, mean that abortion is legally wrong. Abortion is now legal in all states, according to the Supreme Court decision of *Roe* v. *Wade*, previously discussed. However, not all states fund abortion for poor women through Medicaid. Nor does the nurse's belief that abortion is morally wrong free him or her of professional obligations to advise the young woman. The nurse's responsibility is to give the patient objective information and referrals to appropriate resources before, during, and after an abortion.[53] The Division on Maternal and Child Health Nursing Practice of the American Nurses' Association recognizes the woman's right to seek a legal abortion free from the imposition of anyone else's judgments or beliefs. This position is consistent with the American Nurses' Association *Code for Nurses* which says that

> Each client has the moral right to determine what will be done with his/her person; to be given the information necessary for making informed judgements; to be told the possible effects of care; and to accept, refuse, or terminate treatment. These same rights apply to minors. . . .[54]

Clearly, then, the young woman with the unwanted pregnancy has the right to information and counseling, with consideration given to all the alternatives to abortion as the basis of informed consent. The patient who chooses abortion has the right to information and counseling in an environment of mutual respect, trust, privacy, and confidentiality. Referrals are expected to be made to facilities where expert nursing and medical care is provided.

The nurse, too, has a right to his or her own moral and religious values. However, these values and beliefs do not give the nurse license to impose or to influence the already frightened, worried, and vulnerable client to accept the nurse's value preferences. Nor should the client's self-esteem be lowered by implication that her decision is less than morally acceptable. The nurse in any situation, except an emergency where the patient's well-being is at stake, has the

> . . . right to refuse to participate in a voluntary interruption of pregnancy . . . and . . . a right not to be subjected to coercion, censure or to discipline for reasons of such refusal.[55]

A nurse in New Jersey, Beverly Jazelik, assigned to the obstetric floor, refused to participate in procedures related to abortion. The state's law supported her refusal. The hospital then transferred her to another unit where she would have no contact with patients undergoing abortion. Ms. Jazelik objected to the transfer and sued the hospital. The Court ruled in favor of the hospital's right to transfer Ms. Jazelik to a nonabortion area.[56] Thus, the patient's right to interrupt pregnancy and the nurse's right to refuse to participate are both upheld. But moral questions arise if the nurse who opposes abortion is the only nurse available and a patient decides to have an abortion.

Nurses who defend or oppose abortion have similar responsibilities to provide information concerning the alternatives as the basis for informed consent and appropriate referral to resources. Alternatives include prenatal care and adoption.

Clearly, abortion in the case of the college student, as in so many others, is a concern and responsibility primarily for women in our culture. Tragic choices such as this require the utmost kindness and consideration from the nurse in support of the patient's struggle with the decision. Providing conditions of calmness, free from pressures of time and place, in which the alternatives can be thoroughly explored is helpful to the process of deliberation and decision. Few women ordinarily want abortion. Some women are forced into securing abortions because of socioeconomic, psychological, or physiological circumstances unsupportive to a minimum decent life for themselves and the child. For them, there is no alternative. Other abortions are performed because of contraceptive failure. The intent was not to have a child. Increasingly, humans have exercised control of their procreative functions. Much remains to be done in the way of medical research to enable each couple to bring each new life into the world by deliberate choice and design and as a consequence of mutual love, respect, and desire for a family.

The nurse who assists with abortions on a regular basis may understandably be saddened by the loss of so much potential life; yet the nurse's concern properly belongs with the woman who, in the last analysis, must part with a potential life in which she is deeply invested. In most cases of abortion, the woman is the victim of her biological and social vulnerability and deserves the respect and help accorded all human beings by reason of their humanity. Unlimited procreation without controls implies massive starvation, malnutrition, pain, and suffering—all due to the refusal to accept the moral permissibility of abortion.

Beyond the individual level, the nursing profession has the collective responsibility in policy formulation. An example of how this may be done is the New York State Nurses' Association support of the repeal of a restrictive state abortion law. The Association cited two reasons for liberalizing the law. The first is that the law "encourages poor health practices"[57] because the woman is forced to resort to illegal and hazardous abortions. The second reason given is that the restrictive law "deprives certain segments of the population of adequate medical care."[58] Poor women are simply unable to pay for safe and legal abortions. The Association stated unequivocally that it "takes no position on the moral aspects of abortion"[59] and supports the law that protects the rights of individuals refusing to participate in any procedure "contrary to their religious beliefs or conscience."[60]

CONCLUSION

The opposing positions of pro-life and pro-choice, and a spectrum of views between these extremes, reveal the complexity of abortion. Competing ethical models and metaphors are at work. Pro-life supporters claim the principle of the sanctity of life. Pro-choice supporters base their arguments on the human rights to one's own body and the utilitarian principle of maximizing happiness and minimizing harm. Meanwhile, reproductive technology advances increase the significance of abortion to the individual and to society.

Legal restraints on abortion or a lack of them reveal deep moral differences on the abortion issue. On some issues, one or the other side tends to be or is right. On other issues, there is a stalemate. On still other issues, both sides may be "talking past each other." The abortion issue seems to us to be either a stalemate or a case of communicating on different levels. Perhaps when antiabortionists speak of the beginning of life, they refer to the moment of conception whereas prochoice supporters refer to newborns.

In saying this, however, we do not wish to hide behind the banner of neutrality; we have supported the argument on behalf of a woman's right to choose. But we also think it only circumspect to point out that the problem of abortion has not been solved with a conclusively justifiable or morally compelling answer. The reason is that, on such questions, no such answer is forthcoming.

Discussion Questions

1. What conditions make abortion morally and/or legally permissible or impermissible and for what reasons?
2. If abortion were universally regarded as murder and there were no contraceptives, or *using them was universally regarded as immoral,* what consequences would there be to the human race?
3. How does the presence of multiple anomalies among some newborns affect the abortion issue?
4. How does overpopulation affect the attempt to justify a pro-life argument?

REFERENCES

1. *Tabers' Cyclopedic Medical Dictionary.* 14th ed. Philadelphia: FA Davis. 1981; 1206.
2. *Roe* v. *Wade,* 410 U.S. 113.
3. Ibid.
4. Ibid.

5. Ibid.
6. Ibid.
7. Segers MC. *Abortion and the Supreme Court: Some more equal than others.* The Hastings Center Report. 1977. 7(4):5.
8. Ibid.
9. Ibid; 6.
10. Kolata G. Tests of fetuses rise sharply amid doubts. *The New York Times.* September 22, 1987; C1.
11. Ibid; C10.
12. Ibid.
13. Ibid.
14. Ibid.
15. Ibid.
16. Ibid.
17. Ibid.
18. Ibid.
19. Ibid.
20. Ibid.
21. Kolata G. Multiple fetuses raise new issues tied to abortion. *The New York Times,* January 25, 1988; 1, A17.
22. Ibid.
23. Ibid.
24. Regelson W. Letter to the editor. *The New York Times,* October 8, 1987; A38.
25. Ibid.
26. Ibid.
27. Ibid.
28. Dedek JF. Abortion. In: *Ethical Issues in Nursing: A Proceeding.* St. Louis, MO: The Catholic Hospital Association. 1976; 77–78.
29. Ibid; 81.
30. Ibid; 82.
31. Ruddick W. Parents, children and medical decisions. In: Bandman and Bandman, *Bioethics and Human Rights.* 165. Lanham, MD: University Press of America, 1986, p. 165.
32. Thomson JJ. A defense of abortion. *Philosophy and Public Affairs.* 1971. 1(1):47–66.
33. Ibid.
34. Ibid.
35. Ibid.
36. Ibid.
37. Ibid.
38. Ibid.
39. Ibid.
40. Toulmin S. *The tyranny of principles.* The Hastings Center Report. 1981. 11(6):31–39.
41. Held V. Abortion and the rights to life. In: Bandman EL, Bandman B. (eds). *Bioethics and Human Rights: A Reader for Health Professionals.* Lanham, MD: University Press of America, 1986, p. 108.
42. St. Thomas Aquinas. The sin of suicide. In: Abelson R, Friguegnon ML.

(eds). *Ethics for Modern Life*. 2nd ed. New York: St. Martin's. 1982; 25.

43. Held V. Abortion and the rights to life. 105–107.
44. Nozick R. *Anarchy, state and utopia*. New York: Basic Books. 1974; 169.
45. Feinberg J. *Social philosophy*. Englewood Cliffs, NJ: Prentice-Hall. 1973; 54.
46. Ruddick W. Parents children and medical decisions. In: Bandman and Bandman. *Bioethics and Human Rights*. 165.
47. Brody B. Opposition to abortion: A human rights approach. In: Arthur J. (ed). *Morality and Moral Controversies*. Englewood-Cliffs, NJ: Prentice-Hall. 1981; 200–213.
48. Brody. Opposition to abortion. 211.
49. Ibid; 212–213.
50. Jaggar A. Abortion and a woman's right to decide. *Philosophical Forum*. 1973–1974. 5:351.
51. Ibid.
52. Ibid.
53. Executive Committee on the Division on Maternal and Child Health Nursing Practice. *Statement on abortion*. Kansas City, MO: Author. June 12, 1978.
54. American Nurses' Association. *Code for nurses with interpretive statements*. Kansas City, MO: Author. 1976; 4.
55. Executive Committee on the Division on Maternal and Child Health Nursing Practice. *Statement on Abortion*.
56. Curtin L. Flaherty MJ. *Nursing ethics: Theories and pragmatics*. Bowie, MD: Brady. 1982; 254.
57. NYSNA Legislative Bulletin. No. 14. Albany, NY: New York State Nurses' Association. April 27, 1972.
58. Ibid.
59. Ibid.
60. Ibid.

CHAPTER 9

Ethical Issues in the Nursing Care of Infants

Study of this chapter enables the learner to:

1. Utilize ethical arguments for and against saving premature and deformed babies in facilitating the family's decisions regarding alternatives.
2. Formulate the nurse's role as patient advocate for protecting the infant's right to care and safety and the family's well-being.
3. Understand the significance of such moral issues as quorum features and the potentiality/actuality distinction.
4. Discriminate among relevant principles of Utilitarian, Deontological, and Rights-based ethics in relation to each problem infant.

INTRODUCTION

A tiny, helpless infant appeals to the strength and benevolence of adults. The newborn's total dependency on a supportive environment and a loving family matrix for its growth and development evokes adult nurturing and protective responses. The newborn child needs a healthy and friendly environment. Some newborns are premature underweight or defective. For them, one of the best friends is a good nurse—one who cares for them, who can identify and respond to feelings of discomfort from wetness, hunger, and thirst and to the infants' desire for warmth, closeness, and gratification.

Appreciation of the feelings of another with the desire to help that person is necessary to be an effective nurse. Infants, young children, and sometimes even older children and adolescents are unable to express feelings and needs effectively. They are often defenseless against imposition of painful treatments or the withholding of treatment by parents and health professionals. These are opportunities for implementing the nurse's role as advocate of the patient's rights to respect and to receive treatment. These young patients are the most vulnerable to neglect, indifference, rejection, or manipulation and abuse. Equally serious may be the moral conflicts that arise when the child is either physically or mentally abnormal.

Ethical dilemmas arise when the parents want a normal child and the newborn is severely retarded or has physical abnormalities, such as trisomy 18, meningomyelocele, or Down's syndrome. Does the nurse comply with the parents' wishes if they refuse treatment for the child as their right, or does the nurse exert initiative to save the infant's life as the child's right to live?

If family and community resources are scarce, competing moral values may call for other moral values to be given priority over the interests of preserving the life of a severely abnormal newborn. Some people call the failure to save a life "murder." Others condemn the practice of preserving infants that show few or no prospects of becoming independent, self-sufficient persons. The question is: How to decide who lives and who dies, and who is given quality care and who not? The issue of treatment for the abnormal infant is one filled with moral concerns and conflicts and with considerable potential for good or harm. This is another example of the quantity versus quality of life issue.

The pediatric nurse has a special role in evaluating the viability of the infant. Systematic assessments of the infant's functional assets and deficits as well as responsiveness are useful data in the final decisions of whether to care for, treat, or place the infant with the family or in an institution. Each nurse caring for the infant is a vital link in compiling the data to be considered in making that ultimate decision. Nurses' interactions with parents provide data regarding parental perceptions of their ability and desire to cope with the problematic situation. Despair may be profound. Parents may be overwhelmed, guilty, angry, and ambivalent about what to do. Their moral conflicts may be acute. The advice given them may be conflict-ridden. The time for decision may be short and pressured. Parents may turn to the nurse for advice, support, and help.

The nurse's role as advocate of the child's right to live and to be treated under all conditions may conflict with other moral principles holding that the happiness of the greatest number, in this case the family, may be in direct contradiction to saving the child. Careful consideration of all the variables relevant to the infant's capacities and potential as well as those of the family's abilities and willingness to cope with a painful, problematic situation of an abnormal child are determining factors in the final decision. In some situations with which some nurses are in agreement, the principle of the sanctity of life may prevail over all other considerations. Here, again, the nurse may play a significant role.

However, the "sanctity-of-life" principle, that human life is to be preserved under all conditions, conflicts with another principle, "the quality of life." This principle holds that there are conditions, sometimes referred to as *quorum features,* such as the presence of consciousness, that define a worthwhile human life. Thus, not all life is to be preserved if it fails to comply with "quality-of-life" standards. Consequently, five sometimes conflicting principles govern health professionals' first encounters with newborn infants. One principle is to save human life under all conditions (sanctity-of-life principle). A second principle is to promote worthwhile human life with the implication of productivity and independence (quality of life principle). A third principle is to prevent or minimize harm (nonmaleficence principle). A fourth principle is to alleviate suffering. A fifth principle is to seek to do good, as by giving skilled nursing care (beneficence principle). These principles will be considered in relation to examples of moral dilemmas in the nursing of infants.

ARGUMENTS FOR AND AGAINST SAVING PREMATURE AND DEFORMED INFANTS

Infanticide of deformed and even normal female babies was an ancient practice for controlling populations. High infant mortality rates were accepted. The death of a deformed baby was often welcomed and perhaps assisted by midwives sympathetic to women's destiny of uncontrolled pregnancies.

The contrary principle, that life is the highest good, is supported by the Judeo-Christian tradition prohibiting abortion, infanticide, and euthanasia. Significantly, medical technology has now advanced to a level of saving an increasing number of premature, underweight, and underdeveloped infants by means of neonatal intensive care units. The most sophisticated forms of monitoring vital signs and regulating electrolytes, food, and fluid are keeping premature and deformed infants alive at an astonishing rate. The principle of saving all life is respected through routine application of extraordinary means to continue the living processes of these infants. The cost of continuous professional care, high-level technological equipment and supplies, and prolonged hospitalization is more than $1000.00 a day per child in some neonatal intensive care units. In these fully lighted, windowed enclosures, nurses adjust rates of flow of fluids and gases in response to readings of the monitoring devices attached to each infant. The operating principle and the goal are identical. These are to save all life with no regard for the quality of the life saved or the costs to parents and society. The infant is given care, in most instances, without regard for the present and later burden this may impose on families and society or even the suffering of the infant itself from necessary injections and intubations. Once the infant is received in the neonatal intensive care unit, the decision has already been made to treat fully and intensively, with no regard for such long-term consequences as brain damage or chronic cardiopulmonary disease.

However, not all premature or deformed infants are immediately transferred to intensive care units. Two examples of frequently occurring problems in newborn infants illustrate the scope and depth of the moral issues involved in decisions of treatment or nontreatment. These cases point to the usefulness of identifying short-term and long-term goals and consequences to the individual affected as well as the family and society.

The first frequently occurring example of a neonatal problem is the birth of very premature, underweight, underdeveloped babies as a result of spontaneous or induced abortion. On one view, the gasping infant is left to die in a surgical pail. On another view, that infant is admitted to an intensive care unit. On one view, the decision to seek an abortion is an automatic death sentence for the fetus; on another view, the abortion decision is one of ending the pregnancy. On one view, the viable fetus has the right to live and the nurse, as patient advocate, has the duty to protect the fetus's life above all other values. Questions arise as to who decides, and by what criteria, either to save or not to save the infant. Other questions arise as to what difference voluntary versus involuntary abortion makes. Related questions concern the difference socioeconomic status, race, age, and the mother's marital status play in decisions to resuscitate and treat or not to resuscitate and treat.

The second example is that of the infant born with multiple defects that threaten life, such as the baby on a respirator due to respiratory difficulty with evidence pointing to the diagnosis of trisomy 18. This genetic disorder leads to severe mental retardation, failure to grow, and many other abnormalities.[1] Adapting the case somewhat, let's suppose one parent insists that the chief of pediatrics does nothing to keep a four-day-old trisomy 18 infant alive. A pediatric resident points out that another patient who has a mild respiratory difficulty cannot be put on a respirator because the trisomy 18 infant is using the only available machine. Without the respirator, the other infant, "who is otherwise healthy, runs a 50 percent risk of some brain damage."[2] The fact is that 87 percent of trisomy 18 infants die in the first year. At this point two nurses directly responsible for the infant's care interrupt. Nurse A insists that the trisomy 18 infant "has every right to live and should not be allowed to die by human hands." Nurse B disagrees with Nurse A and says that those beings with a meaningful life have the right to be given health care resources, that an infant with a mild respiratory difficulty should not be sacrificed for the trisomy 18 infant. Nurse A supports the principle of "the sanctity of life" under all conditions. Nurse B believes in the principle of "the quality of life"; she believes the trisomy 18 infant has poor prospects. If you are Nurse C, what do you advise the parents and Nurses A and B to do—save the trisomy 18 infant or leave it to die?

Further questions arise as to the original decision to start a life-support system and to continue it. Considering the evidence of multiple defects, a poor quality of life, and an expected life span of less than a year, questions arise as to what criteria for decision are relevant, who the decision makers are, and what the role of the nurse is in facilitating the decision.

A second case involves a baby boy who had Down's syndrome and who also had a surgically repairable duodenal obstruction. The parents, by not consenting to surgery, contributed to the death of their six-day-old Down's syndrome child.[3]

One writer who fictionalizes a similar account points out that "many nurses and physicians thought it was wrong that the baby was forced to die. . . ."[4] This writer adds this fictionalized scenario to the actual case.

> The burden of caring for the dying baby fell on the nurses in the obstetrics ward. The physicians avoided the child entirely, and it was the nurses who had to see to it that she received her water and was turned in her bed. This was the source of much resentment among the nursing staff, and a few nurses refused to have anything to do with the dying child. . . . But one nurse . . . was determined to make . . . [the baby's] last days as comfortable as possible. She held the baby, rocked her, and talked soothingly to her when she cried. . . . But even [this nurse] was glad when the baby died. "It was a relief to me," she said. "I almost couldn't bear the frustration of just sitting there day after day and doing nothing that could really help her."[5]

In actual fact, Dr. Milton Heifitz writes that "the world press in 1971 condemned the 'inhumanity' of a husband and wife and the staff of a major American medical center. A mongoloid baby was born with an intestinal obstruction at John Hopkins Hospital in Baltimore. The parents, who had two normal children, refused to give consent to correct the obstruction. The infant could not be fed and died within fifteen days."[6] According to Heifitz, "the child's death caused a furor in medical and lay circles. It was a major topic at an international symposium concerning medical ethics. Panelists disagreed with parents. They suggested the child's right to life, to the limit of happiness possible, was more important than the years of anguish and burden the child would bring the family."[7] Thus, "the sanctity of life" overrides all other principles on this view. However, arguments for the sanctity-of-life principle do not respond to the opposing view of parents' preference for a life of quality for themselves and their offspring. Nevertheless, proponents of the sanctity-of-life principle can raise the spector of the horrendous evil of the Nazi policy and practice of exterminating population groups they regarded as "unfit."

ETHICAL CONSIDERATIONS IN THE NURSING CARE OF INFANTS

Nurses working with infants, like nurses working with any other age group, occupy a number of roles. Pediatric nurses, however, may perceive themselves as primarily patient advocates for the rights of the helpless, vulnerable infants in their care. They may see advocacy responsibilities as a significant feature in the delivery of quality care to each baby. The American Nurses' Association *Code for Nurses* defines the role of client advocate in sweeping terms.

> The nurse's primary commitment is to the client's care and safety. Hence, in the role of client advocate, the nurse must be alert to and take appropriate action regarding any instances of incompetent, unethical, or illegal practice(s) by any member of the health care team or the health care system itself, or any action on the part of others that is prejudicial to the client's best interests.[8]

This definition of the role of client advocate is tantamount to a mandate or command to safeguard the infant's life against those who would not treat or feed the infant because of a decision using a quality-of-life argument. But a question arises as to whether a nurse is an advocate of the infant client or the infant's parents. This becomes crucial if the infant's parents have conflicting interests between themselves or if their interests are not those of their infant. Pediatric nurses most in contact with the infant may feel the decision by parents to terminate an infant's life to be unfair or to be tantamount to an act of murder. These nurses perceive themselves to be advocates for the infant's right to life.

Patient advocacy may be expressed in a variety of ways. One way is to marshal the facts based on careful, systematic assessment of the infant's status as the basis for arguments favoring the continuation or termination of life on the basis of quorum features. The arguments may then be presented to the physician and family for consideration. Through contact with the parents, pediatric nurses may exert considerable influence on their decision. Sharing of nurses' knowledge of this child's estimated needs for care through the life span and the experience of other parents facing similar demands may be useful information in the parents' process of decision. In some cases, nurses as patient advocates comply with the directive of the *Code for Nurses* for being fully aware of institutional policies and procedures as well as state laws regarding unethical, incompetent, or illegal practice by taking necessary steps to initiate action through appropriate channels. It is important to provide careful documentation and to use established mechanisms for appeal so as to avoid reprisal. There have been instances in which the courts have directed that an infant be fed and treated where parents have refused treatment. Sometimes, custody of infants is taken from the parents at the instigation of a family agency on grounds of neglect when the parents refuse treatment. A counterexample occurred in 1982 in Bloomington, Indiana, where two Monroe County courts and the state Supreme Court all declined to force parents to feed or treat a baby born with Down's syndrome and an incomplete esophagus. The Monroe County prosecutor said he would not file charges in the death of the week-old baby despite plans for an appeal to the Supreme Court.[9] Those nurse advocates who participate in securing legal advocacy for this and similar babies to whom nourishment, treatment, and life itself were denied are committed to the sanctity-of-life principle.

Other nurses may support the quality-of-life principle. Nurses committed to the quality-of-life principle may believe it cruel and unjust both to the child and the family to prolong the suffering of a severely handicapped child. Such nurses may support parental decisions not to treat the deformed infant while giving compassionate care to the hungry infant. Such babies can be kept sedated and comfortable until they die. Parents need the support of nurses and physicians in handling the inevitable guilt feelings concerning their decision not to treat or feed.

In still other examples, parents may not consent to treatment for correction of a minor deformity that will not interfere with the full potential of the infant. The nurse as patient advocate may in this instance be in the very best position to protect the "client's care and safety"[10] by persuading parents to permit treatment on the grounds of the child's right to a full human life. Nurses and physicians, in advocating infants' rights, may consider in extreme cases openly disagreeing with the parents by presenting morally cogent reasons and arguments. Nurses and physicians may also appeal to the courts, if necessary, to protect the right of a minimally deformed child to be fed and treated.

Another issue for the nurse advocate to consider is the principle to do no harm. Such a principle is as relevant for the physician as it is for the nurse. Some research done on infants may be justified in terms of benefit to the immature client. Other research may be done for the social benefit of others at some indefinite time without any benefit to the infant subject. We have all benefitted, after all, from research done on others at an earlier time or at some other place. So, on a reciprocity basis between generations and places, we owe it to others to submit to research, but not as our primary duty. The nurse who secures consent from the parents for research or experimentation involving their child needs to make the clear distinction between benefit to the parents, benefit to the individual, and social benefit. A truthful account would distinguish research for the benefit of one's child and research for the benefit of other children. One argument against research is that research that is of no benefit to the infant is solely an assault against its tiny body. A counterargument is that donation of an anencephalic infant's organs to other babies is an act of generosity by the parents for the benefit of other children.

Those nurses who agree with the quality-of-life argument and the need to minimize the suffering of the affected infant and family appreciate the integrity of the Duff and Campbell study. These two Yale University physicians reported that in a 30-month period, 43 infants judged by parents and staff to have little or no hope of achieving personhood were left to die by withholding essential medical treatment.[11]

The role of patient advocate for handicapped infants became a national issue in April 1982 when a six-day-old infant, "Baby Doe," of Bloomington, Indiana, died from lack of food and water. Treatment of the infant's tracheoesophageal fistula was denied by the parents, who were supported in their decision by the Indiana courts. Presumably the parents refused surgical repair of the condition because the infant also had Down's syndrome.

In response to the public outcry of indignation, the United States Department of Health and Human Services Office of Civil Rights issued a "Notice to Health Care Providers" on May 18, 1982. The notice quoted the Federal Law, Section 504 of the Rehabilitation Act of 1973.

> No otherwise qualified handicapped individual shall, solely by reason of handicap, be excluded from participation in, be denied the benefits of, or be subjected to discrimination under any program or activity receiving federal financial assistance. . . . It is unlawful for a recipient of federal financial assistance to withhold from a handicapped infant nutritional sustenance or medical or surgical treatment required to correct a life threatening condition, if: (1) the withholding is based on the fact that the infant is handicapped; and (2) the handicap does not render the treatment or nutritional sustenance medically contraindicated.

This notice directed that anyone with knowledge of the denial of food or customary medical care should immediately contact the Department's handicapped-infant hotline available 24 hours a day or the particular state's child-protective agency. Telephone numbers were provided, as well as a promise of confidentiality. The notice stated that failure to feed and to care for infants may also be a violation of state criminal and civil laws. Providers of health care to infants were required to post this notice in conspicuous places where such care is given. Thus, nurses, physicians, and parents of handicapped infants were continuously confronted with this reminder of the stipulations of the advocacy role in delivery rooms, nurseries, and intensive care and pediatric units.

A suit against the Department of Health and Human Services and its secretary to prohibit the notice from becoming final was brought by the American Academy of Pediatrics, the National Association of Children's Hospitals, and Children's Hospital National Medical Center. On April 14, 1983, the United States District Judge ruled the Health and Human Services regulation to be invalid because the Department did not follow proper procedures in making public the terms of a proposed law and inviting wide public comment.

The judicial decision simply postponed the inevitable clash of values between proponents of conflicting legal and ethical principles. Later, Judge Gesell, who ruled on this regulation, pointed to elimination of the role of the infant's parents in selecting appropriate medical treatment as an infringement of privacy. Parents presumably know what the infant's best interests are, based on their knowledge of the economic, social, psychologic, and physical aspects of their situation. The judge described the regulation as "arbitrary and capricious." He recommended that "federal intervention in the delivery rooms and newborn intensive care units should 'obviously reflect caution and sensitivity.' "[12]

Medical critics point to several major difficulties in the Department's regulations. First, major handicaps, such as major malformations of the brain along with the absence of kidneys, are a reason for withholding treatment because the child will not benefit from treatment and treatment is not in its interest.[13] The Department responded to this criticism by pointing out that "Section 504 does not require the imposition of futile therapies which temporarily prolong the process of dying of an infant born . . . with anencephaly or intra-cranial bleeding."[14]

In 1983, another infant, known as Baby Jane Doe, was born with multiple defects of meningomyelocele, anencephaly, and hydrocephaly. Following consultation with clergy, neurologists, nurses, and social workers, the parents refused surgery but permitted the use of antibiotics. Pro-life lawyers appealed the case on grounds of discrimination against the handicapped infant in violation of the regulations of Section 504 of the Rehabilitation Act.

In 1986, The Supreme Court struck down the Baby Doe regulations since no evidence of discrimination by hospitals or by the parents of this infant existed. The judicial opinion noted that no law justified federal intervention, unsolicited advice, or requiring hospitals to treat impaired infants without parental consent. The Court returned the major responsibility for making treatment decisions to families and physicians. The Court recommended that hospital infant care review committees be formed.

In 1984, the American Academy of Pediatrics issued a joint policy statement developed with eight other national organizations dealing with the handicapped. The statement read as follows:

> When medical care is clearly beneficial, it should always be provided. . . . Considerations such as anticipated or actual limited potential of an individual and present or future lack of available community resources are irrelevant and must not determine the decisions concerning medical care. The individual's medical condition should be the sole focus of the decision.[15]

The major medical criticism of attempted Federal interventions remains that handicap alone is an insufficient "criterion for distinguishing justified from unjustified deaths. . . . The potential for human relationships or the capacity to survive infancy and participate in human experience may serve better."[16]

Nurses play significant roles in these decisions, both through their participation in the assessment and their participation in the judgment process as members of a team. If open-ended moral dialogue is regarded as an essential condition of the decision-making process, then that process is one of mutual respect. Mutual respect in this context means that the negotiation process is open and encourages reasoned arguments until some approximation of consensus is reached about the infant's right to live versus the benefit to the child, as well as to the family and society, which bear the cost. As caregiver and with understandable feelings of deep compassion for the short and tragic life of the tiny, defenseless patient, the nurse provides for the comfort of the dying infant to whom food and treatment are denied. If the nurse disagrees with this order or is unable to give skilled care and comfort to the infant because of resentment of the family's "dumping of their responsibility," the nurse may refuse to provide care.

Before the nurse takes individual action, he or she might benefit from institutional review. The need is for the development of institutional policies and review processes that apply broad rules to specific cases, such as the priority given to the best interests of the infant, with care not withheld solely because of mental retardation.

When the parents of a seriously ill newborn are disqualified from making decisions by incapacity, disagreement between them, or choices clearly against the infant's best interests, there are currently civil courts, state laws, child protection agencies, and even criminal penalties available to respond to the presumed neglect of the handicapped infants. Until such policies and processes are developed in each caregiving institution, the nurse is the best interim advocate protecting the interests of the handicapped infant.

The *Code for Nurses* states that if the nurse is

> . . . personally opposed to the delivery of care in a particular case because of the nature of the health problem or the procedures to be used, the nurse is justified in refusing to participate.[17]

The *Code* goes on to say that such refusal should be made known in time for other arrangements for providing nursing care to be made. According to the *Code,* the nurse can withdraw from a situation only when others are available to provide the care and comfort needed by the infant as its last demands. But two moral questions arise: (1) What if a nurse does not accept the conventional morality of the *Code* and refuses to participate before any other nurse is willing to help? and (2) What if there are no other nurses available who are willing to comply with the decision to facilitate a dying infant's last moments? There is the understandable moral ground that nurses may not concur with an act they regard as "murder." To such questions there may be no answers, only stalemate and tragedy, which the patients and nurses have no choice but to accept.

ETHICAL AND PHILOSOPHICAL CONSIDERATIONS

Several Philosophical Moves

Moral and philosophical questions arise about these cases such as: Whose rights are to be taken most seriously? Since decisions concerning these cases involve values, either the sanctity or the quality of life, these questions cannot be settled by science, by evidence, or by verifying only what is true or false. Nor can one settle these questions by considering sociological factors, such as: "What do most people favor?" These are philosophical value questions. Value questions, if they are settled at all, are settled by showing that one moral value is more justifiable than another. One way to justify a moral argument that a trisomy 18 infant has fewer rights to live than a mild Down's syndrome or normal infant is to show that the consequences clearly favor one side over the other. Another way to justify a value preference is to show that one belief has more conceptual and practical difficulties than any other.

Quorum Features. Several philosophical moves have recently been developed in an attempt to clarify the right to life and parental, health professional, and nursing responsibilities. One move consists in applying the idea of "quorum features"[18] to the question, "When does a person's life begin and end?" A quorum at a meeting means that a previously agreed-upon number of persons have to be at a meeting for the meeting to take place. So one philosophical move consists in applying the idea of a "quorum feature" to the question, "When does a human life begin and end?" or to the question, "What is a person?" A being who lacks the quorum or majority of essential features of an ordinary person, such as one who has multiple deformities or lacks consciousness, such as a trisomy 18 infant, does not satisfy the quorum features of being a person. What makes the refusal to save the life of the Down's syndrome infant morally questionable to some people and an outrage on the border of "murder" to others is that the Down's syndrome patient is more clearly a person than is the infant with trisomy 18. Some might say that the Down's syndrome infant has some prospects for a meaningful human life, whereas the trisomy 18 infant does not have such prospects.

Tracing and Examining for Appropriate Metaphors and Models. A second philosophical move consists of considering a viewpoint that purports to provide an answer to the question, "What is a person?" One then traces that viewpoint to some deeply acknowledged metaphor, word picture, or pictorial analogy on which defense of the viewpoint depends philosophically. One then examines the metaphor to determine how it applies or breaks down in practical discourse. One may consider next whether supplementary or alternative metaphorical analogies aid in the defense of a given viewpoint. One may, for example, regard any being born to be unconditionally worth preserving on the ground that "life is a gift,"[19] to cite St. Thomas Aquinas's insightful metaphor. One thus traces a viewpoint to a metaphor on which its philosophical defense partly rests. But one may next examine the metaphor to note what conceptual or practical limits or difficulties it implies. A difficulty immediately becomes apparent. Is life always a gift? Is it necessarily a gift, so that there could be no instance of life that was not a gift? One has only to consider some terminal patients or seriously maimed or wounded persons to note that there are exceptions to life always being a gift. Furthermore, in ordinary language, if one gets a gift, one may keep it, give it to someone else, or discard it in the wastebasket. But the gift of which St. Thomas Aquinas speaks, because it is given, may not be taken. This is a strange requirement for any gift. And yet one can appreciate that the recognition that life is a gift spurs health professionals to save it. A metaphor may thus be examined for its illumination as well as for its implied difficulties. Life is not always a gift, as the trisomy 18 case amply shows.

The Potentiality-Actuality Distinction

A related effort to answer "What is a person?" is to regard any potential person as a person. Thus, an acorn is potentially an oak tree and therefore is to be accorded the recognition that someday it will be an oak tree. Similarly, a girl is a potential woman. Since a rock, stamp, or oak tree is not a potential person, one need not confer personhood status to these entities. But even a seriously deformed person enjoys the status of being a person, according to the potentiality principle. This is not true, however, if one shows that the potentiality principle has limits. According to philosopher Stanley Benn, "A potential president of the United States is not on that account Commander in Chief of the U.S. Army and Navy."[20] According to another philosopher, Joel Feinberg, "A dog is closer to personhood than a jellyfish, but that is not the same thing as being 'more of a person.' . . . In 1930, when he was six years old, Jimmy Carter didn't know it, but he was a potential president of the United States. That gave him no claim then, not even a weak claim, to give commands to the U.S. Army and Navy. Franklin Roosevelt in 1930 was only two years away from the presidency, so he was a potential president in a much stronger way . . . than was Jimmy Carter. Nevertheless, he was not actually president and he had no more of a claim to the prerogatives of the office than did Carter."[21] One could, however, criticize this analogy by pointing out that a fetus's becoming a person is a biological process rather than a social or political process, unlike a candidate for president's becoming president. The point nevertheless remains that potentiality does not imply actuality; and the potential person may be discounted from being regarded as an actual person. A trisomy 18 infant who has multiple deformities, while *potentially* a person, is not *actually* a person. The analogy one appeals to is to show that a presidential candidate, who is a potential president, while closer to being a president than a potential candidate who is six years old and therefore under age, is not an actual president, who alone has the rights and responsibilities associated with being a president. The analogy of president to person shows that as a potential president is not an actual president, a potential person is not an actual person.

Traditional Ethical Viewpoints Applied to the Infant Cases

A fourth and last philosophical move one might consider is to examine how the ethical principles previously considered apply to resolving the question of what to do about infants with abnormalities. A Utilitarian, for example, would adopt the quality-of-life principle. In relation to competing demands for the available respirator, the Utilitarian ethicist would say that considering "the greatest happiness of the greatest number," one ought to give preferential treatment to the one normal infant with respiratory difficulties over the infant with trisomy 18. A Utilitarian might even defend the refusal to consent to surgical repair of a duodenal atresia in the case of a Down's syndrome infant. However, on a Christian or Agapist or love-based ethical view, which favors "the sanctity of life," one does all one can to save the life of a trisomy 18 infant or one with Down's syndrome, on the ground that "they are all God's children," to cite yet another metaphor.

One might think Kantian deontological ethics commits one to a similar ethical conclusion, but Kant confines his ethics to rational beings. The point about Kant's deontological ethics is that appeal to universal principles requires the same treatment for all individuals within a given group without exception, allowing exception only if relevant differences are shown.

From a rights point of view, if persons alone have rights, and a seriously deformed being is not regarded as a person, then such a being, including a trisomy 18 infant, is not a person, and hence has no rights. The mild Down's syndrome infant who falls within the quorum feature of being human—that is, satisfies the requirements of personhood—does have rights, including the right to live. The violation of the Down's syndrome infant's right to live is an indication of its moral wrongness.

Since one cannot always reconcile these alternative moral points of view, one has to consider the place both of tragedy in human life and of stalemate in the effort to resolve sometimes unresolvable problems.

Application of Philosophical Moves to Infants with Handicaps

We have seen that the federal regulation issued as a "Notice to Health Providers" on May 18, 1982, required health providers "to meet the immediate needs that can arise when a handicapped infant is discriminatingly denied food or other medical care."[22]

In regard to this handicapped-infant ruling, Goal-based ethics (see Chapter 4) says: Consider the consequences. A consequence to future generations is to be borne in mind. For every pregnancy, two questions are relevant: Who will provide? and How will it be provided for? On an aggregate macrolevel, there must be enough people with the capacity to develop into persons of adequate achievement to contribute to advancing levels of knowledge, science, and technology for everyone. One might refer to the principle to reproduce no more people than there are resources for them as the Principle of the Adequate Distribution of Resources to People. The need to provide persons of social and economic merit is basic to the dictum that people generally have to pay their way in the world. Future health care and human service providers will be decreasingly able to cope effectively with excessive numbers of essentially dependent people.

Infant health care policies consequently cannot be oriented solely toward the principle of saving every infant, no matter how handicapped. Nor, however, can health care policies be oriented toward saving only those some people deem as fit to lead a high-quality life.

A problem for both those who strive to save everyone and those who exclude those with less than optimum human qualities is analogous to having either too many or too few people at the world's dinner table. If there are too many at the table, then everyone will not have enough to eat. If one excludes too many, those excluded will have nothing to eat. Moreover, the principle of selection and the basis for excluding are apt to be arbitrary. A difficulty of including or excluding too many beings is illustrated by having to decide whether to treat infants with myelomeningocele, hydrocephalus, mental retardation, and other serious anomalies.

One can picture this dilemma of distributing resources to people by drawing concentric circles, one inside the other. Let the inner circle represent limited available resources and the outer circle represent people and their needs and desires. The larger the inner circle is made in relation to the outer one by thinning out the resources, the smaller will be the shares for each person. But if the inner circle is kept small, more people will be excluded. One possible resolution of this dilemma is to limit the outer circle, the number of people, keeping the inner circle representing resources as close to the outer circle as possible. A dynamic equilibrium between the world's population and available resources calls for both circles to be as close as possible.

On this ground, Utilitarianism or goal-based ethics seems to have a claim on future societal needs. Decisions have to be made employing fair, rational, and relevant criteria as to whom to help and save. To save blue-eyed infants, for example, seems to be irrelevant and/or unfair. It is fairer to save those who have the best chance of leading socially useful lives. In addition to observing this dictum, one works to achieve a balance between extreme positions, regard for merit and for the equal distribution of socially useful resources.

The appeal to the achievement of merit calls for exclusions of those who show little or no merit. Exclusions of this or that group may be painful. Such exclusions may also be unjust. Including everyone, however, means resources may be too thinly distributed to do much good. A policy, like Section 504, may tip the scale in favor of attempting to save too many infants, and also more infants than can be provided for throughout the life span, because they require continuous medical care, special education, and housing and financial assistance.

One strikes a balance not by ignoring the claims of each position, but by attending to both claims, "prevention of harm" and "caring for quality of life."

There is no innate obligation to favor the prevention-of-harm or quality-of-life principle. Both are good because of the good they bring, in the estimation of people who have good reasons for judiciously applying both these principles.

According to Aristotle, the good is "that at which all things aim."[23] One may amend this to read: The good is that which attempts to reconcile the goods at which people aim. One aim that is believed good is the prevention of harm. Another is fostering the quality of life. One route is to realize that, as with life, there are moral polarities, intermediate positions, priorities, and criteria for selection. Appeal to rational criteria, such as impartiality and consistency, helps resolve disputes between goals. A health care policy, for example, may take the form, "Every baby having features A, B, C . . . is regarded as a person and every baby with features D, E, F . . . (medically untreatable) does not qualify as a person. Every person shall be adequately cared for and treated. Therefore, babies having features A, B, C . . . , being persons, shall be treated; and babies with D, E, F, (and medically untreatable), not being regarded as persons, shall not be treated." Invoking a Kantian appeal to a universal moral principle minimizes (but may not eliminate) arbitrariness as to what counts as a person. Specifying features, such as A, B, and C (drawing a justifiable and useful distinction between these features of a "person" and those without such features), may reduce arbitrariness somewhat.

On this view, a health care policy would be a health care guideline to health providers. Details of the features of persons and nonpersons would be worked out in health care ethics committees by relevant professionals, including nurses, with input from public policymakers, parents, and other representatives of society. A so-called hotline would go, not to a centralized bureaucratic government agency, but to an appropriate impartial patient-advocacy group. Its functions would be to guide present and future decisions effectively rather than to blame or punish health providers for past decisions.

CONCLUSION

Ordinarily, the wonder and joy of human life begins with the birth of an infant. The mother of the new infant is apt to feel the emotion of participating in the creative process of life. But the infant is fragile, helpless, and dependent. It will need the highest quality of nurture a mother and father are prepared to give it in order to grow into childhood, adolescence, and responsible adulthood. Not all newborns, however, are normal at birth. Some are born with minor deviations from health. Others are born with gross abnormalities. Nurses are involved in the health care activities and processes of decision making for all infants. Therefore, nurses contribute their observations regarding the infant's health status when decisions are to be made regarding who lives, who receives special consideration, and who is left to die.

The quorum feature or majority features of a human life, including evidence of consciousness, helps parents and health professionals, including nurses, to make ethically justifiable decisions. The sanctity-of-life principle, under which life is regarded as sacred under all conditions, may conflict with a quality-of-life principle in those instances when not all can be effectively helped to live decent, fulfilling lives. If resources are scarce and not all can be saved, the sanctity-of-life principle may appear impractical, inflexible, and unworkable. If the quality-of-life principle is then invoked, questions of arbitrariness arise. How to decide on just grounds who lives and dies is the question continuously considered by morally reflective people. Therefore, while both principles, the sanctity and the quality of life, have a claim on nurses, neither principle is satisfactory in every case, nor is either quite free from fault, nor is either able to withstand further questions.

Discussion Questions

1. What is the cutoff point for determining the human viability of an infant's life? For example, should lines be drawn at mild, moderate, or severe retardation? What physical and mental attributes are criteria of a viable infant?
2. How do changes in technology affect standards for justly deciding the viability of an infant's life?
3. If an infant is denied all surgery necessary to save its life, is it being discriminated against and are its rights being violated? Why is it appropriate or inappropriate to attribute rights to an infant with multiple mental and physical anomalies?

REFERENCES

1. Brody H. *Ethical decisions in medicine.* 2nd ed. Boston: Little, Brown. 1981; 116.
2. Ibid.
3. Shaw A. Dilemmas of "informed consent" in children. In: Hunt R, Arras J. (eds). *Ethical Issues in Modern Medicine.* 2nd ed. Palo Alto, CA: Mayfield. 1983; 252–258.
4. Munson R. *Intervention and reflection: Basic issues in medical ethics.* 3rd ed. Belmont: CA: Wadsworth. 1988; 114.

5. Ibid.; 114–115.
6. Heifitz MD with Mangel C. *The right to die*. New York: Berkeley. 1975; 59–60.
7. Ibid.; 60.
8. American Nurses' Association. *Code for nurses with interpretive statements*. Kansas City, MO: Author, 1985; 8.
9. The prosecutor closes case in death of Indiana baby. *The New York Times*, April 20, 1982.
10. American Nurses' Association. *Code for nurses*. 8.
11. Duff RS, Campbell AGM. Moral and ethical dilemmas in the special care nursery. N Eng J Med. 1973; 289:885.
12. Annas GJ. *Disconnecting the Baby Doe hotline*. Hastings Center Report. 1983. *13*(3):14.
13. Fost N. *Putting hospitals on notice*. Hastings Center Report. 1982. *12*(4):5.
14. Federal Register 48(129):30846, July 5, 1983.
15. American Academy of Pediatrics. Joint Policy Statement. Principles of Treatment of Disabled Infants. *Pediatrics 73*(4): April, 1984. 559–560.
16. Fost: Putting hospitals on notice.
17. American Nurses' Association. *Code for nurses*. 5.
18. Hospers J. *An introduction to philosophical analysis*. Englewood Cliffs, NJ: Prentice-Hall. 3rd ed. 1988, 122–124.
19. St. Thomas Aquinas. The sin of suicide. In: Abelson R, Friquegnon ML. (eds). *Ethics for Modern Life*. 3rd ed. New York: St. Martin's. 1986; 25.
20. Benn S. Abortion, infanticide and respect for persons. In: Feinberg J. (ed). *The Problem of Abortion*. Belmont, CA: Wadsworth. 1973; 102.
21. Feinberg J. The problem of personhood. In: Beauchamp T, Walters L (eds). *Contemporary Issues in Bioethics*. 2nd ed. Belmont, CA: Wadsworth. 1982; 113–114.
22. Federal Register 48(45):9630–9632, March 7, 1983.
23. Aristotle. *Nichomachean ethics*. Martin Ostwald, tr. Indianapolis: Bobbs Merrill. 1962; 3.

CHAPTER 10

Ethical Issues in the Nursing Care of Children

Study of this chapter enables the learner to:

1. Identify the ethical issues involved in problematic situations involving children's rights to health care, safety, and well-being.
2. Facilitate the parents' participation in shared decision making regarding the well-being of the child in relation to the whole family.
3. Distinguish between a biological and a biographical life as criteria for personhood.
4. Clarify the role of children's rights in relation to parental and societal rights and duties owed dependent children.
5. Evaluate the role of the nurse as patient advocate in nursing practice with children.

INTRODUCTION

Children are almost universally regarded as the hope of the future for a better world. Yet in parts of this globe, large numbers of children are ill-fed; inadequately clothed, housed, and educated, and in dire need of curative, preventive, and rehabilitative health care. Children are perceived in the light of cultural values and mores. It is the culture that defines "the length of childhood, the essential nature of childhood, and the meaning of childhood."[1] At least one writer claims that childhood is a European invention of the 16th century. This means that from that time on children were taken more seriously as distinct beings.[2] But in view of child labor laws and cruelty and abuses inflicted on children since then to the present, this assertion is debatable.

The pluralistic culture of the United States presently supports a wide range of values reflected in child-rearing practices. Children are incorporated into various family models. One model of parent-child relations is that of Ownership. According to this model, children are perceived as being possessions of their parents. A second model, Partnership, implies that children are more nearly equal with their parents. A third model, widely practiced, especially in remarriages, is that of Club Membership. Here, the members of the family are not cared for very much as individuals. They are essentially left on their own. Family socioeconomic differences are usually reflected in the prevalence or absence of family planning, numbers of children, and the desirability of the birth of each child. Middle- and upper-class families in the United States are usually child-centered, attempting to meet each need and foster individuality. Poor families may struggle to provide basic necessities of life with little concern for the special needs of each child. Nevertheless, affluent and poor families may each have difficulty in meeting children's rights, due to the parental tendency to prefer either the Ownership or Club Membership models over the Partnership model.

In response to the largely dependent and vulnerable status of children all over the world, several declarations of rights have been developed. The *Declaration of the Rights of the Child,* developed by the United Nations in 1959, recognizes the worth and dignity of each human being. The *Declaration* recognizes the special protection needed for enabling the immature child's physical, mental, moral, social, and cultural growth and development to proceed. Humankind "owes to the child the best it has to give . . . to the end that he may have a happy childhood and enjoy for his own good and for the good of society, the rights and freedom . . . set forth."[3] The *Declaration* calls for nondiscriminatory entitlement to rights, which recognize the interests of the child. At birth, the child has a right to a name and a nationality. The child has the right to adequate food, shelter, recreation, and health care. The handicapped child shall be given special care, treatment, and education. Every child's need for love and understanding, parents, and security will be supported by state assistance to families and care of children without families. The child has a right to education, at least through the elementary grades, free of cost but on the condition of compulsory attendance. This requirement is purportedly justified by the need for the child to develop his or her abilities and to contribute to society. The child has the right to special protection from neglect, cruelty, and exploitation in the form of traffic or employment detrimental to health and development. Lastly, the child will be protected from discriminatory practices and be reared in "peace and universal brotherhood."[4]

Wieczorek and Natapoff point to the United Nations *Declaration* as omitting rights "to love from a significant adult . . . to a safe environment . . . to reach individual potential . . . to be a wanted child in a situation that has resources . . . to respect the individual autonomy of the child, and . . . to personal space that may include sexual expression."[5] All of the rights listed have the dual function of both enhancing the child's personhood and protecting the child's fundamental needs in its growth and development toward humanity.

ETHICAL ISSUES RELATED TO CHILDREN

Some major ethical issues concerned with children between 1 and 12 years of age involve the principle of informed consent, its scope, and its limits when applied to children. Other issues concern parental control versus the child's growing autonomy. Another moral concern is that of the abuse of children directly and through neglect or denial of the child's rights to the truth, to proper health care, education, and a safe environment, as well as by direct inflicting of harm and injury of children.

Selective cases will illustrate the importance of these issues to the child's survival as a person. As these cases illustrate, there is a continuum of decision regarding children's rights. At one end there is absolute parental control, with complete child autonomy at the other end. This gives rise to conflict in making health care decisions when there is disagreement between parent and child or parent and health care provider regarding the so-called child's best interests. The process of making decisions for and by the child is also related to the quality of child-parent relationships and family values, the age and maturity of the child, the diagnosis, and the significance of the treatment to the future of the child.

Some decisions to treat or not treat are uncomplicated. For example, a pediatrician does not prescribe drugs for a hyperactive child at the request of the teacher or school nurse without parental consent.[6] One might also expect that the decision for tonsillectomy in a 6-year-old would be the sole decison of the parents. On the other hand, one would expect sensitive parents to seek the informed consent of a 10-, 11- or 12-year-old child to the same surgery. Where parents are divorced, the parent with legal custody of the child is legally responsible for informed consent to treatment.[7] Moral considerations, however, are complex when parents, either married or divorced, have an honest difference of opinion regarding the desirability of treatment, such as tonsillectomy or amputation for a malignant tumor. Here the principle of beneficence, that is, to do good, directly collides with the principle of "Do no harm," or nonmaleficence. This is a common problem in the example of tonsillectomy, where the tonsils are not a focus of infection but where frequent colds and sore throats occur. The evidence on either side, for tonsil removal or retention, is inconclusive.

The situation becomes even more complex when the child disagrees with the parents. Holder a legal expert on children, says that when a genuine emergency occurs, the child is to be treated even without parental consent.[8] In a nonemergency, for example, when a 10-year-old wearing glasses requests contact glasses from the ophthalmologist to participate in sports, parental consent is morally indicated. The parents and the child need information regarding the benefits, risks, and costs of the procedure as the basis for informed and judicious consent. In contrast, a 12-year-old with venereal disease seeking treatment who refuses to name or to notify her parents has the moral and legal right to receive treatment, since the consequences of nontreatment to the child, to others, and to society override the rights of the parents to know of the infection and to agree to its treatment. Generally, any communicable disease is an emergency to be treated without parental consent, if necessary.[9] Holder maintains that the physician who refuses to treat a drug-addicted child refusing treatment if parents are notified is "himself guilty of contributing to the delinquency of his patients."[10] The trend appears to favor the consent of the minor to health services. This is reflected in the Statement on Consent by the Task Force on Pediatric Research, Informed Consent, and Medical Ethics of the American Academy of Pediatrics permitting the self-supporting and separated minor to consent to treatment. The statement also calls for treatment of any pregnant, infected, or addicted minor without parental consent.[11]

The Statement provides that any minor with physical or emotional problems who is capable of rational decisions and who refuses help if parents are notified may consent to treatment. The health professional may legally thereafter tell parents or guardians unless it jeopardizes the patient's life or treatment results.[12] If serious health care procedures are to be given without parental consent, approval is sought from another physician. Thus, the Statement seeks to protect the minor's rights to treatment, the parents' right to be informed of the health of their child, and the physician's right to provide treatment without legal consequences.[13] The Statement strives to protect the child's right to privacy and confidentiality.

The following two cases present moral dilemmas. The first case is that of a mass screening program for iron-deficiency anemia in children that requires the direct participation of nurses. The focus of concern is for the nutritional status of lower-socioeconomic-class children whose mothers use food stamps to purchase foods that are less nutritious and contribute to dietary deficiencies. The plan is to secure finger-prick blood samples for hematocrit from the children by requiring the child's blood test in order for the mother to secure food stamps. Anemic children would be immediately provided with free iron supplements.[14] Nurse A argues in favor of the test, since it is the same used in the well-baby clinic. She points to the inadequacy of current detection of iron deficiency of children, the free treatment, and to each child's right to health care. A signed consent form will be requested of each mother. Nurses are the only available health professionals to do this test.

Nurse B argues against the compulsory nature of the screening and invokes other moral arguments favoring truth-telling and the client's moral right to self-determination, in this case the mother's deciding for her child. The issue is whether the coercion used in this screening program is ever morally justifiable, even though the predicted consequences are beneficial to the child.

Another case adapted from Brody is that of 10-year-old Janie, who was admitted for routine observation following a fall against the corner of the fireplace. Her head wound was superficial. No skull fracture was found. On a routine check, the nurse discovered her not breathing, blue, and with fixed and dilated pupils. She was immediately intubated, given drugs, and hooked to a cardiac monitor. The heartbeat returned in a half hour, but the pupils remained fixed and dilated. The evidence points to a considerable period of anoxia of the brain "with irreversible damage, but you cannot be sure."[15] The issue becomes one of treating or not treating by transferring Janie to a respirator in the intensive care unit. Here tests will be made to diagnose brain death or irreversible brain damage. Supposedly, this diagnosis will be followed by turning off the respirator.

The counterargument is that once Janie is on the respirator and treatment is started, it will be continued regardless of Janie's diagnosis or condition. Nurse A argues in favor of pronouncing the child dead for the sake of the greater good of the family and society. Nurse B argues for giving the child every help and every chance regardless of the consequences to Janie, the family, or society. Nurse B favors the sanctity of life, while Nurse A favors the greater happiness.

A third case illustrates the ethical problems of organ donation of one sibling to another. It raises the further issue of whether one sibling or child should be used to help another when there is no benefit to the donor. One of a pair of 8-year-old identical twin girls suffered from a life-threatening kidney disease necessitating the removal of both kidneys. The identical twin sister was the ideal donor. She appeared to understand and to agree with the procedure. The issue for the nurse as a member of the transplant team is on what grounds the healthy sibling is permitted or denied the donation of a kidney to her sick sister at some risk to herself.

Nurse A argues for donation on grounds of the greatest happiness of the greatest number. Nurse B argues against the donation on Egoistic grounds of no benefit to the donor, but certain risk and pain. Nurse C argues for donation on the grounds of the child's autonomy and self-determination. The 8-year-old donor appears to understand the issues and to be closely identified with her sister. The moral dilemma is whether to permit or deny the kidney donation.

Abuse of young children is a frequent problem of deep concern to nurses in emergency rooms, crisis centers, hospitals, schools, and public health agencies. The abuse may be physical, sexual, or emotional. One not infrequent example is that of an intimidated wife and a sexually abused 9-year-old daughter with whom the husband and father is having intercourse. In a routine exam, the school nurse discovers signs of penetration, and upon questioning, the child admits to intimacy. She begs the nurse not to tell anyone of her secret, since the father has threatened to kill mother and child if he is exposed. The child fears her father and is convinced that he will carry out his threats. The nurse is horrified at the exploitation of this child and all other defenseless, vulnerable children who are abused and neglected. She views her role as that of patient advocate with her "primary commitment . . . to the client's care and safety."[16] The nurse is aware of the laws protecting children from abuse and the sad lack of implementation by child and family welfare agencies and child placement facilities. The incest is clearly "prejudicial to the client's best interests" by interfering with the child's normal psychosocial growth and development. The father-daughter relationship will undermine the child's perception of the security and trust expected of parents and other authority figures. The incest may seriously warp the child's future relationships with intimates. Despite these serious misgivings, the nurse weighs the child's present security against an uncertain future in a foster home, separated from the family. The nurse is filled with doubt regarding the pledge of confidentiality to the child and the moral problem she faces.

MORAL IMPLICATIONS IN THE NURSING CARE OF CHILDREN

For the nurse working with children, the role necessarily involves consideration of the parents' significant contribution to the child's well-being. It is the parents who generally carry the lifelong burden of a seriously handicapped child. Parental responsibilities include investment of their energies, emotions, time, and finances in the care of the disabled child. Continuous health care, frequent hospitalizations, and special education are usually indicated throughout the life of the child. Some parents may fear the birth of another defective child and so devote the rest of their lives to the care of this one. Siblings, where they exist, may be deeply hurt and resentful of the disproportionate share of parental involvement and family resources taken up by the afflicted child. Mothers, especially, may be forced to give up career aspirations in order to give continuous care to the child. Parental conflict and even divorce may occur as a consequence of spousal guilt, frustration, and rage in this troubled situation.

Thus, the *Code for Nurses'* description of the nurse as advocate with "primary commitment . . . to the client's care and safety"[17] can be in conflict with other moral principles, such as the greatest good of the greatest number of family members. The nurse may be in a genuine dilemma regarding the conflicts of the infant's right to life and the family's right to a full human life without the lifelong burden of a child with little potential for personhood. The sensitive nurse ponders the identity of the client: Is it primarily the child, the family system, or the interests of the whole society? The nurse can muster persuasive arguments favoring the family system and still other arguments favoring the individual child as the client in need of advocacy. If the nurse gives serious and primary consideration to the children's bills of rights previously discussed, then the role of advocate as "primary commitment . . . to the client's care and safety"[18] is the only morally permissible alternative.

If the statement in the *Code* is to be taken literally, then all deformed children will be treated and no respirators turned off. Moreover, no thought will be given to the burdens of the handicapped child to the parents and the negative consequences to the family. No child will be deprived of the chance to live in the state to which he or she is restored, whatever that may be. Much more can be done by official and voluntary agencies to help families care for the retarded and the handicapped at home. The mother deserves compensation for her care. Allowances are needed for special foods, special clothing, and extra transportation to clinics and schools for the child. The overburdened family would thereby be helped in concrete ways, with considerable saving to the state. Most important, life will be saved, and each child will live to the extent of its potential.

A difficult situation for nurses is that in which the parents have opposing opinions about whether or not to treat. The tendency is for deeply troubled parents to turn to nurses caring for their child with such questions as, "What would you do if this were your child?" The child does not belong to the nurse, of course. Nor can the nurse put himself or herself in the parents' shoes. The nurse does not know the parents' circumstances, their values, commitments, feelings, or relationships as they do.

The nurse can facilitate parents' careful assessment of the relevant facts of the case, the parents' values, family resources, and the deep concerns of each parent. Identification of the problem, facts, values, and concerns are useful steps in helping parents resolve ambiguities and ambivalence in problem situations. Parents can be encouraged to talk together alone and with pediatric or family-practice nurses, physicians, clergy, lawyers, children, and relatives. Other families who have experienced similar problems may be consulted regarding their experiences with a handicapped child. Nevertheless, after all possible help is given parents, there remains the tragic choice of sustaining the fragile life with the utmost commitment to the child's right to life or the denial of that right based on the principle of the greatest happiness for the greatest number. Although some physicians and nurses tend to make that decision to treat or not treat for others, it can be viewed as the parents' rightful decision, since they bear the lifelong burden. If, however, the parents' decision is seen as improper, inappropriate, ethically unjustifiable, or illegal, the nurse as patient advocate has the duty to appeal that decision in the most effective way possible.

The nurse in contact with families in which there is abuse seeks information concerning laws protecting children, local regulations surrounding reporting of abuse, law enforcement agencies, child and family welfare agencies, and measures for protection of the child. The nurse may view his or her role as primarily one of patient advocate committed to the child's care and safety. In that case, the regulatory and child-caring resources can be utilized to the utmost on behalf of the child. If the nurse views himself or herself as an advocate of the family, he or she can then secure the resources of community family agencies in enlisting the family's participation in family therapy or counseling.

As advocate of the child, the nurse has an important role in facilitating the child's participation in ethical decision making regarding its own health care. The Partnership Model of relationship (cited in Chapter 7) recognizes children as full human beings due respect for their thoughts, feelings, interests, and desires in relation to their own health care. Ideally, the Partnership Model of relationships is based on an open, shared decision-making process, in which children's growing autonomy is supported to the extent of each child's cognitive maturation, personality, and thought processes. This model recognizes children's rights to information about their health status and to truthful answers concerning diagnosis, hospitalization, treatment, intensive procedures, chronic disease, and even impending death. Such knowledge is shared in words and at times by persons appropriate to the child's age, understanding, emotional state, and relationship with the nurse and significant others. Wieczorek and Natapoff recommend interviewing children regarding their health status. Some children will readily respond; a few will not. The process reveals whether the parents use the Ownership, Partnership, or Club Membership models of family relationships. Some parents answer for the child. Other parents qualify the child's answers. Parental interference is consistent with the Ownership Model. The ownership model may shield parents who evoke religious or philosophical beliefs to rationalize withholding medical care from their children. For example, a 2½ year old boy died in Boston of bowel obstruction in 1986 after five days of "treatment" by a Christian Science practitioner and nurse. Parents were exempted from legal blame on the basis of religious belief. Some parents support the child's expression of his or her thoughts regarding the health problem; this is consistent with the Partnership Model. The nurse who practices within this model believes it important to find out what children think is causing their health problem and the nature and source of their worries.[19] The child's sense of autonomy is enhanced by responsibility for providing information and sharing thoughts and feelings with the nurse and the physician about the health problem. In turn, the stress for the hospitalized child can be reduced by the warm and sympathetic nurse who supports the school-age child's ability to reason, to generalize, and to understand cause and effect in relation to the illness and treatment. The nurse as partner and child advocate is willing to support the child's autonomy by giving simplified scientific explanations for bodily changes, functions, diagnostic procedures, treatments, and the workings of the various hospital machines. Likewise, the nurse who respects the child gives truthful explanations for illness and treatment appropriate to the child's understanding. Such explanations are significant to children, especially younger children, who believe that their illness is related to their being bad in some way or that it is causing their parents considerable distress. Other misconceptions can be clarified.

The process of nurse-parent-child shared decision making assumes that the child, the nurse, and the parent have the capacity to understand essentials of cause-and-effect disease processes, as well as stages and principles of human growth and development, and that they are oriented toward a Partnership Model.

The nurse who perceives the role of advocate as a meaningful one can then move into shared decision making with the child. The nurse's alliance with the child is supportive of the child's participation in health care decisions. Concretely, the nurse permits as much freedom as possible, and encourages independence. The hospitalized or sick child may be an astute observer, with heightened awareness of bodily changes, and may want to be in control of the self. Enabling children to participate in developing their health care plans, such as making choices about sites of injection, days and times of scheduled visits, or going home to die, is a manifestation of deep respect for children's right to participate in health care decisions. The nurse can assist parents in helping the child express fears associated with dying, such as pain and abandonment, and in providing the necessary comfort, freedom from pain, and security. The nurse supports the child's participation in his or her own health care until the very end by respecting the child's determination of the need for pain medication, privacy, and peer, sibling, and parental visits. The child is respected throughout illness as a person of worth who is intensely concerned with what is happening to his or her body and life, with the nurse perceiving herself or himself as an ally to the dying young patient. Despite the overwhelmingly tragic outcome to the child, when the nurse and child interact in shared decision making together on a mutually benevolent basis, a morally significant human relationship may occur, an example for other human relationships.

ETHICAL-PHILOSOPHICAL APPROACHES TO NURSE-CHILD-PARENT RELATIONSHIPS

Several Philosophical Moves

There are several ethical considerations by way of an ethical check list for evaluating nurse-parent-child relationships. In addition to the "quorum feature notion" cited in Chapter 9, there is a further philosophical move by two recent philosophers, J. Rachels and W. Ruddick. This move consists in distinguishing biological or zoological life from biographical life. Human beings live anatomically and physiologically biological lives. Human beings who fulfill the majority features of being human also give evidence of being conscious. A person with hopes, projects, a history, joys, frustrations, and expectations of the future with plans and prospects, all of which presuppose consciousness, is said to have a biographical life. That person is not just living a biological life.[20]

A prominent Protestant theologian, Joseph Fletcher, restates the biological/biographical distinction by citing several conditions for being regarded as a person. These include a minimum intelligence of between 20 and 40 I.Q., self-awareness, a sense of past and future time, the ability to have human relationships and to show caring and concern for others, and to exercise some self-control over material and psychological conditions of existence. Fletcher's criteria boil down to the presence of consciousness.[21]

One astute commentator and interpreter of Fletcher's view, Margot Fromer, argues for Fletcher's criteria of personhood. Fromer points out that Fletcher's criteria for personhood are the most commonly used.[22] But she concedes that "many people disagree with them."[23] According to Fromer, for Fletcher "the one characteristic basic to all others is the presence of neocortical functioning, without which biologic life may exist but personhood does not. . . ."[24] To Fromer "health professionals are concerned with the quality as well as the sanctity of life."[25] But she thinks it is unlikely that human beings will ever reach agreement about what is an acceptable quality of life.[26]

Whether one refers to "the quality of life" or to a biographical life, to one's rational life plan, as does Rawls, or to one's projects, as Sartre does, or to consciousness, one uses these distinctions to refute the contention that the sanctity of life is unconditional, absolute, and undebatable. Although children cannot carry out all the cognitive functions of adults, normal children are expected to develop capacities that will enable them to fulfill more and more of these cognitive functions as they grow up.

There are advantages and drawbacks to the conception of biographical life. A strength of this distinction is its use as a practical basis, a cutoff point, for deciding who is a person to be helped and who may be medically ignored without public censure. A long-time comatose child, for example, or a child with severe mental and physical anomalies, may be given little or no medical attention without public recrimination.

A drawback to this distinction is that it can be used to decide that some types of humans, social deviants, cripples, and the comatose, are arbitrarily ruled out as persons. Therefore, no charge of genocide or homicide attaches to those who cause these unfortunate beings to be killed. This would be unjust.

A response, however, by the advocates of a biological/biographical distinction, is that the members of any society cannot afford to keep all breathing beings alive if they are not conscious and productive or have any hope of being so. Such a cut-off point, the defenders of this biological/biographical distinciton claim, is not like the Nazi basis for eliminating unwanted human beings with mental illness, epilepsy, or healthy Jews, Slavics, and blacks, since ethnic and religious factors are not relevant to the consciousness or social productivity of the person. Nazi claims about the inferiority of these non-Aryan groups were false, but even if Nazi claims of their inferiority were true, Nazi mistreatment of these groups would not be morally justifiable on biographical grounds.

The Concept of Rights Applied to the Nurse-Child-Parent Relationship

A further philosophical move consists in clarifying the concept of rights that apply to children in a health care context. The question of whether children have any rights has one of four responses and accompanying arguments. One view is that children have no rights at all. Parents, nurses, and other adults may have duties, but children have no rights. A second view is that children have rights to be cared for, to food, clothing, shelter, health care, and education, but no liberty rights to make their own decisions. A third position is that children have limited subsistence rights and liberty rights in relation to their readiness to make responsible decisions. Children, for example, may walk across the street when they show that they are careful. But children do not have the liberty right to stay out all night and imbibe alcohol whenever they wish. A fourth position holds that children have unlimited liberty and subsistence rights shared equally with adults.

Each position has defenders and opponents. The customary philosophical moves consist in arguing on behalf of one of these views. In the process, one may make use of philosophical arguments to clarify the concept of rights applied to children. Several arguments for rights are worth noting. Rights imply liberties; they also imply corresponding duties imposed on other appropriate persons and groups, such as nurses, parents, and schoolteachers. The AIDS crisis imposes serious constraints on children's rights of sexual expression and imply adults' restraints of children's erotic pursuits.

M. Cranston, a prominent writer, points to three requirements of rights: practicability or feasibility, which means a right can be put into practice; universality, or the equal application of the right to all those to whom it applies without arbitrary exceptions; and "paramount importance," or the singling out of these needs deemed vitally urgent to individuals in society.[27] This third requirement of rights of paramount importance confines rights to the most urgent conditions of social life rather than fads and frills. The paramount requirement or value priority calls for a society to have "fire engines and ambulances," for example. "Fun fairs and holiday camps"[28] are luxuries rather than the rights of persons. If rights have no restraints, then rights become everything, and if they mean everything, as with any other term that has no exclusions, rights become frivolous. Applying Cranston's criteria shows that whereas one can speak of a child's right to food, clothing, shelter, health care, and education, the child cannot have a right to be loved in the same way. For every child to be loved may be a desirable ideal, but to refer to a child's right to be loved is, in Cranston's terms, "a utopian aspiration" or ideal, but not a right.[29]

Furthermore, morality may be separated into agent or character morality, act or decision morality, and the critics' or judges' morality. The first concerns classical and contemporary virtues, such as wisdom, courage, compassion, love, generosity, kindness, devotion, and loyalty. The second, act or decision-making morality, is about decisions made or acts or actions agents make. Act morality concerns declarations of rights, duties, justice, equality, and fairness. The third morality, that of the critics or judges, consists in applying critical canons in evaluating both agents and actions as being either courageous or cowardly, wise or unwise, trustworthy or not, and judging actions as fair or unfair, or as respecting or violating rights.

There can be no right to love, then, because love belongs to agent morality rather than act morality. Rights belong to the class of acts that are either just or fair; violations of rights are their opposite. Around rights, boundaries can be drawn in which this act is fair and that not, but in which love, being a character trait, is too vague to qualify as a right.

Dependency, Paternalism, and Freedom

One difference between adults and children that needs to be considered in ethical decision making and in ascribing rights to children is that children, while potentially adults, are dependents. As dependents, children are not always able to make effective decisions. There is a three-way child-health professional-parent relationship, in which parents or health professionals, including nurses, have the role of deciding on behalf of a helpless, dependent child what therapeutic intervention is presumably best for the child.

The point is that a child between ages one and six has health care measures, such as injections, vaccinations, and prescribed drugs, and operations, such as tonsillectomy, done for it, often without asking its permission. The doctrine of informed consent does not apply to children in the earliest years of life. This general exemption is connected to the principle that to have rights presupposes consciousness or the capacity for rational behavior. Yet children are expected to become conscious adults who have the capacity to make decisions. The place of children is between other sentient beings governed more by feelings and instincts and those beings who have a rational capacity.[30] This immature state presents a dilemma: How to regard children?

One way out of this difficulty of either denying that children have rights, thus treating them as inferiors with paternalistic intervention, or attributing the same rights to children as to adults, is to carve out a special class of rights for children. These are called "rights-in-trust." These rights-in-trust for children are the rights they will have when sufficiently mature to exercise those rights. Rights-in-trust are held in safekeeping by relevant adults, who in the appropriate time will turn those rights over to the children to whom they properly belong.[31] Appropriate adults, including nurses, have the role of safeguarding children's rights. In that role, appropriate adults are guardians, protectors, trustees, and advocates of the children in their charge.

The question arises, however, as to whose rights nurses and other health professionals protect, the parents' rights or the child's rights. If parents are clearly abusive, the nurse's role is to protect the child's right. But if a parent, such as a Jehovah's Witness, intends no harm but insists on no blood transfusion for a child seriously hurt and in need of blood, nurses may feel they are in the middle of a conflict. One consideration for the nurse is to invoke the prevention-of-harm princi-ple. The harm to the child from an unnecessary death gives the health professionals a strong reason to override the parents' right to decide to withhold a blood transfusion.

On the other hand, if a child of 10 or 11 has a certain form of cancer which only a leg amputation can arrest, and if the child refuses the operation, the parent, invoking the principle of preventing the greater harm, has the moral right to override the child's right to refuse. The parent has the legal right to decide in favor of amputation as well.

There are fairly clear cases of benign versus malignant Paternal-ism. The abusive parent falls into the malignant Paternalism category. The parent permitting amputation to arrest cancer in the hope of preventing greater harm falls under the benign Paternalism category. Since the term "Paternalism" is and will be used in succeeding pages, a definition of the term may be helpful. Paternalism comes from the Latin word *pater,* meaning father, and refers to the idea that father knows best and has the authority to decide.

There are obviously cases and arguments in which Paternalism is defensible, such as the parent who orders a stomach pump for a three-year-old child who has just swallowed household cleaning fluid. The nurse's role in such a case is solely to aid the parent in saving the child's life, even if the procedure is painful to the child.

There are other cases and arguments in which Paternalism, exer-cised by parents more powerful than their children, is clearly indefen-sible. Examples are parents who abuse their children by putting them in scalding hot water, beating them into insensibility, or putting them into a hot oven. In such abuse cases, the nurse's role is to intervene on behalf of the child.

Two sometimes complementary models of patient advocacy may be consulted. One is the model presented by Robin Hood, who fights and overcomes oppressors. There are no conflicts between children and adults on this model. Considerations of justice and fairness determine whose rights the nurse protects. A second nurse-advocate model is presented by the example of Antigone in Sophocles' play of the same name. Antigone directly confronts and defies Creon, king of Thebes, who has decreed that Polynices, her brother, is a traitor and to be left unburied, contrary to custom. Antigone demands the right to bury her brother, even though her power is no match for the king's.[32] We may call this the *direct-confrontation* model of patient advocacy. Some nurses treat their patients in that way, doing what they regard as right, regardless of consequences to themselves. Other nurses use in-stitutional channels to protect children who are victimized by anyone. On a higher, macrolevel, professional organizations are also advocates of children through the organization's sponsorship and support of legis-lation and social policy affecting children's rights and welfare.

CONCLUSION

Children, the proverbial hope of the future, are developing persons. To become mature persons, children need the nurture parents and health professionals can give to support their growth into adolescence and adulthood. The health and well-being of children places a pleasurable obligation on parents and health professionals to provide maximum resources.

One way to recognize the importance of children is to attribute health care rights to them. An advantage of attributing rights to children in place of imposing duties on parents alone is that rights give force to the duties imposed. But the kinds and quality of rights children have also leaves us with difficulties. The rights of children cannot include the right to drink alcohol, use drugs, spend their parents' money without restrictions, or absent themselves from school. Children's rights call for constraints.

Most importantly, children have not the capacity to decide what is in their own interests in health matters. So children cannot have such rights as the right to informed consent until they reach an appropriate degree of maturity. To offset these difficulties, the concept of "rights-in-trust" is applicable to children. Such rights, however, presuppose that children are beings who have not only a biological but also a biographical life, one with plans, projects, hopes, expectations, and realizations as well as failures and disappointments. These aspects of one's biographical life give evidence of human consciousness, a necessary condition for being regarded as a person.

The challenge to the nurse working with children is to support the growing independence of the child. One way is by encouraging the child's responsibility for and participation in his or her own health care. The child's growing awareness of his or her bodily processes, recognition of the fragility of a state of wellness, and a relationship of trust with the nurse can all be strong forces in the sick child's return to health. This child can be an articulate participant in planning and implementing his or her health care.

The role of the nurse working with very young or abused and neglected children is largely that of patient advocate. Such children need protection and help. Sometimes, for the sake of the child's very survival, the child needs to be taken out of a home with abusive or incestuous parents. The nurse can effectively advocate for every kind of help available, such as the use of police and referral to child and family welfare agencies.

Discussion Questions

1. Parents are told by physicians that their 3-years-old child has a malignant form of leukemia that may respond to an experimental

drug with highly unpleasant and possible fatal side effects. All health professionals recommend the treatment to the parents in the "best interests" of the child. The parents refuse the drug in the "child's best interests" and to avoid needless suffering from the side effects. Who is right? What does this example show about appealing to the "person's best interests" doctrine?

2. Using the same case, how is appeal to the substitute judgment doctrine also begging the question?

REFERENCES

1. Wieczorek RR, Natapoff JN. *A conceptual approach to the nursing of children.* Philadelphia: Lippincott; 1981: 31.
2. Ariès P. *Centuries of childhood: A social history of family life.* New York: Vintage; 1962: 128.
3. United Nations. *The declaration of the rights of the child.* New York: United Nations; 1959.
4. Ibid.
5. Wieczorek and Natapoff. *A conceptual approach to the nursing of children.* 33.
6. Holder AR. *Legal issues in pediatrics and adolescent medicine.* New York: Wiley; 1977: 137.
7. Ibid.; 138
8. Ibid.
9. Ibid.; 143.
10. Ibid.
11. Brown RH. Consent. *Pediatrics.* March, 1976; *57*(3):414–416.
12. Ibid.
13. Ibid.
14. Brody H. *Ethical decisions in medicine.* 2nd ed. Boston: Little, Brown; 1981: 253.
15. Ibid.; 233.
16. American Nurses' Association. *Code for nurses with interpretive statements.* Kansas City, MO: Author; 1985: 8.
17. Ibid.
18. Ibid.
19. Committee on Bioethics. American Academy of Pediatrics. *Pediatrics.* January, 1988. *81*(1):169–171.
20. Wieczorek and Natapoff. *A conceptual approach to the nursing of children.* 810.
21. Ruddick W. Parents, children and moral decisions. In: Bandman EL, Bandman B. (eds.). *Bioethics and Human Rights: A Reader for Health Professionals.* Lanham, Md.: University Press of America, 1986: 165–170.
22. Fletcher J. *Four indicators of humanhood—the enquiry matures.* Hastings Center Report. 1974. *4*(6):5.
23. Fromer MJ. *Ethical issues in health care.* St. Louis: Mosby; 1981: 12–14, 31–32.

24. Ibid.
25. Ibid.
26. Ibid.; 32.
27. Ibid.
28. Cranston M. Health rights, real and supposed. In: Raphael DD. (ed). *Political Theory and the Rights of Man.* Bloomington, IN: Indiana University Press; 1967: 50–51.
29. Cranston M. *What are human rights?* New York: Taplinger; 1973: 67.
30. Houlgate L. *The child and the state.* Baltimore: Johns Hopkins Press; 1980: 50.
31. Feinberg J. A child's right to an open future. In: Aiken H, LaFollette H. (eds). *Whose Child? Children's Rights, Parental Authority and State Power.* Totowa, NJ: Littlefield, Adams; 1980: 125–126.
32. Cranston. *What Are Human Rights?* 9–10.

CHAPTER 11

Ethical Issues in the Nursing Care of Adolescents

Study of this chapter enables the learner to:

1. Distinguish the rights of adolescents in relation to physiological, psychological, social, cultural, and legal dimensions of capacity and maturity.
2. Define the role of the nurse as patient advocate of the adolescent client seeking health care.
3. Develop the role of the nurse in controversies between parental authority and adolescent autonomy.
4. Recognize the adolescent's duties and responsibilities to self, family, and society as a dependent, independent, and interdependent person in a Partnership family model.

INTRODUCTION

Adolescents differ from other minors in the degree of autonomy they claim and exercise. Some middle- and upper-class segments of this society support adolescents in prolonged dependence on parents. Adolescents exercise decision-making rights as well as rights to be cared for. These include rights to support, education, clothing, and recreational funds. Poor adolescents are forced to earn their own way. Nevertheless, the emphasis is on the differences of adolescents from all other age groups in matter of dress, communication, music, drug and alcohol consumption, sexual activity, life-styles, and values. A paradox of adolescent culture is the conflict between claimed independence and actual reliance on parental and other forms of community support in the name of rights.

The spectrum of goods and services to each adolescent passenger in the metaphorical lifeboat is anchored by the concept of rights. Adolescents tend to claim rights and liberties restricted to adults. These rights include such activities as sexual freedom. This single issue raises many questions regarding parental responsibility for such adolescent problems as pregnancy and care of the ensuing child, abortions for an unwanted pregnancy, compliance with contraceptive measures, and medical care for sexually transmitted diseases. Thus, a central issue of adolescent health care is the extent of the autonomy of an adolescent in relation to the duties, responsibilities, and rights of parents and other significant adults.

A related issue is the extent of adolescent rights and the duties of society to protect and to provide for those rights. The United Nations' *Declaration of Children's Rights* lists rights to be provided by society and parents. Despite its good intentions, the *Declaration* may be seen as either a Paternalistic or utopian doctrine, since it places the fundamental responsibility of the child on his or her parents.[1] Moreover, its provisions are in some cases far-fetched—desirable ideals perhaps, but not practical or feasible. There is a doubtful presumption here that adolescents lack interests that they are able to identify, express, and evaluate independently of the interests and values of their parents, teachers, and others in authority.[2] Arguments can be put forth that adolescents generally are competent to defend their own interests. Other arguments show that the adolescent is still immature and inexperienced. Therefore, in important matters of health, parental concern for the best interests of the child may be in direct conflict with the values, moral principles, and autonomy of the adolescent. This may place the nurse in the middle of adversarial camps, which he or she may seek to reconcile on behalf of continuing parental-child dialogue concerning rights, duties, responsibilities, trust, fairness, and other moral principles.

ETHICAL ISSUES

Selected cases illustrate ethical issues that may be confronted in the nursing care of adolescents.

Karen, age 16, Catholic, the second of seven siblings, was hospitalized for chronic, active glomerulonephritis in 1968. Her kidneys were removed following two years of intense but unsuccessful treatment. A transplant of her father's kidney was unsuccessful. Hemodialysis before and following surgery caused her to have "chills, nausea, vomiting, severe headaches and weakness."[3] Psychiatric evaluation and treatment was provided for Karen and her parents before and following the transplant. In April 1971, it was obvious that the transplanted kidney was not functioning. "Karen and her parents expressed the desire to stop treatment."[4] This decision was unacceptable to the medical staff. Psychiatrist and social worker attempted guidance toward continuation of medical care. The family agreed to home care, which Karen found isolated and restricting. She was fatigued and uncomfortable. She was then hospitalized for high fever and removal of the transplant; the shunt became infected, clotted, and closed. At this point, Karen and her parents again refused dialysis and shunt revision. The staff was angry and frustrated and of the opinion that this was an unsound, immoral, and inappropriate decision for a 16-year-old. Karen discussed the decision with the hospital chaplain. She decided that hell and possibly heaven were nonexistent, but that "nothingness would be far better than the suffering which would continue if she lived."[5]

On consultation, the child psychiatrist found Karen not psychotic and her decision to be a carefully reasoned, rational one. The nephrologist agreed. The staff was then to make her life comfortable "with daily counseling in the event she changed her mind."[6] The alternatives of taking the case to court to force treatment or requiring the parents to take Karen home to die so as to avoid the staff's assistance in what they thought to be a suicidal act were considered. A dialysis nurse visited Karen and insisted on further dialysis. Staff members who had witnessed Karen's prolonged suffering were more supportive.

Karen's spirits and appetite improved following her decision. She thanked the staff, picked a burial place near her home, wished her parents happiness, and supported them in their doubts about the decision. She died on June 2, 1971, suddenly and peacefully, with both parents at her side.

Since there was no consistent parental opposition to Karen's decision, the issues appear to be her autonomy and right to die in conflict with the staff's view of this act as suicidal and immoral. Some staff members, such as the hemodialysis unit nurse, were strongly opposed to Karen's decision and in favor of intervention on a Paternalistic basis.

A case that complements that of Karen is the case of Phillip Becker, age 12, a mild Down's syndrome person. He needed heart surgery, but his parents refused to consent. Phillip's parents said in court that in their opinion he was better off dead than alive. They appealed to the "best interests" doctrine. Fortunately, foster parents, following the lead of George Will,[7] came to his rescue and provided the needed surgery for Phillip. The parents regarded him as an "embarrassment."[7]

Less clear-cut are examples of 13- to 18-year-old adolescents living dependently under the parental roof who seek abortions without the knowledge and consent of their parents. These minors do not qualify

for the status of emancipated minor, since they are neither independent, self-supporting, nor married. One moral stance is that the nurse
must protect the privacy and confidentiality of these young patients on
grounds of the adolescent's right to her own body. Another issue is
that of the parents' rights to be informed of the health concern and to
decide for the immature offspring.

Another type of case involves Martin Sieferth, 14, who had a cleft
palate and harelip in need of surgery. Martin's father, unlike Phillip
Becker's father, showed signs of parental affection. The father believed, however, in "mental healing" and in letting "the natural forces
of the universe work on the body!"[8] Therefore, he refused surgery
to repair his son's seriously deformed and unattractive jaw. Martin
agreed with his father.[9] Martin was consequently disfigured as an adolescent and will need physical and emotional relief if he is to flourish.

THE NURSE'S ROLE IN ADOLESCENT CARE

Working with adolescents is particularly challenging. Adolescents tend
to shift between determined independence and exercise of autonomy
and the delayed recognition that the situation is fraught with problems and possibly peril. This developmental phase is one in which
high value is placed on acceptance by peers. Another characteristic of
this adolescent phase is behavioral and role experimentation within
the peer group. Thus, the adolescent may experiment with drugs and
sexual and criminal activity in response to peer pressure. It is ex-
tremely difficult for most adolescents to separate from the values of
the peer group with which they identify.

Acceptance of peer values, such as positive regard for sexual activity with resulting pregnancy, abortion, sexually transmitted disease or
AIDS, can, for example, be the source of considerable conflict between
adolescents and parents. The nurse can be caught between the anger
and duties of the parents and the defensiveness and vulnerability of
the adolescent. Each believes that his or her choice is the right one.
Each expects that the nurse will advocate and actively support his or
her position. For example, the 13-year-old seeking an abortion without
parental knowledge expects unconditional support from the abortion
unit as patient advocate. This adolescent insists on carrying the burden of guilt or regret regarding the abortion decision and of her fear of
the procedure without the parental support she might otherwise receive. The nurse tries to help the young person identify and analyze
her perceptions of her family in the hope that parents will be viewed
in a positive light. The adolescent's negative reasons may be substantive, including abuse and incest. The pregnant adolescent may fear
both punishment and rejection from a family that has forbidden pre-

marital sexual activity. The nurse as patient advocate and in accordance with the *Code for Nurses* supports such a patient's self-determination while giving information relevant to making an informed judgment. Such information includes the possible helpfulness of parental support and participation in the decision, the alternatives to abortion of full-term delivery and adoption, the steps and effects of the procedure, and the patient's right to receive or to refuse treatment. Relevant information also includes referrals to family planning for counseling and information regarding contraception. Supportive nursing care includes concern and interest for the tragic choice faced by the young adolescent. Anticipatory guidance is directed toward prevention of future unwanted pregnancies, along with adolescent evaluation of personal values expressed in behavior and in relationships.

The second level of advocacy is for a nurse to refer a sexually active adolescent to a family planning unit or physician for contraceptives or individual counseling. Such agencies aim to counsel, educate, and guide the adolescent toward control of pregnancies and of matters of general health. Care is usually free or low-cost.

A third level of advocacy is appeal to the courts. The Department of Health and Human Resources has regulations requiring that all family planning projects receiving federal funds make "services . . . available without regard for religion, creed, age, sex, parity, or marital status."[10] A 15-year-old whose family was receiving Aid to Families with Dependent Children sued the Planned Parenthood Association of Utah for denying her contraceptives without parental permission. A three-judge federal court in Utah held that the parental-consent requirement was in conflict with federal requirements. To deprive the adolescent of contraceptives from agencies receiving federal assistance was therefore unconstitutional. The court further ruled that the requirement for parental consent was a violation of the minor's right of privacy. Therefore, the federal regulations were to be enforced.[11]

The controversy between parental authority and adolescent autonomy continues. At times, the nurse's role may be much like that of a broker, trying to reconcile the adolescent's insistence on rights to sexual activity, contraception, abortion with parental authority, parental concern for the adolescent's welfare, and such consequences as unwanted pregnancies. The parent may argue justifiably that the adolescent's rights are limited by her inability to care for a child and her dependence on parental support, or that sexual freedom, contraceptives, abortion are wrong and therefore undesirable. The nurse may suggest to parents the unrealistic expectations for adolescent sexual abstinence. The nurse may then be in the position of advocating the adolescent's right to contraception as a lesser evil than unwanted pregnancies, abortion, and AIDS.

The dilemma of adolescent sexual activity, contraceptive use, abortion, and childbearing without marriage is a serious and persistent problem. "There were nearly 600,000 infants born to adolescents nineteen years or younger in the United States in 1975."[12] Obviously, the adolescent is asserting her right to sexual freedom. A counterargument is that the exercise of a right requires a correlative duty of someone to provide for that right. According to this argument, it is the duty of a parent to provide decent conditions for a fulfilling life for the child produced. Most adolescents cannot do so. The issue for the nurse then becomes one of presenting rational alternatives to adversarial parents and adolescents, if possible. Moral and social consequences of behavior are elicited and analyzed together by parents, adolescent, and nurse. Assumptions of parental support by providing the necessary goods and services to the adolescent regardless of life-style and choices need examination and evaluation by parents and adolescent together.

Adolescents, too, can engage in the process of morally justifying their major decisions. Little recognition is given to adolescent responsibilities for analyzing and evaluating the moral dimensions and consequences of behavior. In the public media, particularly, the adolescent is regarded as glamorous and exciting when experimenting with drugs, alcohol, sexual activity, music, dress, and deviant life-styles. The central issue for the nurse becomes one of supporting those adolescent rights that facilitate a decent, fulfilling life, or, as in the case of Karen, the right to die as a release from excessive or pointless suffering. This is the role of the patient advocate in support of the individual's moral right to rational decision making or autonomy. As problems of adolescent sexual activity in the form of pregnancy, abortion, AIDS, and other sexually transmitted disease, childbearing, child abuse, and substance abuse illustrate, there are morally justifiable limits to adolescent rights. The boundaries to adolescent rights may come from several sources. Compulsory driver education has in some states made a significant statistical difference in the accident rates of adolescents. In family relationships, the development of responsibilities and trust goes with the exercise of rights. This shows the relation of rights and virtues. To paraphrase on Kant, rights without virtues are empty; virtues without rights are blind. One without the other is incomplete. Thus, the adolescent learns to be both a provider and a recipient of goods and services rather than a mere rightholder in a world of rapidly increasing rights and shrinking resources.

ETHICAL CONSIDERATIONS IN THE ADOLESCENT-NURSE-PARENT RELATIONSHIP

The fact that one shares social life with others has an important bearing on adolescent development. A socially worthwhile life calls for an adolescent to recognize not only rights but also responsibilities commensurate with the growing physical power to do good or harm to the self and others. The moral education of an adolescent includes the point that social life is shared and people depend on one another. Human relationships call for reciprocal give-and-take, the mutual recognition of rights and responsibilities.

One may consequently argue that the moral-correlativity thesis of rights might well apply to adolescents. This means that for them to have rights, they must demonstrate the capacity to live up to corresponding responsibilities. Driving a car calls for an adolescent's ability to drive safely. It may well call for the adolescent to earn part or all of the cost of driving. The adolescent may also be expected to refrain from drinking alcohol while driving. Similar constraints govern the use of drugs. These are constraints imposed equally on adult members of society who are expected to fulfill social and economic responsibilities. The new rights adolescents gain, then, such as driving, may be said to be "earned rights," which depend on appropriate assumption of responsibilities. Similar constraints may well govern sexual activities. Adolescents of school and college age who are not yet ready to assume adult responsibilities in bearing and rearing children are not free to engage in sexual activities without appropriate constraints, such as the proper use of condoms.

The governing principle in determining the rights and responsibilities of adolescents is whether such rights and responsibilities are conducive to leading a socially worthwhile life. This ideal rules out socially destructive behavior such as unsafe sex, unsafe driving, drug experimentation, vandalism, violence, and lack of concern for others. The point is that one does not want adolescents to become veritable savages, like those portrayed in William Golding's *Lord of the Flies*. When shipwrecked on a deserted island, these boys become cannibals. Such behavior is unacceptable.

The role of the nurse, along with other health professionals, is to be a health educator and therapist in reinforcing positive social values. The nurse supports values that help an individual adolescent become a responsible, upstanding member of society. The nurse helps the adolescent learn both to contribute and allocate, and facilitates individual adolescents' functioning together. In this connection, the concept of physical, social, psychological, and economic well-being becomes a decidedly important nursing model.

A socially worthwhile life also calls for appropriate recognition of and training in standards and skills of sustained intellectual judgment. Such judgment requires a common understanding of the methods and results of cognitive disciplines with appropriate regard and familiarity with rules of evidence in the sciences. The relevance to ethics is that enormous good or evil comes by either considering or ignoring rules of evidence.

The biological/biographical/social/cognitive distinction rules against regarding an adolescent who has been comatose for a long time as a person on the grounds that he or she lacks a biographical life, a life with conscious activities. These distinctions also rule against identifying an adolescent as a person if he or she has extreme physical, intellectual, social, or psychological handicaps, such as substance addiction or criminal or antisocial behavior. These biographical and social distinctions also support an adolescent's right to terminate her fifth pregnancy on grounds that she is unlikely to provide a worthwhile human life for yet another child. The biographical/social/cognitive distinction also rules against a biology major's refusal to dissect animals in the course of study. The social/cognitive distinction rationally counts against a nurse's refusal to participate in surgical repair of a boy's cleft palate or in an abortion indicated by social and cognitive considerations. By implication, the cognitive requirement, respect for and familiarity with scientific methods and results, gives a reason against a nurse's recommending Laetrile or faith healing as a rational alternative to scientifically verifiable health care measures.

Some people ask: "Who decides?" or, "Who shall have the justifiable authority to decide whether an adolescent's life is no longer worth sustaining?" One move in philosophy consists in rephrasing the question to ask: "What criteria does a rational person appeal to in deciding nurse-adolescent-parent issues?" or "What counts as a good reason or as evidence?" In some types of cases, such as the faith-healing issue, appeal to scientific evidence is appropriate because it works; and the reason it works is that it has a truth value that appeal to faith healing lacks. The reason for believing in the truth value of cleft-palate surgery over faith healing is that the verifiable evidence favors the results—a clear victory for Utilitarianism.

In other kinds of cases, such as saving the life of a Jehovah's Witness by giving needed blood, one effective and wise appeal is to conventional or "common morality."[13] While it is true that conventional morality is not the whole of morality, it does address itself to the common moral sentiments and virtues, such as honesty, affection, generosity, wisdom, courage, and happiness, and to the survival and well-being of people.

A distinction made earlier between various models of health care by Szasz and Hollander applies to the issue of restraints versus the freedom of infants, children, and adolescents. Their first model, activity-passivity,[14] holds that a health professional is active and a patient is passive. Their second model, "guidance cooperation," involves the health professional's guiding but not exclusively directing or coercing the patient. Their third model, "mutual participation," makes health professional and patients equal partners in the effort to achieve health.

Applied to the nursing of infants, children, and adolescents, the first, the activity-passivity model, aptly applies to the role nurses have in caring for essentially dependent and helpless infants and children. Children need to be told when to take their medicines, when to go to bed, and what to eat and drink.

As children grow into adolescence, the guidance-cooperation model increasingly applies. Young adolescents will need to learn how to develop increasing degrees of independence and self-sufficiency. The adult, including the nurse, will be analogous to the driver education teacher who sits next to the student and guides the student's driving activities.

The third model, mutual participation, is the goal sought for in a democratic society, a society of equals. This goal guides and orients the adolescent on its way to and through adulthood.

CONCLUSION

The main moral problems in each developmental span—infancy, childhood, and adolescence—are different in some aspects and similar in others. Adolescents are similar in concerns to other human beings throughout all phases of growth. They are self-respecting persons; they learn to respect others; and they live by sharing social life. As such, young people are brought up to be not only dependents or independent. The adult, and the nurse as health educator, who brings up a child only to think of himself or herself is overlooking a crucial reality consideration that governs social life. For example, adolescents who cough without covering their mouths in a public place are inconsiderate. The role of the nurse as health educator is to teach children and adolescents appropriate health behavior. There are other rules of social life in which the development of a person is aimed not only at independence but at interdependence. These rules admonish a child to eat a nutritious breakfast, to have wholesome physical, intellectual, cultural, and emotional activities, to avoid drug and alcohol abuse, premature and unsafe sexual activity, crime and violence.

The development of persons with rights and reciprocal responsibilities constitutes goals that apply from birth to death and do not vary from infancy to childhood and adolescence. As Harry Stack Sullivan, the eminent American psychiatrist, said, "Everyone is much more simply human than otherwise."[15]

The moral differences in the three phases of growth are many, but they center on dependence in infancy, development of independence in childhood, and developing interdependence in adolescence. Each phase brings moral problems, some of which have no completely satisfactory answers, as in the attempt to decide whether to save an infant, child, or adolescent with few or marginal prospects of living a full human life. Moral problems are thorniest at the fringes. The core of morality is fairly well settled. Phillip's foster parents were morally right to insist on his cardiac surgery. Karen was not wrong to choose to die. Martin Sieferth's father was clearly wrong.

In the nurse's role as health educator, patient advocate, agent of reality, and therapist, the nurse is not alone. Because of the common morality, one that generally aims at the well-being of everyone, the nurse has many allies and resources to call on for help while coping with the admittedly real hindrances and obstacles of adolescence.

Discussion Questions

1. On what grounds did Karen, the adolescent kidney patient, have a right to refuse dialysis and thus end her life? Give reasons for and against your position.
2. What reasons might one give both for and against Martin Sieferth's father refusing surgical repair of his son's cleft palate? Which reasons outweigh which others?
3. What health care rights and responsibilities does an adolescent have? May adolescents rationally refuse to drink milk and eat the nutritious foods their parents serve them at home?
4. Which doctrine, if either, best applies toward guiding adolescent decision making in health care, the "substitute judgment" doctrine (put yourself in the other's shoes) or the "best interest" doctrine (doing or not doing X in your child's best interests)? Critically evaluate the application of either of these doctrines. From a caring perspective, what are the strengths and weaknesses of "substitute judgment" and the "best interest" doctrine?

REFERENCES

1. Young R. In the interests of children and adolescents. In: Aiken W, LaFollette H. (eds). *Whose Child? Children's Rights, Parental Authority and State Power.* Totowa, N.J: Littlefield, Adams; 1980: 179.
2. Ibid.; 180.
3. Schowalter JE et al. The adolescent patient's decision to die. *Pediatrics.* 1973; *51*(1):97–103.
4. Ibid.; 98.
5. Ibid.
6. Bandman E, Bandman B. The nurse's role in protecting the patient's right to live or die. *Advances in Nursing Science.* 1979; *1*(3):21–35.
7. Will G. *Newsweek,* April 14, 1980; 112.
8. In the matter of Sieferth. In: O'Neill O, Ruddick W. (eds). *Having Children.* New York: Oxford University Press; 1979: 139.
9. Holder A. *Legal issues in pediatrics and adolescent medicine.* New York: Wiley; 1977: 284–286.
10. Ibid.; 271.

11. Ibid.
12. Golding W. *Lord of the flies*. New York: Putnam; 1954.
13. Donnegan A. *The theory of morality*. Chicago: University of Chicago Press; 1977: 6, 7, 28–31, 102, 172, 210–243.
14. Szasz TS, Hollander MH. The physician-patient relationship. Arch. Intern. Med. 1956; 97:585.
15. Sullivan HS. *The interpersonal theory of psychiatry*. New York: Norton; 1953: 32.

CHAPTER 12

Ethical Issues in the Nursing Care of Adults

Study of this chapter enables the learner to:

1. Understand adult development in relation to the moral issues significant to this phase of human development.
2. Apply ethical principles of the prevention of harm, truth-telling, informed consent, the right to receive and to refuse treatment, and the right to privacy and confidentiality in practice with adult clients.
3. Utilize patients' bills of rights in development of the nursing role as patient advocate.
4. Facilitate the patient's right to self-determination and well-being through shared decision making in relation to the client's life goals, rational plans, and values.

INTRODUCTION

A person's passage from childhood and adolescence to youth or early adulthood is one of the most exciting times of life. Romantic love and attachment to another person marks this period as a peak experience in life. Vigorous health is the norm for youth and young adults. Therefore, serious or chronic illness is devastating to life-styles, educational and social goals, careers, family planning, and realization of hopes.

ADULT DEVELOPMENT

Adulthood is the longest and most productive phase of human development. The process is one of continuing change characterized by growth, development, and slow decline. The rate of change differs considerably among individuals. Consequently, all divisions of the adult life span are somewhat arbitrary and apply only generally to a particular individual.

Young Adulthood

Young adulthood is regarded as the years up to age 35. In this period, persons are establishing themselves in occupations and in situations of interpersonal intimacy, including marriage.

Customary developmental tasks of young adults include gradual independence from parents with progressive involvement in the world of education and work. The young adult is concerned with a role in the community and in selected groups. Marriage, childbearing, and child rearing are characteristic of this phase of development.

The young couple are expected to provide for the health, education, and care of their children and for their own welfare and future. Serious illness at this age is unexpected and catastrophic to all members of the family system. Chronic illness in a spouse can be disruptive to the marital relationship and to the security of children. Ethical decisions regarding life-prolonging measures of comatose spouses can be especially difficult at this age, since they involve a healthy spouse and children in need of social, emotional, and financial resources. If however, the young family enjoys good health and good fortune, the couple gradually moves into the developmental tasks of middle age.

Youth. In contrast to this traditional path of development, there are those young adults unable to accept the traditions they were taught without reexamination and anguish. Kenneth Keniston has defined an emerging developmental phase called "youth." He describes it as an "optional stage, not a universal one. . . . Most young Americans who enter this stage of life tend to be between the ages of 18 and 30."[1]

The term describes a new generation born in the nuclear age and usually of college and graduate-school age. They refuse to settle down in traditional ways and "often vehemently challenge the existing social order."[2]

A central concern is the issue of individual autonomy expressed in a variety of ways. One expression is that of living and working arrangements that seek independence from the money economy of the larger society. Mass and local protests against the use of nuclear power and the use and disposal of toxic substances is another expression of autonomy.

This group assumes moral responsibility for the dwindling resources of the planet by conservation measures. Consequently, nutritional patterns are often vegetarian. Another issue is concern for the second-rate status of women, racial and ethnic minorities, and other disadvantaged groups. The attempt is to bring about fundamental change in society's distribution of goods and services on the basis of fairness and need. If such youth were successful in their efforts to create basic change in social institutions, a system free of war-making machines and ideology and of greed and corruption, society would be vastly different in its goals and processes. This may mean more support for holistic health approaches and for health care as a right enjoyed equally by everyone. These new ways of youth include home deliveries and natural methods of healing. These young people will question the reasons for care provided. They expect to participate fully in the decisions affecting them and to reserve the privilege of deciding the ethical issues for themselves.

Middle Age

The years of middle age, from age 35 up to age 65, are regarded as the most productive. In these years, individuals consolidate and expand their financial and occupational security. These are years of focus on the rearing, education, and enjoyment of children. There may be additional responsibilities for aged parents. In these years, nursing plays a role in ongoing health education. There is less obstetric care and more care for growing children, in emergencies and in crises. The nurse can be a significant influence in facilitating the processes of moral deliberation in health care that guide the family in its choices of action.

Middle-aged women and men recognize that theirs is the most powerful age group, that it is they who make most decisions and carry forward social norms. Although this society is oriented toward youth, it is under the control of the middle-aged.[3] The middle-aged have most to lose from ill health, incapacitation, and death. This phase of life is the period of maximum competence in self-assessment and cognitive problem-solving abilities. The middle-aged person has developed a wide range of coping strategies. New appreciations come from in-between relationships with younger and older generations. Middle-aged persons find themselves in control and in the driver's seat, in contrast to their youth or to their expectations of old age.

Middle age can also be seen as a period of losses and crisis. Some women see menopause and the departure of grown children as tragic. Other women celebrate the launching of children into adult independence. Members of both sexes may regard the inevitable decline in youthful good looks, strength, energy, and sexual appetites as a cause of bitterness. Other individuals see these as turning points toward serenity and tender expressions of touch and caress.

The occurrence of unexpected events such as sudden serious illness, forced retirement or unemployment, or death of the spouse or of a child out of the natural sequence is highly traumatic for either young or middle-aged individuals and families. Nurses can play a supportive role by helping the family in anticipatory grieving when there is time, or by encouraging appropriate grief after an unanticipated loss. Nurses can be helpful to clients in working through feelings of unrealistic self-blame. It is the unanticipated event that is likely to cause major stresses, ". . . events that upset the sequence and rhythm of the expected life cycle."[4] Consequently, serious illness, impending death of self, or actual death of spouse or child, accidents, and loss of job or income are severe stresses to the middle-aged adult especially. The nurse can help alleviate this stress through helping the family identify its strengths and values.

Widespread social change in the form of increasing longevity for both sexes along with the inclusion of nearly half of all women in the work force emphasizes values of personhood and self-actualization for the middle-aged individual. Values of respect for self and others are expressed in demands for accessible health care oriented to the needs and rights of the adult. Women, particularly, are seeking health care that respects their sensitivities and special needs of combining a career, parenthood, marriage, homemaking, and possible further education. Women are not only living longer than men, but are expressing a new sense of freedom in their increased status, reproductive control, economic independence, and the assumption of new career and civic roles.[5]

SELECTED CASES AND PRINCIPLES

Selected cases illustrate the major ethical issues that affect the adult developmental phase. Major issues are the enforcement of patients' rights.

Prevention of Harm
Herbert, age 28, a depressed suicidal patient, tells Ms. M, the nurse, that he has a right to jump out of the 22nd-story hospital window, that he has a right to die, and that Ms. M has no right to restrain him.[6] The issue here is the patient's autonomy and self-determination versus the principles of "do no harm" and "do good," which the nurse may invoke as guides to action.

The Allocation of Scarce Resources
Phillip, age 57, an alcoholic, derelict patient claims a right to unlimited medical care, including three dialysis treatments a week at over $200.00 per treatment or more than $31,000 a year. Phillip has now applied for a kidney transplant and is on the waiting list. Should a good match occur, is it fair to give Phillip the scarce and precious organ while others go without? Phillip is not a young person making a

useful social and economic contribution to society. The issue here is whether or no any person who is noncontributing with a self-destructive life-style has unlimited rights to health care and to the community's scarce resources.

Allan, a 19-year-old college student, rode his motorcycle without wearing a helmet. One Saturday night Allan was hit by an uninsured drunken driver and sustained severe head and spinal injuries. Although employed part time, health care costs were so high that Allan qualified as a medical indigent eligible for public aid. Allan is but one of 105 motorcyclists in Washington state whose medical care was 63 percent ($1.9 millions of dollars) subsidized by public money, state and Federal, mostly Medicaid.[7] The ethical issue is over the conflict between the freedom not to wear helmets and the heavy cost to the public of medical care for injured riders. What moral reasons, if any, are there for motorcyclists to be legally forced to wear helmets and carry insurance? What moral reasons are there for the public to be forced to subsidize Allan's very costly treatment and care for the remainder of his life?

Truth-Telling and Deception

Robert, age 27, is a handsome, successful account executive on Wall Street. He seriously considers marriage to a beautiful, 21-year-old recent graduate of an "ivy league" university nursing program. His application to an exclusive health club required a comprehensive health examination. Tests and retests of his blood show him to be unmistakenly positive for the human immunodeficiency virus (HIV). Nevertheless, Robert sees advantages in marrying and not telling his nurse friend the truth. He believes that she will care for him devotedly as her husband when the disease becomes symptomatic. She has useful scientific, medical, and nursing knowledge of the treatment of disease that may prolong his life. Once infected, she will have less reason to abandon him. The examining physician and the nurse practitioner reflect on the morality of notifying the girl friend and other possible contacts of the facts of Robert's health status. Should they tell? Not to tell, while not a falsehood, is a deception.

In a case adapted from Dan Brock,[8] Edward, a high-anxiety cardiac patient with several previous near-fatal heart attacks, refuses tranquilizers. The head nurse, in consultation with the attending physician, gives Edward tranquilizers, but without Edward's knowledge or permission. The nurse does this for life-saving reasons, thus setting aside the patient's right to know what is being done to his body.[9] The other nurses, Ms. C and Ms. G, are instructed to lie about the real content and effects of the drug given. Ms. C believes the head nurse, the authority figure, knows best. Ms. G thinks the patient has the right to decide what is done to his body. Who is right?

Another example of the patient's right to know the truth about diagnosis, prognosis, proposed treatment, alternatives, risks, and benefits is a case adapted from H. Brody.[10] A 54-year-old mother of four grown children, Ms. Jones, is admitted complaining of severe abdominal pain. She fears cancer. Surgery reveals advanced cervical cancer and distant metastases. The five-year survival rate is less than 20 percent. The chief resident avoids the word "cancer." He believes that a diagnosis of incurable cancer will prompt the patient to jump out the window. The resident later tells the patient that the malignant process has been removed. The patient then confronts the nurse with the statement, "I really have cancer, don't I? And they don't want to tell me the truth." The nurse evaluates the patient's situation and her need to prepare her children, husband, and herself for dying and death. The nurse considers the possible but unlikely event that the patient will react in a self-destructive fashion to the news, and ponders the assignment of guilt and responsibility for such an act. The nurse then analyzes his or her own responsibility and loyalty to the chief resident as a member of the team in need of support in a difficult situation, and a nurse's vulnerable status in contradicting a physician's word to a patient. The nurse weighs the use of meaningful silence and verbal reflection of the patient's concern for her diagnosis and prognosis. Finally, the nurse is able to separate the issue of whether to tell the truth or not from the issues of what truth shall be told by whom and in what words and circumstances. The ethical issue has priority. The ways and means are secondary.

The Principle of Informed Consent

Another major issue is the patient's right to informed consent regarding proposed medical, diagnostic, or surgical procedures. Informed consent includes diagnosis, prognosis, and the risks, benefits, and alternatives to the proposed measures in words the patient can understand. Few patients know or are told that a second opinion before consenting to surgery is not only a form of insurance against unnecessary surgery but is paid for by such major health insurance plans as Blue Cross of New York.

Glaring examples of the failure to seek informed consent include the coercive consent of parents of mentally retarded children in the Willowbrook hepatitis experiments and the use of 600 United States Army servicemen for an LSD experiment without their knowledge.[11]

The Right to Receive and to Refuse Treatment

Another major ethical issue in the adult development phase is the right to receive and to refuse treatment.

An example is the case of John, age 32, married and with two children. His wife is unable to tolerate oral contraceptives or intrauterine devices. The couple finds condoms unsatisfactory. On the recommendation of the nurse family practitioner, the couple considers a vasectomy among the alternatives. John and his wife conclude that the best method of contraception for them is a vasectomy, since their family is the ideal size. John's request for a vasectomy is refused by the urologist who feels that John is too young and might change his mind or remarry and that the operation is irreversible.[12] The urologist may argue that the right to life includes the right to reproduce. This right is inalienable, which means John may not renounce the right to reproduce through vasectomy. The nurse family practitioner is in a dilemma concerning relationship with the family and the urologist. As patient advocate, the nurse's loyalty is to the family's autonomy and self-determination. In that case, he or she would support John's decision and furnish him with the names of other urologists. The nurse considers the possibility that in the future, after a vasectomy, the patient may remarry and bitterly resent the irreversibility of the procedure and the nurse's advice. The nurse also considers the refusal of the urologist to perform the vasectomy as an infringement on the patient's right to receive treatment. Since this urologist is the only available one in the surrounding community, the patient will have difficulty and incur financial cost in securing the services of a urologist in a distant large city. The nurse's dilemma is that of upholding the patient's right to treatment or agreeing with the urologist's right to refuse treatment on grounds of the patient's best interests.

Despite the best-intentioned and well-planned strategies, psychiatric nurses are still confronted with young, deeply disturbed psychiatric patients who refuse neuroleptic medications. An example is that of Jane, a 22-year-old, unmarried, beautiful girl who does not want to risk repulsive side effects such as tardive dyskinesia, in the form of uncontrollable grimaces, which appear in some patients. Jane, a graduate student, also regards drugs as a form of intrusion and control. She may also refuse drugs on the basis of their effects on mental acuity, the "snowed-under" or "zombie" effect. If Jane is a voluntary patient, the refusal is honored. Jane may be discharged, however, if she continues to refuse treatment and fails to improve. In extreme cases, the patient's status is converted to involuntary admission and the patient is declared incompetent and forced to take prescribed medication.

The nurse, in possession of all of the facts surrounding the use and misuse of medication and side effects of tardive dyskinesia and dystonias, may be in a genuine dilemma in relation to Jane's refusal. The nurse may deplore the sleepiness and sealing over of acute anxiety that comes from the use of medication. On the other hand, the nurse may, out of loyalty to fellow nurses and workers who prefer quiet patients, feel strongly motivated to influence or coerce Jane to

take the major tranquilizers. Another dimension of the nurse's dilemma is that of the community's desire for conformity to social norms
and laws. Community pressure on nurses and the mental health estab-
lishment to tranquilize troubled or troublesome patients raises questions concerning the nurse's role. The psychiatric nurse is placed in
the role of double agent—for the community's good versus the patient's good. In this example, what began as simple truth-telling about
the intended effects of drugs to facilitate a patient's compliance with
the drug regimen became a genuine dilemma when the psychiatric
patient refused medication on reasonable grounds.

Another case is that of Virginia, age 26, a Jehovah's Witness,
mother of three, who is wheeled into an emergency room, unconscious
and hemorrhaging as a result of a car accident. Her husband refuses
blood transfusions on religious grounds. Again, two nurses have the
problem of deciding, along with the interns, what is to be done to
either save or not save Virginia's life. What is the right thing to do,
and how would you reason to a conclusion?

The Right to Privacy and Confidentiality

A patient example that involves the nurse in a dilemma of confidentiality is also adapted from H. Brody. Jim, a young man of 26, is
brought into the emergency room following a seizure in a movie the-
ater. Jim is known to the emergency-room nursing staff because he
has previously been treated for seizures due to failure to take prescribed anticonvulsive drugs. Meanwhile, Jim drives his fellow workers in a car pool one week out of four and drives twice monthly to a
neighboring town to visit his mother. Under the licensing requirements of that state, an individual with uncontrolled seizures is ineligi-
ble for a driver's license. The patient begs that the nurses not report
him, since he depends on his driver's license and jobs are very scarce.[13]
The nurses debate the patient's right to confidentiality and privacy
versus the right of others to a safe driver who will not endanger
innocent human life.

George is a 25-year-old homosexual patient hospitalized in a large
medical center on the East Coast. He is seriously ill with AIDS related
disease and wishes to see his parents before he dies. When George left
his home on a sheep ranch in Montana at the age of 18, his parents
had no knowledge of his life-style; nor have they seen him since.
George does not want his parents to know the cause or the seriousness
of his illness or the nature of his life-style. He asks the staff to respond to his parents' questions regarding his illness as some form of
leukemia or other exotic disease of which they have no knowledge.
After three days of visiting their obviously dying son, the parents ask
the nurse "Does he have AIDS?" Should the patient's right to privacy
and confidentiality take priority over the parents' right to the truth?

Responses to AIDS related moral issues. There are three types of responses to the ethical issues raised by the AIDS epidemic. One is to reject AIDS patients as outcasts to be shunned, villified, or ignored. Some proponents of Legal Moralism claim that AIDS is a just retribution for the life-style of AIDS patients who engage in drug abuse, homosexuality, or sexual promiscuity. A difficulty with this argument is that innocent people—adults transfused with infected blood and infants born of infected mothers contract, suffer, and die of the disease. Moreover, punishing AIDS patients does not minimize the disease or its tragic consequences.

A second type of response to AIDS patients is to quarantine them; isolate them from the public. Other victims of dreaded diseases such as typhoid fever, cholera, and measles have been quarantined with the aim of saving others from contracting the disease. By placing AIDS patients in quarantine, their liberty rights, their rights of informed consent, of confidentiality and of privacy are violated. Yet the very difficult question remains of what to do with the known AIDS-infected person who actively practices prostitution without informing his or her customers of the hazard. What reason, if any, are there for violating that person's liberty rights and quaranteeing him or her?

A third response is to intervene, treat, and interact with the victims and carriers of the AIDS disease. Although health professionals incur a very slight risk of contracting AIDS by treating infected patients, active intervention is the course leading to the control and cure of this disease. Active intervention also poses risks of infection to the general public that works and socializes with unidentified AIDS and HIV positive individuals. Public education through mass media, educational institutions, and individual counseling appear to be the only alternatives to mandatory blood testing for AIDS, public exposure, and the unnecessary but certain stigma that attaches to this dreaded disease.

Intervention has the advantage that one takes care of problems by dealing with them, not by evading them. Treating AIDS victims, who require enormous amounts of highly skilled nursing care, requires demonstrations of nurses' commitment to the ethical principles of care, compassion, and altruism. The nurse, therefore, should interact with the dying son and parents mentioned earlier in a compassionate manner that facilitates their communication.

ETHICAL AND PHILOSOPHICAL CONSIDERATIONS

Reason and Freedom as Marks of Personhood
Several philosophical concepts help to clarify the cases presented. In the adult years a human being is preeminently a person who has

rights and responsibilities. In Joel Feinberg's terms, a person is said to have consciousness, a self-concept, self-awareness, the capacity to experience emotions, to reason and to acquire understanding, to plan ahead, to act on plans, and to feel pleasure and pain.[14] One could add other features of personhood, such as the capacity to form significant human relationships evident in long-term, harmonious marriage and parent-child relationships and friendships. In addition to Feinberg's conditions, H. T. Engelhardt adds a further characteristic of a person, the capacity to develop moral relationships.[15] A person, for Engelhardt and for Kant before him, is also a moral individual. A moral personality is one who lives in freedom in the sense that he or she has an internalized sense of freedom, is a rational being, and is not constrained or coerced into his or her actions, since reason, not compulsion or coercion, governs a rational person's actions. The police officer's or holdup person's pistol is not the motivating force of a free individual. He or she acts by reason.

Openness and Self-Corrective Feedback

To the extent that information is available to health professionals and is communicable and understandable, the principle of *informed consent* applies. Informed consent means that patients and subjects alike are entitled to updated information on which to base their consent or dissent to a proposed health care procedure. The publicness test once proposed by J. Rawls is relevant. According to Rawls, a procedure of justice is fair if, among other conditions, it conforms to the test of publicity.[16] This means that procedures used are openly aired. We may call this the "fishbowl" view of health care, in which procedures and processes such as x-rays are subject to public scrutiny. The growth of health care in doctors' offices may be a trend away from openness and publicity of procedures. The publicness principle or fishbowl metaphor point to the advantages of the teaching hospital, in which mistakes are used as a source of health care learning in the form of self-corrective feedback.

The Right to the Prevention of Harm

One cannot possibly guarantee the right to prevent harm in a world filled with dangers and vicissitudes. Natural catastrophes, as well as human misjudgments and foibles, do not make the world safe from chance and fatality. Instead, one has the right to live in a society that seeks to practice the prevention, or rather minimization, of harm. The concept of doing no harm figured prominently in Plato's concept of justice. To do justice consisted in not doing harm to anyone. To fail was to countenance injustice, an intolerable obstacle to being civilized. Thus, a standard was set, however woeful or deficient in practice. The prevention of harm in health care also includes the alleviation of suffering. This brings us to the case of Herbert, who believes he has a right to jump out of the 22nd-story hospital window. Ms. M, his nurse, sensing that there is a viable life in Herbert, attempts to restrain him, and succeeds. One may wonder if Ms. M is right or wrong.

A central issue of nurse-patient relationships concerns the role of negative and positive rights. Negative rights are those rights to be left alone, to choose regardless of consequences to oneself. If a person is helpless, too bad for him or her. On this view, no one has a right to be given help.

This view has recently been called the "will" or "choice" view of rights,[17] an unduly stout form of anti-Paternalism. That view seems morally impoverished, for it fails to account for a person's incapacity to express option or autonomy rights if a person is too poor, too sick, too unenlightened, and too powerless to express those autonomy or self-determination rights. There are cases in which a person does not know best and in which he or she needs help to make the wisest decision.[18] This provides a counterexample against a client's right to do whatever the client wants to do at the moment. The example of restraining Herbert shows that to identify one's autonomy right with one's choice of the moment is a faulty moral practice in nursing. Ms. M, the nurse, was justified in interfering.

There are limits to one's self-determination. Identifying one's rights with one's will and desire exclusively is not the only way to determine one's most vital rights. One may also connect one's rights to one's rational best interests. There are grounds of justified interference with one's liberty both for one's interest and for the good of others. One may be restrained from unknowingly harming oneself, as by taking medically inadvisable forms of treatment. One may also be counseled to take appropriate measures to prolong one's life where the evidence on behalf of the viability of life warrants doing so.

Recently, D. N. MacCormick developed a distinction between a "will"-based view of rights, which emphasizes values associated with freedom, and an interest-based view, which emphasizes benefits conferred equally on all persons, regardless of the capacity to exercise one's will.[19] *The United Nations Declaration of Human Rights* shows that Articles 1 to 21 are oriented by a will-based view, whereas Articles 22 to 27, which include the right to a decent standard of living and the right to health care for everyone, are oriented by an interest-based view. These newer positive rights to be cared for are rights of another kind. Such rights are not recognized by those who believe that rights are only negative rights to be free from interference by others. These newer rights include the right to food, clothing, shelter, education, and health care.

The Right to Truth-Telling and the
Avoidance of Deception

To show how rights to be cared for may have priority over liberty rights in certain cases, some examples given earlier will be considered. Robert, age 27, about to be married, does not tell the truth about his HIV positive status to his intended bride. Edward, a high-anxiety cardiac patient, is given a tranquilizer, and Ms. Jones, a woman with cervical cancer who the physician fears will jump out of the window, is not told the truth. The right to truthful information and avoidance of deception is ordinarily an important part of the right to be treated as a rational person. The truth enables a person to decide for himself or herself what course to follow. Ordinarily, a person's will-based negative rights are a vital feature of one's complement of human rights. Paternalism, too often practiced, undermines an essential aspect of one's complement of human rights. Having rights to decide shows respect for a person as a rationally autonomous being. These rights to decide include the right to be told the truth and not be brainwashed, told falsehoods, or deceived by having information withheld. For health care team members to withhold information from Robert's intended bride is a gross violation of her right to know the truth about his condition as the basis for informed consent to the marriage. The withholding of the fact that he is HIV positive interferes with his future and that of his intended bride.

According to Brock, "medical advisability" does not override a patient's precious autonomy rights by "withholding relevant information from the patient. . . ."[20] Brock appeals to "our right to control what is done to our body" to justify being given "relevant available information."[21] Brock, too, appeals to the metaphor of ownership of one's body as the basis for the right to truthful "relevant available information." The right to truthful information, in turn, serves as a moral standard for criticizing lies, deception, and withholding of information. One cannot be morally free without access to truth about one's body. The case of Ms. Jones, with cervical cancer, who was told, "We got it all," is an example of a lie and a violation of her right to know the truth about her body. In the absence of demonstrable morally compelling reasons for overriding her right, such a lie is reprehensible.

In a pinch, however, showing how rights to be cared for may have priority over liberty (autonomy) rights leads one to consider the case of Edward, the high-anxiety cardiac patient. If one believes in the moral priority of the right to prevent harm, even over truth-telling, a case may be made showing that the health team respects the fundamental interest-based rights of the patient by withholding information. The concept of medical advisability, cited in *The Patients' Bill of Rights*, may in some cases give grounds for overriding a patient's autonomy rights. Therefore, Brock rather than *The Patients'*

Bill of Rights may be mistaken. The right to live and not be seriously harmed, on an interest-based view of rights, is in a pinch prior to the right to self-determination. The health care team members may know in some selected types of cases, such as the case of Edward, that the only way to save a patient's life is not to tell him that he is being given tranquilizers. If a wise nurse believes that there is still a viable and enjoyable life to be lived in which the patient who is prevented from harm or death could retrospectively say after a time, "Thank you for not listening to me when I wanted to refuse help," then we do not think such a nurse wrongs the patients. Such a patient may become grateful for his life.

On the self-determination view, the nurse will be apt to perceive himself or herself as the servant and instrument of the patient, willing to assist the patient and to take the client at his or her word. It may be better, however, for the nurse to perceive himself or herself as a friend of the client in Aristotle's sense—one who cares with intelligence and wise judgment. One could set aside a patient's will-based rights in such cases by considering a person's more fundamental, deep, interest-based rights that are preemptive and compelling, and that shine over all else. Truth-telling is precious, but in a pinch, prevention of harm overrides truth-telling. This does not mean, however, that truth-telling is canceled, only that truth-telling has a few justifiable classes of exceptions. The Biblical injunction, "The truth shall make you free," is not vacated by a small number of morally certifiable exceptions.

Informed Consent

Truth-telling and the right to informed consent are close cousins that overlap. Nevertheless, there are differences. One difference is that truth-telling, more generic than informed consent, covers accurate information governing all health care states, processes, and procedures. Informed consent enables patients to have the right to decide whether to undergo medical procedures before they occur. Informed consent implies the patient's permission for surgery and stipulates the extent of morally permissible procedures.

Informed consent is an example of a patient's special right to adequate relevant information prior to medically invasive procedures or interventions. The infamous Tuskeegee syphilis experiment and the shameful Nazi Holocaust experiments are examples of violations of the right to informed consent. Similar violations occur when prisoners are offered early parole or other bribes in exchange for their willingness to be subjects of medical experimentation with untested drugs. Such consent may be termed consent by coercion.

But even on the principle of informed consent, there are marginal cases that give rise to legal and moral issues. One such case is the

Canterbury case. According to one writer, the *Canterbury* case involved a laminectomy "that led to unexpected paralysis, the possibility of which had not been disclosed." Judge S. Robinson reiterated the powerful moral appeal to the right to self-determination in these words:

> The root premise, fundamental in American jurisprudence[, is] that "every human being of adult years and sound mind has a right to determine what shall be done with his own body." True consent is held in this case to be contingent upon the informed exercise of a choice and thus the physician's disclosure must provide the patient an opportunity to assess available options and attendant risks. As to sufficiency of information, the court holds "The patient's right of self-decision shapes the boundaries of the duty to reveal. The right can be effectively exercised only if the patient possesses enough information to enable an intelligent choice."[22]

Thus, the right to informed consent cannot easily be overridden, according to principles of our common morality.

The Right to Respect and to Receive and to Refuse Treatment

The rights to prevention of harm, truth-telling, and informed consent imply a trilogy of patients' rights: the right to respect, the right to receive treatment, and the right to refuse treatment. The right to respect is manifested in giving kind, considerate, quality care and in honoring every patient's right to receive and to refuse treatment.

In the vasectomy case, the urologist violated the patient's right to decide whether to reproduce or not. It is, again, the patient's body.

In the case of Phillip, the 56-year-old alcoholic who demands too much, the right to receive treatment has to be weighed against the rights of others and so cannot be an absolute, unchallengeable right, for the concept of rights involves the equal rights of all. Since rights are limited by resources, no one individual can have rights to unlimited medical resources.

The case of the beautiful 22-year-old graduate student, Jane, presents a no-win situation, an unsolvable dilemma from the point of view of knowing what is best. Although the behavior-modifying drugs are indicated, some of the side effects are unknown. Since, however, no compelling moral reason, such as prevention of harm, clearly presents itself, and Jane is competent, Jane's right to refuse cannot be overridden. To override her right to refuse is to violate her autonomy rights. If Jane's symptoms worsen with danger to herself or others, her autonomous rights to refuse might be overriden in favor of her interest-based rights.

On just such grounds as the interest-based rights, one may consider the case of Virginia, the Jehovah's Witness, who is unconscious in the emergency room. Her husband refuses blood transfusions on her behalf. Is he her advocate, however? In a life-and-death situation, she, were she able to speak, might prefer to have a blood transfusion and live rather than die without one.

To respect a patient's right is to know when to honor the patient's right to refuse treatment and when to override that right. A precedent for overriding the husband's substitute decision in the Jehovah's Witness case is given by the apostle of liberty right, J.S. Mill, who writes:

> If either a public officer or anyone else saw a person attempting to cross a bridge, which had been ascertained to be unsafe and there was no time to warn him of his danger, they might seize him and turn him back without any real infringement on his liberty; for liberty consists in doing what one desires, and he does not desire to fall into the river.[23]

Mill goes on to point out that people may act to prevent a crime before it is committed and if the only function of poison were murder, "it would be right to prohibit [its] manufacture and sale."[24] There is a tacit presumption in society that life is precious. Therefore, the right to seek prevention of harm overrides the right of personal choice. So, by a parity of reasoning, one might similarly safeguard a Jehovah's Witness's real desire to live. If, however, Virginia were conscious and in need of blood transfusions, but on the basis of her religious beliefs refused, the nurse has to consider whether Virginia really prefers no blood and resulting death or prefers to have her life saved at the expense of her religious belief. Virginia's autonomy rights cannot be discounted. They may have to give way in the face of the stronger rights invested in protecting life, endorsed by the common morality. People and subcultures, as Plato long ago observed, are not islands isolated from human relationships with other people. Neither the right to receive nor to refuse treatment is sacrosanct. These are important rights, however, and cannot be ignored or sidestepped. Weighty moral reasons have to be given for overriding either the patient's right to receive or to refuse treatment. Such reasons will involve every person's equal right to respect on behalf of everyone's freedom and well-being.

The Right to Privacy and Confidentiality

Our last case is that of Jim, who drives fellow workers to work in a car pool. Jim gets seizures because he does not take prescribed medications. He begs the emergency-room nurses not to report him to the motor vehicles department. This type of case is in some ways like the *Tarasoff* case, in which a patient reportedly told his therapist that he would murder a young woman who spurned him. The patient did murder the young woman, Ms. Tarasoff, whom the psychiatrist had failed to warn on grounds of patient-therapist confidentiality. The psychiatrist might have prevented this murder.[25] Joseph Fletcher recounts a similar case to that of Jim, that of an English doctor's patient.

> A railway signalman suffers with [such] severe asthmatic attacks that he blacks out altogether. . . . The man works alone in a signal box, regulating fast, express passenger trains. At any time, he may lose consciousness and let a train be wrecked. The doctor would like to warn the company but his patient threatens to sue him for libel.[26]

The rights to confidentiality and privacy, again being crucial autonomy rights, merit high moral consideration. But there are extenuating circumstances in which the paramount right to the prevention of harm overrides even the right of confidentiality and privacy. Therefore, in the *Tarasoff* and Jim examples, the right to confidentiality and privacy may be overridden. This does not mean due regard is not given to these important autonomy rights. As with the rights to receive and to refuse treatment, they can in rare classes of justifiable exceptions be overridden, and only by demonstrably compelling reasons in which the equal freedom to live well is a central factor.

THE NURSE'S ROLE

The American Hospital Association's statement of *A Patient's Bill of Rights* may be one response to public criticism of the lack of active meaningful patient participation in hospital care. The various professional codes, such as the American Nurses' Association's *Code for Nurses with Interpretive Statements,* are another answer to the patient's need for an advocate who will defend the patient's autonomy. Malpractice and negligence suits against physicians, hospitals, and sometimes nurses are another patient response to perceived neglect, errors, or omissions of care. Another response is the hiring of a patient advocate by community health boards; this advocate functions independently of administrative control in hospitals. Other hospitals have employed persons, usually nurses, called patient relations coordinators, who respond to patient complaints and problems. The most effective hope for patient advocates, however, is in nurses intelligently involved in patient care. Although participants in hospital technology and bureaucracy, nurses are the main source of personal, intimate, and continuous contact with patients. More than any other health professionals, nurses have frequent opportunities to facilitate and manifest respect for patients' rights. Modern hospital care and medical technology have largely developed into a team effort of highly specialized members. Nurses are that part of the team implementing the delivery of that care to a particular individual. This provides the nurse with frequent opportunities to inform and to educate the patient, to tell patients the truth about the procedure that the nurse or another professional is about to do in terms the patient can understand. The nurse has many opportunities to inform patients about special diets and the indications for those diets. The nurse who gives medications can inform patients about drugs given, dosages, and expected effects and side effects. The nurse can convey accurate information concerning the patient's body temperature, blood pressure, and laboratory reports.

These nursing practices of health teaching and counseling function to convey truthful information to patients and to facilitate the individual's responsibility for his or her own health.[27] The patient's possession of information regarding health status enhances the patient's independence and self-determination in decisions of health care. Accurate information contributes to the possibility of the patient's choice of the best option among alternatives.

The nurse's respect for persons extends beyond self and patient. It includes others who share in care, such as physicians, social workers, and family. Ideally, therefore, nurses jointly resolve such major issues as telling a young or middle-aged adult the truth about a fatal diagnosis. One goal is to seek consensus among team members concerning how the truth will be communicated to the patient, who will be the bearer of bad news, and what hope can realistically and honestly be given to the patient. In this way, each member of the team is prepared to support the patient's exploration of what it means to receive a diagnosis of a serious, life-threatening, or fatal diagnosis. Since nurses have the most intimate and continuous contact with patients receiving such news, nurses are in the forefront of those who show respect for the patient and for the patient's right to receive and to refuse treatment. Nurses respect the patient's right to information by answering all of the patient's questions, explicit as well as implicit, in a relevant, accurate, sympathetic, and understandable way, as friends of the patient. This means that the patient is not burdened with technical or anatomical details in which he or she has no interest. When, for example, the patient asks how irradiation or chemotherapy will affect him or her, this indicates a knowledge deficit about the side effects, which the nurse fills with relevant facts only.

If the patient inquires about life after a colostomy or similar radical surgery, the nurse again shows respect for patients by sharing relevant information and experiences helpful to educating the patient. The nurse is sensitive to feelings and what are perceived as unstated questions, such as "Can I have sex after a colostomy?" A nurse who lacks up-to-date knowledge has the obligation to tell the patient that he or she doesn't know but will find out or communicate with others who do know. The nurse's duty then is to return to the patient with the latest information or to refer the question to someone more capable of response.

Respect for persons imply patients' rights to know as well as not to know diagnosis, prognosis, treatment alternatives, risks, and benefits. An individual may simply say, "I don't want to know what I have. Just do what you think best. You're the experts." But does the right to know imply the right to decide not to know. There are two possible responses the nurse might give to such an individual. One is to offer unconditional support for the patient's right not to know—a statement such as, "It's your right not to know, since this is your body, after all, and you'll decide when you want to know what is happening and being done to your body." This statement supports the patient's right not to know, while clearly indicating that the choice to receive or to refuse treatment is almost always up to the patient. In this way, the nurse indicates the patient's strong right to seek knowledge when, where, and from whom the patient wishes. The nurse's statement defines and supports the patient's autonomy. As time passes, the patient's defense-mechanism processes of denial lessen. The patient then becomes concerned about what is happening in and to his or her body and seeks to regain control on the basis of relevant information.

A different nursing response is that given by Mary Kohnke, who recommends confronting the client with the consequences of not knowing. Kohnke's experience is that the client agrees to know certain things and not others. The nurse then records what the client has and has not been told and why.[28] The patient's family is often the first to know the presence of cancer, for example, from the surgeon, while the patient is still in the intensive care or recovery room. Some families specifically request that the patient not be told of the cancer, or of the extent of its life-threatening properties. There are several objections that nurses in contact with the family can offer to this position. One argument is that not all cancers are fatal. Some cancers may be cured. Other cancers may be treated with good life expectancies for the patient. Only a few cancers are immediately fatal. The second argument is that the patient will naturally want to know the outcome of the surgery and the reason for such treatments as irradiation or chemotherapy. It is the patient's right to know. A third argument is that the nurses' and physicians' primary relationship is with the patient. The relationship is based on trust and honesty. The patient has the right to a truthful answer to the question of "Did you find cancer?"

Educating and informing the patient of his or her diagnosis, prognosis, proposed treatments, risks, benefits, and alternatives tends to raise questions in the patient's mind—such questions as "Do I want to suffer the side effects of chemotherapy for the small and remote possibility of a short remission of my leukemia?"

Another moral issue for the nurse is the question of supporting the patient's right to receive and to refuse treatment. The example of the young father of two whose wife agreed to a vasectomy as the best method of contraception is a case in point of the importance of the nurse's role in supporting patients' rights. Despite the nurse's own misgivings regarding the possibility that the client might change his mind about having more children and the urologist's denial of that right, the *Code for Nurses* supports the client's moral right

> to determine what will be done with his/her person; to be given the information necessary for making informed judgments; to be told the possible effects of care; and to accept, refuse or terminate treatment.[29]

In accordance with the Code, once the nurse is satisfied that the patient has a complete understanding of the procedure, including the fact that it is irreversible, and that the wife concurs, the nurse is obligated to refer the patient to another physician or facility for a vasectomy in as helpful a way as referring a patient for surgery, such as a herniorrhaphy. It is the patient's right to receive treatment of his choice.

The right of psychiatric patients to refuse treatment is more complex because exercise of this right may delay the patient's recovery and return to the community. The use of neuroleptic drugs carry the low probability of undesirable side effects, some of which are irreversible. The possibility that a young woman may develop unsightly muscular movements of her lips, mouth, face, or extremities is an unhappy one. The possibility that the same young woman will languish in a mental institution without treatment and become progressively disturbed over a long period of time is also an unhappy one. The situation becomes one of trade-off—the drugs versus prolonged illness. In these cases, the nurse depends on an accurate store of knowledge of the particular drugs prescribed, the possible side effects, and the effectiveness of the measures used to control side effects. The nurse supports the patient's participation in regulating the dose, the timing of administration, and the possibility of drug holidays in conjunction with the physician and the goals of the treatment plan.

The alternative is for the nurse to support the patient's refusal of drugs, with disclosure of the full range of consequences to the patient and possibly to the nurse. Kohnke recommends that the advocate support the patient's decision without "falling into a defending or rescuing position, in which responsibility for decision making belongs to the advocate and not the client . . . supporting a client's right to make a decision does not mean giving approval for the decision."[30]

One could disagree with Kohnke's position on the grounds that the patient's perception of the nurse's support of refusal of surgery, of neuroleptic drugs, or of electroconvulsive therapy is one of approval. Colleagues may share the same perception. Even some nurses view their role as one of rescuing patients who are victims of the excesses of medical technology in the form of radical surgery and radical drugs. In such examples, patients tend to react globally to the physician as omnipotent and lifesaving or to the nurse as one who really knows the qualifications of the physician and the merits of the case.

The effective nurse tries to avoid the position of broker or intermediary between physician and patient. Instead, the nurse informs and educates the patient regarding measures designed to restore health and prevent illness. The nurse recognizes the physician as a valuable ally in attempting to reach the patient's health goals. The nurse seeks to involve the physician in the process of the patient's deliberations in every possible way.

One way of supporting the patient's right to receive and to refuse treatment is to inform the physician that the patient has questions and doubts bearing upon prescribed treatment. Another way to involve physicians in patients' deliberative processes is to suggest that the patient formulate and write down relevant questions for discussion over the phone or during a visit. The patient's right to a consultation or second opinion is part of what it means to have the right to know.

The nurse who informs patients of the content and therapeutic purpose of nursing actions as their right to know effectively helps demystify medical and hospital infallibility. The nurse is an approachable person who shares expertise and encourages the patient to ask questions of nurses, physicians, and technicians relevant to the patient's illness and recovery.

Unlike the nurse's advocate role in protecting infants and children from harm, the nurse working with adults promotes the autonomy and self-determination of his or her patients. Through nursing activities aimed at case finding, educating, and counseling the patient, the nurse consciously seeks to facilitate the patient's exercise of rights to information concerning diagnosis, prognosis, treatment, risks, benefits, costs, and alternatives as the basis for informed consent and the right to receive and to refuse treatment. In this respect, a nurse functions as a health educator, which is a valuable form for expressing nurse advocacy.

CONCLUSION

Adults are more independent and also more interdependent than other persons, including children and the elderly. Nursing care correspondingly is more verbal and interactive with adults than with younger and older age groups. The adult span is the longest, most significant aspect of personhood and the standard for judging qualities and degrees of personhood. Cases were cited illustrating the centrality of ethical issues. These were discussed under several topics: prevention of harm, truth-telling, informed consent, the right to receive and to refuse treatment, and privacy and confidentiality. These cases dovetailed with key provisions of *A Patient's Bill of Rights* and the *Code for Nurses*.

The ethical issues considered in these topics and cases centered on the values of freedom and autonomy, rationality, well-being, and optimum health care. These ideals are buffeted by world social and economic realities: a growing population with more demands than resources. There are also conflicts within these goals. Prevention of harm, for example, may collide with freedom of expression of a Jehovah's Witness. There are other moral conflicts. New, hard cases sometimes refute entrenched principles.

The relation of principle to practice shows that, to paraphrase Kant, principles without nursing practices are empty; but nursing practices without principles are blind. For moral principles are like the stars or beacons that guide the nursing and health care navigators through the shoals of ethical and clinical challenges. These moral principles are part of the common morality, which function as moral standards and a steady rebuttal that all values are solely relative to time and place. It is frustrating that there is no one principle, but rather a plurality of them, requiring thought and choice without certainty. That, however, is the price one pays for being human and working in the ethics of adult health care without surrendering to dogma.

Nursing implications show how the principles of the common morality are implemented in daily health care practices. These nursing practices, in turn, show how the principles are strengthened or weakened in accord with Kant's principle that he who agrees with the ends also agrees with the means.[31]

Discussion Questions

1. What moral reasons, if any, are there for persons in high risk groups to be subject to mandatory testing?
2. Are insurance companies entitled to test applicants of high risk groups? Why or why not?
3. What moral reasons are there for arguing that helmetless motorcycling is morally permissible or impermissible?

REFERENCES

1. Keniston K. Youth and its ideology. In: Arieti S. (ed). *American Handbook of Psychiatry*. Vol. 1, 2nd ed. New York: Basic Books; 1974: 422.
2. Ibid; 403.
3. Neugarten BL, Datan N. The middle years. In: *American Handbook of Psychiatry*. 596.
4. Ibid: 606.
5. Ibid: 593.
6. Bandman E. The dilemma of life and death: Shall we let them die? *Nursing Forum*. 1978. *17*(2):118–132.
7. Study cites public expense of injuries to motorcyclists. *The New York Times*, July 14, 1988: B7.
8. Brock D. The nurse-patient relation: Some rights and duties. In: Beauchamp T, Walters L. (eds). *Contemporary Issues in Bioethics*. 2nd ed. Belmont, CA: Wadsworth; 1982: 144.
9. Bandman B, Bandman EL. The nurse's role in an interest-based view of patients' rights. In: Spicker S, Gadow S. (eds). *Nursing: Images and Ideals*. New York: Springer; 1980: 135.
10. Brody H. *Ethical decisions in medicine*. 2nd ed. Boston: Little, Brown, 1981: 46–47.
11. Bandman EL, Bandman B. Rights are not automatic. *Am J Nurs*. 1977. 77(5):867.
12. Brody. *Ethical decisions in medicine*. 41.
13. Ibid; 53.
14. Feinberg J. The problem of personhood. In: *Contemporary Issues in Bioethics*. 108–116.
15. Engelhardt HT. Medicine and the concept of person. In: *Contemporary Issues in Bioethics*. 95.
16. Rawls J. *A theory of justice*. Cambridge, MA: Harvard University Press; 1971: 133.
17. Hart HLA. Bentham on legal rights. In: Simpson AWB (ed). *Jurisprudence*. New York: Oxford University Press; 1973: 170–201.
18. Bandman E. *The dilemma of life and death*.
19. MacCormick DN. Rights in legislation. In: Hacker P, Raz J. (eds). *Law, Morality and Society: Essays in Honor of H.L.A. Hart*. New York: Oxford University Press; 1977: 188–209.
20. Brock D. *The nurse-patient relation*. 145.
21. Ibid.
22. Beauchamp T. The disclosure of information. In: *Contemporary Issues in Bioethics*. 172.
23. Mill JS. *Utilitarianism, liberty and representative government*. London: Dent; 1948: 151.
24. Ibid.
25. California Supreme Court, *Tarasoff v. Regents of the University of California*, 131 California Reporter. In: *Contemporary Issues in Bioethics*. 204–210.
26. Fletcher J. *Morals and medicine*. Boston: Beacon; 1954: 58.

27. American Nurses' Association. *Nursing: A social policy statement*. Kansas City, MO: Author; 1980: 18.
28. Kohnke MF. *Advocacy: Risk and reality*. St. Louis: Mosby; 1982: 18.
29. American Nurses' Association. *Code for nurses with interpretive statements*. Kansas City, MO: Author; 1976: 4.
30. Kohnke. *Advocacy: Risk and Reality*. 5.
31. Kant I. *Fundamental principles of the metaphysics of morals*. Indianapolis: Bobbs-Merrill; 1949: 34.

CHAPTER 13

Ethical Issues in the Nursing Care of the Aged

Study of this chapter will enable the learner to:

1. Understand the developmental tasks of the aged in relation to ethical problems of health care.
2. Identify ethical issues of special relevance to the aged, such as the macro and micro level of allocation of scarce resources, rights, competence, and quality of life.
3. Formulate the role of the nurse as patient advocate in facilitating the aged person's participation in shared decision making on the basis of goals, values, and rational life plans.
4. Utilize Utilitarian and Kantian principles to analyze lifeboat, triage, cost/benefit, and lottery methods of allocating health care.

INTRODUCTION

According to one viewpoint, growing old is and ought to be a special time to anyone fortunate enough to have reached old age. Old age is a time for savoring and evaluating life's myriad experiences of people, places, and events shared with intimates and with strangers. One's older years provide an opportunity to reflect on the time left rather than regret the time of life spent. Life goals and processes take on special significance, like the last brilliant colors of autumn.

DEVELOPMENT OF THE AGED

Since the passage of federal Social Security legislation, the age of 65 has become a developmental landmark. It marks the entry point into old age. Time has, however, different meanings for the aged. Some predominantly grieve the death of a spouse, relations, and friends, and mourn the passing of happier years. Others mainly look forward to the time with optimistic anticipation. All fervently hope for health and independence.

Some persons at the age of 65 are little changed from the middle years, except for differences in their use of time and perhaps money. If they have been fortunate enough to escape disease, they look upon themselves as competent, complete, and capable of independence and self-care. Physical changes such as lessening of the sexual drive occur without diminishing desires for intimacy and affection expressed in touch and caress. As men lose some muscularity and women lose their rounded contours, both sexes look more alike. Likewise, men "become less aggressive and women more assertive as they enter old age and both tend to diminish their activities and become less involved with people."[1] Old friends, relatives, and family become more important, since new friends tend to be less involved. Spouse relationships become more interdependent as the need for help increases. Sexual activity may continue into advanced old age in some cases. The wife regards the growing number of widows with alarm and guards her husband's health jealously.

Lidz reports research done by Reichard[2] and her collaborators in 1962 identifying personality types among men who adjusted well or poorly to retirement. Reichard identified the mature type of man who accepted himself realistically and found satisfying activities and relations. The dependent type of man freed of responsibility also found compensation for old age and retirement. Another well-adjusted group protected themselves against their fear of decline and death by keeping active and maintaining strong defenses.

There are several modes of adjustment to old age. Lidz favors the elderly person's acceptance of limitations such as diminished physical capacities, income, and significance to the lives of others. In his view, old age can be a time of growth through sharing the individual's experience, knowledge, and wisdom in ways useful to others. Growth can be achieved by developing new interests and neglected talents. The indispensable element of time is available to "contemplate, observe, and join the many strands together."[3]

Advanced Old Age

Advanced old age is viewed as beginning at the age of 75. Persons of this age hope "to live out their lives with dignity, to remain capable of caring for themselves and their spouses, to continue managing things between themselves."[4] These elderly people hope to be useful, if not significant, to others. They also hope not to become burdens through illness or senility. Some are serene and content, despite the ever present fear of needing a nursing home or mental hospital care.

The Frail Elderly

Eventually, the elderly become frail and must depend on others, including nurses. Such dependencies can provoke family conflict and apprehension in the elderly individual in need of help.

The nurse caring for elderly patients in the community or in health care facilities can play a significant role in maintaining respect for each person by the time, attention, and quality of nursing care provided. Medical technology such as improved cataract operations with implanted contact lenses, electronic hearing aids, and motorized wheelchairs can be of great assistance to the elderly with such needs.

Hospitalization may be a threat that becomes actualized for the elderly fearing separation, mutilation, pain, and incapacitation. The hospital may be seen as a last resort from which the individual is transferred to a nursing home because of the inability to care for himself or herself. Here home care nursing has a role.

The Person with Dementia

For the aged person living in the community with assistance, the hospital and surgery experience may necessitate transfer to a nursing home. A radical prostatectomy for a man of 80 to 90 years who is confused and forgetful may emphasize his growing dependence on others for what was formerly part of self-care. It may then become obvious to everyone that the critical integrative functions of memory, judgment, and problem solving are seriously impaired. That individual must be given full-time nursing care and supervision. On the other hand, all elderly persons may be completely but temporarily disoriented by the toxic effects of drugs, anesthesia, dehydration, anoxia, diabetes, and urine retention, to name but a few possible causes. As soon as the illness is cleared up, the individual becomes oriented and rational, and is discharged with community nursing supervision. It follows, then, that each elderly person, no matter what the diagnosis, requires respect and attention. A prejudgment of dementia may be premature or inaccurate.

The most characteristic feature of dementia is memory failure regarding recent events, with only memories of childhood left. Demented persons then both live and act as if in the past, and are unable to care for themselves. Such persons are disoriented as to time and place and need monitoring.[5] There is some loss of control of emotions. Impulses, suspicion, and anger are freely expressed. Loss of inhibitions and judgment may occur, followed by masturbation and sexual advances to children. The onset of dementia may be gradual or suddenly precipitated by circulatory deficits, drug toxicity, trauma, death of a spouse, or a move to a new and complex environment.

The quality of health care and human services given in these homes is a direct reflection of the respect for the rights of the aged person to a decent, fulfilling life. A society that rejects its old and consigns them to brutalized care in virtual warehouses suffers from ethical insensitivity and moral callousness. However, no previous society has been faced with the numbers of aged persons now living and the responsibility for providing for them.

A sad story is told about a prison physician who amputates a prisoner's mutilated finger and, as he throws it into the garbage can, says to the prisoner, "You won't be needing that anymore." Such a remark captures the belief that old people are symbolized by the amputated finger, fit only for waste disposal. Some old people feel acutely that they will not be needed any more, and that they no longer rate having their needs satisfied. The television play *Patterns* presents a biting portrait of a vice-president who is older than other executives and is not wanted any more by the firm's president. A dilemma for society is meeting the needs of the elderly, with all the utilization of health care resources this implies, or limiting this utilization of these resources on grounds of fairness to other age groups.

PROBLEMS AND PROSPECTS FOR THE AGED

Erik Erikson views old age as the ripening period for the fruits of earlier stages. It is, he says, the result of taking care of things and people, of bearing and rearing children, or generating products and ideas, and of adjusting to the inevitable triumphs and disappointments of life. He calls this ripening process "ego integrity. It is the acceptance of one's one and only life cycle as something that had to be and that . . . permitted of no substitutions. . . ."[6] Lidz characterizes Erikson's "integrity" as the phase that "requires the wisdom to realize that there are no 'ifs' in life; that one was born with certain capacities, a set of parents, . . . the past cannot be altered. . . . It is too late to start out on a new life."[7] Integrity means one recognizes one has fewer "ifs," fewer options. In later life one rounds out one's goals and way of life, but does not start anew. To Erikson, even for the poorest of human beings who understands that birth into a particular culture at a particular time is an historical accident, but who has lived by its precepts with the awareness of integrity, death has no sting. The one and only life cycle is accepted as final, and death is not feared. For those persons living with integrity, old age can be a harvest of contentment and pleasure. Lidz points to the relief from striving and struggle that comes from the lessening of the passions and of unful-filled ambitions. Leisure can be rewarding, as can be the achievements of grandchildren or the societies and organizations one helped develop. It can be, in Lidz's words, "a time of relaxed closure of life that still contains much to experience and enjoy."[8]

In comparison, Butler views this picture of the tranquility and serenity of old age enjoying the fruits of labor as mythical. It does not square with the values of the general public and its disdain and ne-glect of the elderly. He sees ageism as a national prejudice based on a systematic stereotyping and discrimination against older people. Older people tend to be classified as ugly, rigid, senile, garrulous, and as less than full human beings. As with any form of prejudice, the aged victims believe this negative definition to be true, place a negative value on themselves, and expect and accept the discriminatory treat-ment given them. Other negative societal attitudes stem from the high values placed on productivity, with contempt given the nonpro-ducer. Significantly, this society places positive values on youth and negative values on the aged. Prejudice against the old may be a mani-festation of the inability to face the inevitabilities of one's own aging process and death.[9]

The personal realities of one's own aging process may be psychoso-cial, others economic, and still others may be reflections or symptoms of the advent of disease. The majority of the aged are women, of whom more than half were widows in 1975. The imbalance between men and women increases with age.[10] Twenty-six percent of the elderly live alone, 36 percent with a spouse,[11] and 95 percent are able to live in the community. Eighty-six percent of the elderly have one or more chronic health problems.[12] It is with this 86 percent of the aging population, plus the 5 percent of the institutionalized aged, that nurses are involved. It is with this 91 percent of the aged, primarily, that moral issues and dilemmas arise.

Siegel notes the social and economic implications for health serv-ices related to the aged in this society. An obvious finding is that the elderly are the largest users of health resources.[13] Demand and need rise with age. It follows, therefore, that an increasing amount of health care resources will be utilized for an increasing number of aged persons. This raises ethical issues of the allocation of limited re-sources. Moreover, as health care and medicine improve their technol-ogy, such as drugs, organ transplants, surgery, and dialysis, the elderly will increase their utilization. Additionally, the availability of insurance plans, such as Medicaid and Medicare, support more equal and thereby increased utilization of health care resources by all in-come groups. However, the scarce distribution of health care resources remains problematic to the elderly in inner cities and in nonurban areas.[14]

Another problem is the need to gear health services toward aged women because of their much higher proportion among the elderly population. With declining birth rates, the aged person will have fewer siblings or relatives and less of a family support system. This raises ethical issues of enabling aged persons to die if they choose, versus requiring them to prolong their lives. The plight of these elderly persons also raises issues regarding the obligations of their offspring, who may be supporting their own children. The proportion of smaller kinship networks also raises issues concerning a greater role for government in providing health and human services to the elderly and raises problems of the allocation of limited resources. Some writers, like N. Daniels, advocate a life-long rationing scheme into which one contributes, analogous to social security.[15] Another aspect of the allocation of limited resources concerns the quality of care given the 5 percent of the elderly who reside in nursing homes and other group-care facilities. These persons may be institutionalized to provide needed care for their incapacities or for social convenience. The moral issue is the provision of care that enhances the human dignity and health status of the aged. Some elderly persons in nursing homes have been neglected, exist on substandard food, and in unsafe environmental conditions. The provision of adequate and appropriate nursing services could make a significant difference in the care of the elderly.

Moral problems of distributive justice arise in acutely felt ways for the very old and frail and for those who are terminally ill. Do they have a right to decide to live with dignity and to choose when to terminate life support systems? Or are they required to live as long as they breathe?

SELECTED CASES AND PRINCIPLES

We will consider eight fairly typical cases that involve moral issues in the health care of the elderly.

Case 1: Allocation of Scarce Resources. Mr. H, a 23-year-old motorcycle accident victim, is seriously injured and requires a life-support system in the intensive care unit. There are no empty beds. Ms. K, 66, in coma following a major stroke and on a life-support system, is the oldest patient in the intensive care unit. The nurse must recommend which of these two patients will be given the cardiopulmonary support unit.

Case 2: Assisting the Patient with Suicide. "Suicide rates for males are higher after age 65 than in younger men. That is because male suicide rates increase from age 15 to 85 in a straight line."[16] There is a substantial increase in suicides of both sexes in the age category of 75 and above.[17]

Ms. A covers the night shift for an ill member of the regular staff. One of her patients is Dr. D, age 75, a well-known neurosurgeon and a retired member of the medical school faculty. He has recently been admitted for severe, intractable back pain with increasing difficulty in walking. His wife is dead, and his three children are successful medical practitioners. Dr. D lives alone with domestic help in the same large home in the suburbs and attends medical meetings. Since his radical prostatectomy for a malignancy, his medical practice ceased. There is every reason to believe that examinations performed on this admission will reveal extensive metastatic cancer to the spine. Dr. D may well suspect his true prognosis despite the professionally cheerful and respectful manner staff members accord to him. Ms. A gives him the prescribed injection of narcotics in response to his request. As she turns to leave the room, the patient asks the nurse to open the window wide for ventilation. The room is on the 18th floor, and the window is without a screen. The possibility of suicide crosses the nurse's mind. She wonders if it is not Dr. D's right to determine what shall be done with his disease-ridden, pain-wracked body. She also thinks about the sanctity of every life and the irreversibility of this act. What reasons are there for the nurse either to open or not to open the window?

Case 3: A Patient's Right to Decide. Mr. M was an unmarried 82-year-old resident of a nursing home, independent in self-care but needing assistance in dressing, and able to ambulate with a walker. Despite occasional episodes of memory loss and confusion, he continued to care for himself. His loss of hearing interfered with social activities, but he resisted the use of a hearing aid. The development of dysuria led to the diagnosis of benign prostatic hypertrophy and the recommendation of a transurethral prostatectomy operation. When informed of the necessity for surgery, Mr. M readily consented. His nephew and only relative, however, refused to consent to surgery on the grounds that due to the uncle's mental status, his life was without dignity and should not be sustained by extraordinary means. The nephew believed that the uncle had already lived a long life anyway. The nurse appealed for consent for surgery, but to no avail. Without the surgery, Mr. M's condition rapidly declined, and he died unnecessarily of uremic complications within six weeks. What of the patient's right to decide to accept or to refuse treatment and the nurse's role as patient advocate?

Case 4: Competence and the Patient's Right to Refuse. George Annas relates the case of a 60-year-old woman, Ms. Yetter, who had been involuntarily committed to a mental hospital with a diagnosis of schizophrenia. A lump in her breast was discovered and a biopsy ordered, to be followed by a mastectomy if the biopsy showed malignant tissue. Ms. Yetter refused permission for the procedure on the grounds that she was afraid of the operation because her aunt had died following a similar procedure. Moreover, she believed the surgery would interfere with her genital system and prevent her from having babies and a career in the movies. The judge decided that although she was delusional, she consistently refused the surgery even in lucid periods. Therefore, the court found Ms. Yetter competent to refuse the biopsy.[18] What reasons would justify continuing attempts to persuade Ms. Yetter to consent to the surgery or to refrain from attempting to persuade her on the grounds that the patient is "competent"?

Case 5: A Conflict of Rights. Another related case reported by G. Annas involves

> a 77-year-old woman who suffered from gangrene and who refused to undergo a recommended amputation. Although the court found that the patient was combative, . . . that her train of thought wandered and her conception of time was distorted, it also found that she demonstrated a high degree of awareness and acuity. The patient made clear that she did not wish to have the operation, even though she knew that decision would probably lead shortly to her death. . . .[19]

She made a choice fully aware of the consequences and was therefore "found to be competent."[20] The court said, "The law protects her right to make her own decision to accept or reject treatment, whether this decision is wise or unwise."[21] The moral issue is whether the nurse is to educate the patient regarding the nature of gangrene and the importance of amputation as a condition for the patient's survival or simply supports the patient's decision as an act of self determination?

Case 6: A Case of Truth-Telling. Ms. G, a 68-year-old active, independent, cheerful grandmother who smokes heavily, is admitted to the hospital for an acute bout of pneumonia requiring intensive care. Her diagnostic tests reveal a widespread metastatic inoperable cancer of the lungs. She is expected to live but a few months. Her devoted children and husband are told the diagnosis while the patient is in intensive care. The family insists that the patient not be told the truth so that the patient's remaining time at home will be as happy as possible. When her nurse comes into the room to prepare her for discharge, Ms. G speaks to the nurse. She says, "I know that I've had a lot of special tests and x-rays of my lungs. I have the feeling that something important is being kept from me. I believe that I have the right to know what's wrong with me." The issue is the patient's right to know the truth.

Case 7: The Nurse as Patient Advocate. This example is adapted from V. Barry.[22] It involves a 78-year-old, independent, nearly deaf convalescent-home patient named Ms. R. The patient had suffered a cerebrovascular accident (stroke), and her prognosis was uncertain. She was a difficult patient to please. Her family was devoted and concerned. Ms. R contracted a case of flu and the family demanded reasons of the nurse as to why Ms. R seemed to be getting worse and why she had not been seen by her physician. On admission, the physician reportedly told the family that with rest and physical therapy, Ms. R would soon be her old self. The nurse knew, however, that when the head nurse called the doctor for medication and treatment, "he instructed her simply to have us make" R "as comfortable as possible because she wasn't going to last very long anyway."[23] The nurse concluded:

> I knew, of course, that professionally I should keep my mouth shut and not make anybody look bad. But I felt sorry for R., and I thought the daughter-in-law was getting the runaround.[24]

Barry then asks what the reader would do if he or she were the nurse. Barry then cites some alternatives, one of which is to tell what the nurse knows. Another alternative for the nurse is to put on the professional hat and "stonewall" the daughter-in-law. Another alternative is to refer the daughter-in-law to one's superiors, again the professionally approved route. There is also the problem of not saying anything derogatory about a doctor, fellow nurse, or hospital. There is also the moral issue of the nurse, as patient advocate, informing the daughter-in-law that the physician has not seen the patient for two months despite being notified of the patient's illness and decline. What is the nurse justified in doing?

Case 8: Allocation of Nursing Resources. Barry reports an essentially true case. A, a law professor, aged 84, was considered to be a "brilliant jurist and legal scholar." He was a giant of a man, and he had an admirable "sense of independence," which even "bordered on conceit."[25] He was married to Kate for over 50 years. They were childless but proud of their independence. At 82, he first suffered from diabetes. By 84 he lost his sight and hearing. He then suffered a total heart block and needed a pacemaker. His independence vanished by painful degrees. He was diapered and put on a waterbed mattress. Professor A's self-esteem suffered, in addition to the pain of his physical losses.

Adapted somewhat from Barry's account, the scenario continues. The hospital physician concluded that Professor A no longer needed the facilities of an acute care setting. Much against his wife's wishes, he was transferred to a facility giving highly skilled nursing care. His wife visited him every day. She was at his bedside from early morning to early evening. Although she participated in and observed the high level of skilled nursing care he was given, she respectfully but continually interrupted the nurses' work with other patients because of her extreme solicitude for her husband. She held his hand, watched his face, and rang for the nurse every time he moved or made a sound. Some nurses on the unit felt that Professor A was receiving more than his fair share of the available nursing care on that unit and gave reasons for curtailing the time and resources spent on him. These nurses argued for the Utilitarian concept of the greatest happiness of the greatest number. Other nurses on the unit argued that this patient and his wife needed and deserved that care, as should every other patient on that unit. These nurses argued for the Kantian principle of treating every patient as an end and not solely as a means. The problem was to determine what was a fair distribution of limited nursing services.

ETHICAL-PHILOSOPHICAL CONSIDERATIONS IN THE NURSING CARE OF THE AGED

Five Methods of Allocating Health Care
There are five alternative methods of distributing health care: (1) the Holmes lifeboat method (Egoist); (2) the triage or some cost/benefit calculation of worth (Utilitarian); (3) the lottery method of treatment; (4) equal shares; and (5) equal consideration.

The Lifeboat Method
The Holmes method stems from a shipwreck in 1846 in which the officer in charge of a lifeboat, Mr. Holmes, ordered the "unfit" thrown overboard. Rescue followed shortly, and the moral question remains to this day whether Holmes should have been charged with the murder for which he was found legally guilty. The lifeboat method is the Egoist solution, sometimes called "survival of the fittest." The lifeboat method does not, however, save or serve a maximum number of persons. Nor does it work in the long run by helping a large-scale, complex culture to flourish. Among those thrown overboard, for example, may be some who are physically unfit but intellectually more fit to help the whole group survive. On this ground, the nurse's decision in Case 1 is to allocate the life-support system to the younger person and in effect throw Ms. K overboard.

The idea that old people belong on the scrap heap, illustrated in examples of neglect and ignoring the needs of the elderly in Cases 3 and 7, is morally callous. One argument against lifeboat morality is the classic "is-ought" fallacy that what is, such as existing power, does not by itself justify what ought to be. In effect, the is-ought fallacy exposes the invalidity of the claim that "might makes right." There are additional powerful positive moral arguments on behalf of allocating limited health care resources to the elderly. One argument is the appeal to Rawls's "veil of ignorance,"[26] in which one agrees to rules without knowing one's life circumstances.

The Utilitarian Method

A second method of allocation to the elderly is addressed in ethics by Utilitarianism. The Utilitarian emphasis is on providing the greatest happiness for the majority. Since the elderly constitute only 10 percent of the population, one might argue that they do not, on that ground alone, have much claim to limited social and economic resources. If one adds another Utilitarian argument to the previous one, that the elderly are less likely to grow to be as productive and creative as children, adolescents, and young adults, one may conclude that the elderly deserve less than younger people. A rejoinder to this point is that the elderly as a group helped the young and adults to achieve; therefore, the elderly now merit the allocation of health care resources that they helped make available. The elderly also collectively contribute to the quality of human life through their experience and their wisdom. A variation of this view holds that society owes the elderly for what they contributed in the past.

Readers of Mill's version of Utilitarianism will appreciate Mill's conception of the quality of human life as more than the quantity of pleasure. The quality of human life for Mill means that it is better to be "a human being dissatisfied than a pig satisfied; better to be Socrates dissatisfied than a fool satisfied.[27] A patient who wishes not to be kept alive under all conditions appeals to the "quality of life argument. A refined form of Utilitarianism recognizes the equal right of each individual to happiness regardless of age, sex, race, color, or creed. This view is expressed in Bentham's famous rule cited by Mill that "everyone is to count for one, nobody for more than one.[28] The emphasis on equality, on the equal right of everyone to count, implies a restraint on crude Utilitarianism, which either rules by a hypothetical majority that old people do not deserve ample resources or that it is enough to repay old people for what they did. For if everyone counts equally, no persons, young or old, are likely to pursue happiness by voting against their interests.

A similar principle is expressed by Kant's substantive principle "to treat humanity, whether in thine own person or in that of any other, in every case as an end, never as means only."[29] Kant's principle—to treat people as ends—along with his categorical imperative to act so that one's action is at the same time a universal moral law calls for equal treatment of all people, regardless of their intellectual, cultural, or economic contributions or age.

A practical Utilitarianism health care goal calls for a maximum number of persons, but not everyone, to be helped. The "optimum number" and "everyone" may make a telling difference, especially in crunch cases in which the only practical moral solution is to apply triage. Triage serves the maximum number. Triage in health care emergencies means that one sorts people out into three groups: the worst off, who will die anyway; the best off, who will be most likely to recover on their own or with little help; and the median group, those to whom maximum medical and health care attention will be most likely to make the most difference. Since one has limited health care resources, one serves the largest number by distinguishing them into these three groups and singling out the median group on whom to confer benefits. Triage implies the general Utilitarian formula called cost/benefit analysis and cost-efficient analysis. This means: Serve the largest number most effectively.

This Utilitarian formula is identified with "diagnostically related groupings" (DRGs) and similar methods of federally funded reimbursement programs for the aged. According to DRGs, patients are allocated hospitalization according to their diseases rather than according to their individual hospital needs. Triage provides more widespread distributive benefits for the cost expanded, and triage is also more cost-efficient than any other method of distributing health care under limited conditions.

The Lottery Method

The lottery method allocates health care on the basis of equal chance for treatment. The lottery method has a serious difficulty. The losers get no care. One can appreciate the general unserviceability of the lottery in deciding, for example, which of 30 emergency patients to care for first or whether to help Mr. H or Ms. K with the pulmonary lifesaving unit, for one of them will be untreated. A key premise in having a life-choosing lottery is that of scarcity. This premise may rest on a fallacious moral assumption that allocating adequate health care for the elderly is not worthwhile in relation to other social values. Like musical chairs, the lottery may begin by allocating too few resources, thus compelling small numbers of winners and large numbers of losers. The method may seem fair, but not if the initial allocations are unfairly limited. If a member of the best-off or worst-off group picks the lucky straw, health care resources will have been wasted. The lottery method is based on luck. Yet in some kinds of cases, the lottery method is regarded as the fairest when resources are limited and there is near equality of conditions among candidates.[30] The lottery treats individuals equally in some situations, providing that resources are also limited. For example, the shortage of vaccines and drugs in experimental cancer and AIDS research shows the difficulty of achieving distributive justice by using the lottery method. A practice may seem fair, but not be wise. In deciding whether to use a lottery or triage in some non-acute resource-limited situations, the Utilitarian triage method is the wisest. In other types of cases, such as deciding to save the most intelligent person, a form of Elitism or Egoism or Paternalism may be the best solution. In a battle, one helps the general officer before helping a soldier.

The lottery leaves to chance what may be unwise. Some shortages are genuine. Others are artificial. One alternative to the lottery, lining up on a first come first served basis, may seem to eliminate the difficulty of having losers; but those who line up too late suffer health care deprivations similar to those who do not pick the lucky straw.

The Principle of Equal Shares

The principle of equal shares can be interpreted to mean either equal chance, equal shares, or equal consideration. Equal chance was discussed as the lottery method. Its serious deficiencies were identified. The principle of equal shares means that everyone gets the same amount of health care resources. For the person in robust health, this method of distribution may be eminently satisfactory. For the person born with serious congenital malformations or for the person with chronic disabling illness, this method may be tragic. Their share of health care resources is grossly inadequate. The advantages are that people are given equal shares, but their needs are different. This method only works if people are all equal. People are not equal. Therefore, the method does not work.

The equal shares argument has as the basis of the right to health care several serious objections. One objection is that those who have not worked as diligently, as long, or as effectively as others would rate equally in having their health needs met. This is the objection expressed by supporters of individual merit, and it cannot be discounted. For example, people who save for sickness in old age and who go without better homes, vacations, and entertainment believe that it is not right that those who spend their earnings receive equal shares. One version of this argument is that if health care resources are distributed equally, the nonsmokers, nondrinkers, and weight watchers may have to pay the bills for the smokers, alcoholics, and the obese. This antiequality argument is sometimes referred to as the "anti-freeloader" argument.

A second serious objection to the equal shares argument is that people's value to society is unequal. The idea that all people are equal, if it is unqualified by some such phrase as "in the eyes of the law," is a myth. In some societies, the oldest people are the least economically valuable. As proponents of the "is-ought" fallacy point out, however, that fact is not a justifiable basis for a moral policy that deprives aged persons of needed health care.

A third difficulty with the equal shares argument is that all health care cannot be satisfied with available limited resources. Veatch has pointed out that those most in need,

> the incurably ill . . . would end up with all the medical resources. This is. . . .inefficient. Furthermore, if they do not benefit from the commitment of resources, it is hard to see why it is just that they get those resources.[31]

To say "X has a need due to old age" does not translate into "X has a right due to old age." Needs, unlike rights, are refusable without contradiction. If one were to say, however, that X has a right due to old age, X's right would not be refusable without a reason. The needs argument, therefore, does not have many teeth in it. All people have many health care needs, but needs are not a sufficient ground for distributing limited health care resources.

Appeals to love, charity, and to one's obligations to others, even appeals to decency, are morally refusable in a way that appeals to the survival of the race or to a well-established right are not. One has to reach for stronger reasons to cancel the application of a right. One can refuse a beggar without being morally blamed for doing so. For however great the beggar's need, being given to is not the beggar's right. In contrast, if a patient has a right to health care compensation or if nurses have a right to be paid their due, to refuse to give the patient compensation or to pay nurses their due is morally and also legally blameworthy. The appeal to the moral sentiment that old people have needs will not by itself carry the day. Their needs are also morally refusable.

Another problem is that health care resources may be inadequate. The health care everyone gets may be too little to be effective, like dividing a slice of bread into 25 parts. Distributing equal shares in health care practice means that if health care resources are distributed equally, health care resources are distributed too thinly.

The Principle of Equal Consideration

If the aim of distribution is social justice, then everyone must receive equal consideration rather than equal shares. For example, nurses give more care to acutely ill patients than to ambulatory patients. This does not imply that the ambulatory patient is neglected or abandoned. It is just that she or he needs less care.

A presupposition of equal consideration is that there are ample health care resources including personnel of intelligence, experience, and merit. The problem is that, in health care situations, there are not sufficient resources to give everyone with a health care need equal consideration. Equal consideration does not work if hospitals have too few nurses and too many seriously ill patients. Currently, this society is unwilling to allocate the necessary resources to provide equal consideration to everyone.

Equal consideration depends upon ample resources, human and material. The quality and often the quantity of these resources depends upon human intelligence and talent, including persons of merit.

The problem of providing distributive justice in health care is to combine the principle of equal consideration with appropriate development and recognition of merit. What Jesus ostensibly did in multiplying the loaves and fishes and Edison did by inventing the electric light bulb is a combination of equality and merit. Appropriately rewarding persons of merit, such as expert nurses, developing trained intelligence and supporting medical technology can provide enough intensive care units so that young and old patients do not have to compete for a life support system. The combination of equality and merit has already been achieved in the production and distribution of antibiotics, making them no longer scarce. One can then give effective equal consideration to each elderly patient with a need for antibiotics.

In giving equal consideration to everyone's health care, one appeals to the reciprocity of everyone's needs, like living under a large-scale insurance plan called the social contract. According to the "Veil of Ignorance" or Golden Rule argument, one is to treat others as one wants to be treated. This means that one lives by giving and taking on a roughly reciprocal basis. One practical solution then is to have health care insurance plans into which subscribers pay a fair share throughout their lives. This response means that the beneficiaries share the burdens, in accordance with J. Rawls's principle that benefits and budens be shared equally. On this view, the health care right Professor A has in Case 8 is a limited right. He cannot have unlimited health care resources, such as a private room. And he may have to stand in line like everyone else, not only literally but also figuratively, as when he must wait his turn for a rare but highly desirable drug or specialist's attention.

In geriatric nursing practice, scarcity of personnel, facilities, or resources may rationalize inadequate and negligent treatment of patients who need help. This is illustrated in the case of Ms. R who suffered from lack of medical attention and negligence. The use of Kantian ethics supports the principle of equal consideration. A strength of Kantian ethics is to remind us of ideals, principles, and rights that ought to govern human conduct. This strength of Kantian ethics is illustrated by the case of the nurse who advocates Mr. M's right to a prostatectomy, despite the nephew's refusal to sign a consent form.

Truth-telling provides a further example of the strength of the Kantian orientation. Truth-telling is a vital obligation nurses have to elderly patients, along with other patients, according to this moral point of view. Treating a patient with respect, which is the patient's right, rather than as a mere symptom bearer to be diagnosed and treated, is another example of applying a Kantian principle to geriatric nursing. To paraphrase Kant, a policy of health care benefits to the elderly without appraisal of costs is empty; a health policy without widespread decent benefits is blind.

Appeal to either equality or merit is inadequate if taken alone. Yet each, in pointing to the weaknesses of the other, reveals moral considerations worth taking seriously. For example, a society cannot function or flourish without merit. But a society that fails to make large-scale provision for legitimate human needs would be heartless and inhumane, and, in a very important sense, immoral. To adapt a statement attributed to Dostoevsky, one can judge a civilization by how it takes care of its prisoners. So one may judge a society by how it takes care of its elderly. The problem remains to reconcile the moral relation between the appeals to needs and merit in a world of limited resources.

A Trilogy of Elderly Patients' Rights

Despite controversies over the meaning of elderly people's rights, three important rights emerge on the basis of the general human rights of all persons. These provide a basis for hope, love, justice and wisdom in considering the allocation of health care resources to the elderly. These rights are the client's (1) right to respect, (2) right to receive treatment, and (3) right to refuse treatment. Each of these rights has an impact on nurse-client relations and issues in the care of the elderly. The elderly patient's right to respect includes the right to dignity and regard as a rational person, and as an end, not as a means or instrument of someone else's will only. The right to respect of an elderly person implies the right to be treated on the basis of informed consent. The right to informed consent is the client's right to know what treatment is proposed, what its procedures and processes are, and what its expected results are. The right to respect also implies the right to privacy and confidentiality.

The right to receive appropriate treatment implements the right to respect. The right to receive treatment is the right to effective diagnosis and treatment by qualified health care persons, including nurses. A social, political, and economic issue about the right to receive treatment is that of receiving treatment free of individual cost, or on an individually payable basis. Since this issue is controversial, one may refer to the right to receive treatment in either of two senses, as (1) the right to receive treatment on an individually payable basis, and (2) the right to receive nationally paid-for treatment, as yet unavailable.

The third right in the trilogy of health care rights is the client's right to terminate or refuse treatment. There are several views on whether to override an elderly patient's right to refuse. One position is the Libertarian one, which says to respect a patient at face value and comply, as long as risks of failing to act are carefully explained. "It's his or her life, after all." Another view is the Paternalist view, which holds that patients' rights may be overridden in their own best interests or in the best interests of the state. A third position, a Utilitarian view, holds that a patient's right may be overridden on the grounds of cost/benefit analysis, which may include the patient's good or the good of society.

Competence and the Rights of Elderly Patients

A difficulty arises if a patient refuses treatment that will aid him or her to achieve the autonomy a rational patient would prefer. Macklin gives a reason for overriding a psychiatric patient's right to refuse. A compelling reason for the apparent arbitrariness is that a patient's rational powers and autonomy would be increased as a result of treatment when the patient's consenting organ is affected.[32]

According to G. Annas, to be mentally ill, a psychiatric concept, is not necessarily to be incompetent, a legal concept. Annas cites an example of a 60-year-old woman, Ms. Yetter, presented as Case 4, who refused a breast biopsy and was found competent to refuse surgery, since she consistently opposed it in lucid periods.[33] The court was assured that she understood that she might die as a result of having refused.[34]

A moral and philosophical issue raised by the case of Ms. Yetter is to consider under what conditions to override an elderly patient as incompetent. In Plato's *Republic,* Socrates uses the example of whether to deprive a patient of the right to be given back a weapon the patient has lent someone. Socrates points out that if a person lends one a weapon and then goes mad and demands the weapon back, one would be quite justified in not returning the weapon, out of concern for preventing harm.[35] One ground, then, for overriding elderly patients' rights to refuse treatment is to prevent harm, either to themselves or to others. Socrates has quite formidably presented the obvious paradigm for the morally right action in that type of instance and has identified one meaning of "incompetence" as doing harm.

There are, however, other borderline ambiguities that make judgments of competence unclear. In this connection, one may consider several distinctions J. Feinberg has recently proposed that may help clarify the concept of competence.[36] Feinberg cites three scenarios, the first two of which shows that a patient is incompetent, while the third shows the patient to be quite competent. In the first scenario, the patient, a layperson, disagrees with a physician about the properties of drug X, which the physician refuses to prescribe. The patient is *factually* incompetent. In the second scenario, the patient is told that drug X, which the patient wishes the physician to prescribe, will be harmful. The patient says that is exactly what he or she wants. In this scenario, the patient is *normatively* incompetent. In the third scenario, the patient wants drug X, realizing the harm, but says that X will give the patient enough pleasure to make it worthwhile running the risk of physical harm. In this scenario, according to Feinberg, the patient is competent. For the patient shows recognition of risk and, in doing so, reveals an awareness of making value judgments in the real world.

Unnecessary drug use, alcohol dependency, smoking, driving too fast, eating too much, and eating the wrong foods are examples of the third scenario. This scenario shows that one can disagree morally without being incompetent.

The question is to determine which of these three scenarios, if any, appropriately applies to Ms. Yetter's refusal of a biopsy. Ms. Yetter is delusional about a Hollywood career and having children at 60. If there is adequate evidence that her biopsy would lead to effective lifesaving treatment, then one would have a rational consideration for overriding her right to refuse. If a form of treatment a patient refuses leads to worthy health values that the patient wants, then, in that case, one would have a reason for overriding the patient's right to refuse. The appeal to a patient's own best interests might also be used to override the 77-year-old woman in Case 5 who refused to have her gangrenous foot amputated. The patient's own good might again be cited as a reason for Ms. A's morally justifiable action in saving Dr. D., the would-be suicide in Case 2, from jumping out of the 18th floor window. However, in the case of a woman who requests not to be resuscitated so that her kidneys may be donated to a suitable recipient, the nurse may be justified in supporting the patient's wish. The reasoning is Libertarian. One's liberty rights offer an initial presumption of a person's rights as a person. One's *prima facie* liberty rights are normally honored, unless there is a morally strong reason to override one's liberty rights by other moral considerations, such as prevention of harm to oneself or others. The reasonable moral grounds for honoring this lady's wishes when her life no longer seems viable to her or anyone else seems to place a moral stop sign on all overriding reasons. Even to override an elderly patient's right to refuse treatment does not mean one refuses the patient's right to respect. The reason for overriding, as a nurse might do in a case like that of Ms. Yetter if her chances for living longer would rationally be improved by surgery, shows more rather than less respect. Even if one overrides an elderly patient's right to refuse treatment, this does not overrule the right to respect. If, within the trilogy, the right to respect is accorded priority or is preemptive, an elderly patient's right to treatment or the right to refuse may be overridden. The right to respect means one would do for the patient what the client would, if rational, retrospectively want to have done. The right to respect gives one moral grounds for overriding or preempting Ms. Yetter's right to refuse a breast biopsy, providing a breast biopsy is medically indicated and that she will be helped by it.

NURSING IMPLICATIONS

Role of Patient Advocate

The nurse plays a pivotal and, in some cases, an indispensable role in providing health care for the aged. The elderly are in the majority on most nursing units of a general hospital. They are in need of daily blocks of nursing time for bathing, dressing, medications, treatment, getting out of bed, and various therapies. The elderly in surgical and intensive care units are a particular source of concern for the nurse. Every aspect of their care over a 24-hour period is provided by nurses.

Nursing care plans and goals are set by nurses. The success or failure of these plans is the outcome both of the wisdom of the plans and goals and the quality and quantity of nursing care given in support of those goals. Elderly homebound persons for whom nursing services are the main source of health care are also dependent on the appropriateness, frequency, and effectiveness of that care for survival. The nurse is not only indispensable to the delivery of nursing services, but for coordinating other health and human services on behalf of the patient. Therefore, nurses identify and secure whatever other health services the patient needs. It is the nurse who identifies shortness of breath, irregular pulse, untoward effects of medication, and signs and symptoms of pain and secures medical help both in a home and hospital setting. The nurse identifies deficits in the delivery of effective care. The nurse safeguards the patient from an unsafe environment as well. The nurse then connects with those parts of the system responsible for satisfying patients' particular needs, which have the duty of correcting personnel or environmental hazards.

This view of nursing care as a total responsibility for the elderly patients' health care by coordination of nursing services with medical care and with diagnostic and therapeutic services presumes the role of the nurse as patient advocate. In no other client group except children are patients so vulnerable to outside influences, neglect, and abuse.

Several definitions of the role of patient advocate may clarify this concept and its application to the nursing care of the aged. Kohnke defines the role of the nurse advocate working with conscious patients able to speak or act as twofold. The advocate's first function is to inform the patient by providing information "in a way that is meaningful to the client."[37] One might ask whether the nurse informs the patient of essential knowledge regarding the client's health and welfare or regarding the patient's rights, or provides answers to the patient's questions. The second function Kohnke views as the nurses' support of whatever decision the client makes. "The role of advocate comprises only two functions: to inform and to support."[38] A common example of nurse-patient interaction that provides the nurse with an easy, natural opportunity to be a patient advocate is "Must I have this surgery?"

The patient advocate's function here, according to Kohnke, would be to inform. Since this patient requested information, she deserved an honest, direct answer informing her that she had both a moral and legal right to refuse surgery. If the patient then refused surgery, the nurse as patient advocate is bound to support that decision, in Kohnke's definition of the role. Evidently, Mrs. K's nurse assumed that others, such as the physician, would not want Mrs. K to be informed regarding her right to refuse treatment. However, since many states, hospitals, and nursing homes have adopted variations of the American Hospital Association's *Patient's Bill of Rights,* first proposed in 1973, the nurse may have been incorrect in that assumption. Nurses may well be supported by institutions in informing patients of their right to refuse treatment. Some nurses are unduly intimidated by the presumed authority of physicians over nursing practice. As a consequence, such nurses misperceive the situation as one in which their continued employment is threatened when the facts are otherwise.

Kohnke recommends that the nurse learn how to support the client's decision without either defending the decision or rescuing the patient. Her reasoning is that clients are responsible for their decisions, which the nurse supports without necessarily approving. Nor, in Kohnke's view, is the advocate obligated "to fight their battles for them."[39] Such behavior may be regarded as disloyal to colleagues and family members, who also claim to give priority to the patient's best interests.

The nurse who seeks to be effective as patient advocate becomes familiar with the policies and goals of the institution, the supervisory and administrative practices of the staff, and the provisions of the law. This kind of knowledge enables nursing staff members to develop and test strategies for developing the role of patient advocate and for coping with the risks that may come with implementation. Some groups of nurses have become enormously creative in advocating for patients' rights by pointing out the legal pitfalls of less-than-informed patient consent or unsafe conditions of patient care. Utilizing the provisions and protection of a nursing contract with the facility in which the patient-nurse ratio is specified, or specifying the American Nurses'

Association code of ethics as a guideline to practice, may be useful to the nursing staff striving to develop the role of patient advocate. The ethical orientation examined in this book may serve as the basis for principles stated in the plan of nursing governance and the body of ethical principle in support of that governance. If, for example, support of patients' rights is considered to be an essential feature of nursing care, then the role of patient advocate follows naturally. Hopefully, it results in dialogue and resolution without coercing the patient to consent to or to refuse treatment.

The American Nurses' Association develops the concept of the patient advocate as that of guardian of patients' care and safety. In this role, the nurse is expected to "take appropriate action regarding any instances of incompetent, unethical or illegal practice(s) by any member of the health care team or the health care system itself, or any action on the part of others that is prejudicial to the client's best interests."[40]

Informed Consent

The patient's problems become the nurses' problems, as patients turn to nurses as the persons most involved in their care and closest to them in socioeconomic status and the level of language used. As patient advocate, the autonomous nurse has the duty to remedy the patient's knowledge gap, preferably before the surgery or treatment so that there is time for discussion. The nurse notifies the physician and surgeon of the patient's questions so that the information gap will be closed in ways most useful to patients and families. This may prevent lawsuits.

A further ethical problem for nurses is to respect the patient's right to decide in giving nursing care that involves drug studies, electroconvulsive therapy, or surgery for elderly and possibly brain-damaged patients. One example of this problem was that of Mr. M in Case 2. He needed surgery, but his nephew refused to consent. His life could have been saved. Yet this and similar decisions to operate or not to operate, or to resuscitate, are made for the patient by the family and physician. The rationalization is that the family, not the patient, will sue if dissatisfied with care provided, so that it is their wishes that are honored, not the patient's rights. Advocacy groups for the elderly are formed to prevent just such abuses. The American Nurses' Association clearly states that "each client has the moral right to determine what will be done with his or her person."[41]

The issue of whose consent is to be respected and whose passed over is a major problem that requires vigilance by nurses individually and collectively, so that prompt action may be taken through the appropriate nursing, medical, and legal channels of the health care facility. One example of the failure of vigilance was in the case of elderly residents of a nursing home in Brooklyn, New York. They were asked to participate in research, and they agreed. These elderly patients were then injected with live cancer virus. At the time of the injection, the effects of these live viruses were unknown. Clearly, informed consent means more than the act of a nurse witnessing the patient's signature, which is the extent of the nurse's legal commitment. As advocate, informed consent means the nurse's moral commitment to the patient's clear understanding of the procedure, surgery, medication, or research being proposed. This can be done best by the nurse's presence and participation in the physician's explanation to the patient. The nurse can then ask in the presence of the physician, as in Case 5, "Do you understand what the word 'amputation' means?" If no response is forthcoming, the nurse may say, "Dr. Smith is talking about cutting off your leg to save your life. Your leg is not healing because there's no circulation. The gangrene will spread and threaten your life. But you can learn to walk again using an artificial leg. We'll all help you." Thus, the nurse actively facilitates dialogue between the patient, the nurse, and the physician. In this way, the nurse can be a patient's advocate and health educator who willingly witnesses the signature of the patient in the secure knowledge that the patient understands what procedure will be done, with what consequences, and consents on that basis. Then the nurse is free to do all of the patient teaching helpful to that situation. If the nurse works in the community, a phone call or a visit to the physician's office might facilitate a clear understanding of the procedure and the need for patient education. The easily remediable problem is that not all elderly patients are given the necessary respect, time, and effort needed to give them an understanding of the proposed treatment. Aged persons easily accept and expect the lack of interest shown in their welfare as a necessary part of being old; they view themselves as discards. The caring nurse expects that her aged clients will be given sufficient information, help, and time to consider consequences and alternatives as the basis of informed consent.

The Sanctity of Life versus the Quality of Life. One of the most difficult dilemmas for the nurse to face is between advocating courses of action that favor as primary considerations the sanctity of life and those that favor as primary considerations the quality of life of the elderly person. Nurses working in intensive care units must sometimes rank patients in terms of prognosis, so that a new admission may be given a bed, as in Case 1 involving Mr. H, aged 23, and Ms. K, aged 66. Age and prognosis are factors to be considered. The dilemma is in assigning weights to the variables as the basis of decisions that are fair. This poses ethical problems for the nursing staff of the intensive care unit having to decide or to recommend a transfer of someone out of the unit who is aged so as to give a young person a chance. The question is whether it is fair, if the young person was injured as a result of drunken driving, to condemn the old person to certain death. If, however, the aged person's time is short anyway, the question is whether her life is less precious than the younger man's. There is no easy answer to these questions. They call for careful consideration of ethical principles.

The dilemma of the sanctity of life versus the quality of life arises also in deciding whether to resuscitate. Some aged patients with pain and a fatal prognosis specifically request that they not be resuscitated. If that patient's family wants "everything done for the patient," as might be the case with Professor A, and the hospital has no policy, the question is to determine the moral basis on which the nurse makes the decision. A patient advocate would press for respect and consideration of the patient's wishes. Before the particular event, it is easier to work with colleagues for a clear and unequivocal policy on resuscitation, which calls for written "no code" orders. It is morally indefensible to accept tacit and sly orders such as "Make haste slowly" in cardiac arrest or pencil-written orders not to resuscitate, to be erased on the patient's death for the purpose of defense against malpractice suits. The opposite situation, which also presents a dilemma, prevails on some intensive care units in which a patient is repeatedly resuscitated by an exhausted, frustrated, and perplexed staff. Annas cites one example of a 70-year-old woman who was resuscitated over 70 times within a few days.[42]

Truth-Telling. The question "Am I going to die?" raises an important issue of truth-telling. Aged persons long in touch with their body functions and feeling states are sometimes knowledgeable about their terminal conditions. Such individuals gain great comfort in discussing the disposition of their property, their funeral arrangements, and the living arrangements for a surviving spouse. Visits from family members and friends are cherished and eye contact maintained even when the patient is unable to speak. The nurse's confirmation of the patient's knowledge of impending death may be simple assent to the patient's question. Some patients, however, steadfastly deny the obvious decline of their bodies and neither ask nor wish to hear information regarding their condition. Perhaps all patients, even the most curious and determined individuals, need time and preparation, assuming one can prepare for death, before hearing the most profound truth, "You will soon die." Therefore, even the nurse advocate who supports truth-telling may, out of consideration, surround this final truth regarding dying with sufficient focus on the "here and now" of reality to enable individuals to reach their own conclusions. Harsh, naked truth can be destructive to the aged person's capacity to face this last test of ego mastery and control in the face of the "unthinkable" loss of one's only life. The decision to tell the truth needs the seasoning of compassion and wisdom.

CONCLUSION

To grow old is also to grow in "integrity," in Erikson's term. Older age sharpens one's awareness of where one has been and who one is, even though one becomes vague and unsteady around the edges. Old age is a time of irony. One is both sharper and aware and yet more forgetful and slower. There are reasons to value and also to disvalue old age. Wisdom, long associated with old age, goes side by side with infantile regression.

Attitudes toward the elderly are also paradoxical. The old are castigated, reviled, and regarded with contempt by some. Yet others see and appreciate successful old people as exemplars and models for others to follow. Great old women and men are cited and looked up to with admiration. These opposing attitudes are reflected in allocating health care to the elderly, and in dealing with the tough problems of deciding who gets what and how much. Like a seesaw, striking a balance between what a society can provide for its elderly and how much to allocate to the young, to adults, and for other human goals, such as environmental concerns, and education, leaves deep questions and moral uncertainty.

Geriatric training for nurses implies a common set of moral principles, culled from various ethical views. One principle implicit in geriatric nursing is the prevention of harm. Another principle is truth-telling. Other moral values include respect for equality and fairness, autonomy, regard for merit, and recognition of individual rights. These common values have an initial presumption of soundness. On this view, nurses ought, for example, to prevent harm, tell the truth, and respect the elderly patient's autonomy. Nurses also ought to treat patients fairly and equally. Compelling reasons need to be given for overriding these values. The purpose of this chapter has been to clarify some of the ethical considerations that arise in deciding on the amount and quality of nursing care for the elderly.

Discussion Questions

1. In Case 6, what reasons could the nurse give for telling the patient the truth or for withholding the truth?
2. What reasons are there for a nurse to assist or refuse to assist an elderly suicidal patient?
3. As science and technology make more health care possible, the

aging want more and more, with never enough to go around. What just rationing scheme provides the maximal health care needs for the elderly without bankrupting the rest of society?
4. What do you think it feels like to be an elderly person? How does your sympathy help or hinder your responses to your elderly patients?
5. What is the relation between individual freedom and the conditions for forming and maintaining attachments among the elderly?

REFERENCES

1. Lidz T. *The person.* Rev. ed. New York: Basic Books; 1976: 512.
2. Reichard S, Livson F, Peterson P. *Aging and personality.* New York: Wiley; 1962.
3. Lidz T. *The person.* 518.
4. Ibid.; 521.
5. Ibid.; 525.
6. Erikson EH. *Childhood and society.* 2nd ed. New York: Norton; 1963: **268**.
7. Lidz T. *The person.* Rev. ed. New York: Basic Books; 1976: 512.
8. Ibid.; 514.
9. Butler RN, Lewis MI. *Aging and mental health.* 2nd ed. St. Louis: Mosby; 1977: ix.
10. Ibid.
11. Robb SS. The elderly in the United States. In: Yurick AG et al. (eds). *The Aged Person and the Nursing Process.* New York: Appleton-Century-Crofts; 1980: 35.
12. Butler and Lewis. *Aging and mental health.* 24.
13. Ibid.; p. 21.
14. Siegel JS. Recent and prospective demographic trends for the elderly population and some implications for health care. In: U.S. Department of Health and Human Services: Second Conference on the Epidemiology of Aging. Washington, D.C., The Department; 1980: 309.
15. Daniels N. *Just health care.* Cambridge: Cambridge University Press; 1985: 14–15, 90–96.
16. Atchley RC. Aging and suicide: Reflection on the quality of life? In: Second Conference on the Epidemiology of Aging. 141.
17. Ibid.; 143.
18. Annas G et al. *The rights of doctors, nurses and allied health professionals.* New York: Avon Books; 1981: 80.
19. Ibid.; 81.
20. Ibid.
21. Ibid.
22. Barry V. *Moral aspects of health care.* Belmont, CA: Wadsworth; 1982: 3.
23. Ibid.
24. Ibid.
25. Ibid.; 266–267.

26. Rawls J. *A theory of justice.* Cambridge: MA: Harvard University Press; 1971.
27. Mill J.S. *Utilitarianism.* Indianapolis: The Liberal Arts Press; 1957: 14.
28. Ibid.; 76.
29. Kant I. *Fundamental principles of the metaphysics of morals.* Indianapolis: The Liberal Arts Press; 1949: 46.
30. Childress J. Who shall live when all cannot live? *Soundings 53,* 1970: 339–355.
31. Veatch R. What is a "just" health care delivery? In Veatch R, Branson R. (eds). *Ethics and Health Policy.* Cambridge, MA: Ballinger; 1976: 134.
32. Macklin R. *Man, mind, and morality: The ethics of behavior control.* Englewood Cliffs, NJ: Prentice-Hall; 1982: 90, 91–95.
33. Annas et al. *The rights of doctors, nurses and allied health professionals.* 80–81.
34. Ibid.
35. *Plato's Republic.* Grube translation. Indianapolis: Hackett; 1974: 5–6.
36. Feinberg J. *Social philosophy.* Englewood Cliffs, NJ: Prentice-Hall; 1973: 50–51.
37. Kohnke M. *Advocacy: Risk and reality.* St. Louis: Mosby; 1982: 5.
38. Ibid.; 2.
39. Kohnke. *Advocacy: Risk and reality.* 5.
40. American Nurses' Association. *Code for nurses with interpretive statements.* Kansas City, MO: Author; 1976: 8.
41. American Nurses' Association. *Code for nurses.* 4.
42. Annas G. Remarks on the law-medicine relation: A philosophical critique.

CHAPTER 14

Ethical Issues in the Nursing Care of the Dying

Study of this chapter enables the learner to:

1. Apply ethical principles of respect for the dignity and worth of the dying person and for the individual's right to accept, refuse, or terminate treatment.
2. Evaluate ethical principles for the relief of suffering versus the principle of double effect, ordinary versus extraordinary treatment, the active vs. passive distinction, voluntary vs. involuntary euthanasia, and suicide.
3. Counsel clients in the provisions of the Living Will and organ donation.
4. Distinguish between definitions of circulatory and respiratory death.
5. Respect the religious values and practices of the patient and family.
6. Implement supportive physical and psychological care to the dying patient.

INTRODUCTION

Everyone dies at some time or other. Although nurses are intimately involved with the care of the dying, to be a nurse in every important sense of that term is to be on the side of life. The profession and the activities of nursing support the most fundamental value beliefs of human beings. These values are twofold:

1. We want to live as persons.
2. We want nurses and physicians to help us live a long, healthy life.

This simple means-ends belief was a reasonable goal throughout nursing and medical history. Until recent times, intense and continuous skilled nursing care was the only hope of saving lives. (Currently, the care of AIDS patients is largely a nursing responsibility since neither cure nor immunization is available.) There were no miracle drugs, radical surgery, or life-sustaining machines. Beyond using heat, cold, food, fluid, rest, and a sanitary environment, nurses and physicians relied on the natural healing powers of the body. If the body failed to be healed and the patient died despite the efforts of nurses and physicians, the conditions of the professional means-ends value statement had been met. Nurses and physicians fulfilled their moral obligations on the side of life. Their power was simply not equal to the strength of the disease. And their sense of moral obligation was reinforced by the nature of the struggle against death.

Except for the care of AIDS patients, the then prevailing patterns of communicable diseases, early deaths, and home care have changed dramatically. The leading causes of death are now heart diseases, cancer, and cerebrovascular disease. These diseases are progressive and occur in later life. The individual concerned is usually receiving health care and medical interventions. With the advent of miracle drugs, radical surgery, and life-sustaining technologies available in hospitals, persons with heretofore life-threatening prognoses are now seeking restoration of health and function. The capacity to prolong life and to ease the plight of dying patients has improved to the extent that almost all acutely ill and seriously ill persons are hospitalized. As a consequence, most deaths now occur in institutions.

> By 1949, institutions were the sites of 50 percent of all deaths; by 1958, the figure was 61 percent; and by 1977, over 70 percent. Perhaps 80 percent of the deaths in the United States now occur in hospitals and long-term institutions, such as nursing homes.[1]

Increasingly, death comes quietly within the blinking lights of the monitors, the pumps, the drips, and the suctions of critical care units. Death is impersonal under such conditions. Death can seem to be a separation of body from tubes and machines. Death is due to someone's decision rather than the failure of the heart to pump blood. There is only a deteriorating organ system present. In some cases, the person of the patient has long been absent. The family has exhausted its grief during the prolonged period when the patient was neither responsive nor dying, seemingly neither dead nor alive. The family aches for resolution of an ambiguous situation in which neither grief nor hope is appropriate. The family longs to resume normal feelings, responses, and living.

Nurses are central characters in these dramas who are intimately and continuously involved with the dying patient and significant others. This care involves the coordination of nursing with health care services of other disciplines, medicine particularly, on behalf of the patient. Care of the dying may require prolonged close contact with the dying person's family and friends. Those who are concerned may look to the nurse for guidance or information helpful to reaching decisions of life-and-death proportions. Thus, one function of the nurse is to facilitate communication and the dissemination of information among all the participants involved in the care of the dying person. Another function of the nurse is to be an advocate for dying patients, who quite often are unable to talk or to fend for themselves.

SELECTED CASES AND PRINCIPLES INVOLVING NURSING JUDGMENTS AND ACTIONS

We cite cases to illustrate moral issues in the care of dying persons.

Case 1: The Johns Hopkins Case of Active/Passive Euthanasia. A baby with Down's syndrome "was born with an intestinal obstruction at Johns Hopkins Hospital. The parents . . . refused to give consent to surgical repair of the duodenal obstruction. The infant could not be fed and died within 15 days."[2]

Two issues arise in this case: (1) If Nurse A believes in the infant's right to life, and Nurse B believes that the parents have a right to decide, what argument is there for either side? (2) Is passive euthanasia morally equivalent to active euthanasia?

Case 2: Sandy, 5: A Case of Active Euthanasia. Sandy, aged 5, had a malignant brain tumor. There were three major operations. The scars on her head looked like zippers. "She got worse and worse and slipped into a coma." Her mother, distraught, attempted suicide. "One night, Sandy stopped breathing . . . and some nut jumped on her chest and her heart started beating again." She was put on a respirator. When she got infected, the doctors gave her antibiotics. Nurse A said the child's arm looked "like a pincushion. She was black and blue. Nothing worked. She smelled like decaying flesh. She had been such a pretty little girl. . . . I went into her room to bathe her. This time, I closed the door, took her off the respirator, bathed her and powdered her. I hooked her up again, but her heart had stopped. I felt relief."[3]

In this case, Nurse A committed active euthanasia. If you were Nurse B and learned about Nurse A, what would your response be?

Case 3: Jack, 14: Should the Plug Be Pulled? Jack, 14, was injured in a football accident and comatose for two months. Jack's mother asks the nurse to "just unplug the respirator. . . . The physician who has not discussed this case with the parents . . . has adopted a 'wait and see' attitude because he knows of a similar case where a patient on a respirator is now back in school."[4]

This case illustrates a conflict between the mother and the physician. Nurse A believes her role is to inform the mother that she has a right to know the patient's diagnosis, prognosis, treatment, risks, and alternatives as the basis for accepting, terminating, or refusing care. The physician is the best source for this information. Nurse B believes that she should not comply with the mother's wishes.

Case 4: Carolyn, 21: Leukemia: A Patient's Right to Know the Truth. Carolyn, 21, is dying of leukemia. She wants to know what is happening to her. However, her devoted mother believes in shielding Carolyn from this prognosis. Nurse A believes her client, who repeatedly asks about her worsening signs and symptoms, has a right to know the truth. Carolyn's mother, a wealthy, influential woman, threatens to sue the hospital if her daughter finds out that she's dying. Nurse A wishes to support the patient's right to know the truth. Nurse B wishes to acquiesce to the mother's wishes.

Case 5: Tom, 26: The Right to Suicide. Tom, 26, is a brilliant and handsome young man who has contracted Acquired Immune Deficiency Syndrome (AIDS). His family, friends, and lover have abandoned him because of fear of contagion. Tom is still ambulatory. One day he walks to an open window on the 17th floor and starts climbing onto the ledge in a suicidal move. Should the nurse stop him?

This case illustrates a conflict for both the patient and the nurse. If Nurse A believes in the self-determination rights of patients, she may perceive her role as letting the patient jump and die. If, however, Nurse B sees herself as protecting the best interests of the patient, then she may see her role as restraining Tom. What should the nurse nearest the window do?

Case 6: Mr. C, 40: An Adult's Right to Die. Mr. C, blind, a severe diabetic on renal dialysis, wants to die. When Mr. C. has a cardiac arrest, he is resuscitated, in accordance with hospital policy. Despite his protests, Mr. C is resuscitated several more times. The hospital authorities contend that life must be preserved and these are their policies. Mr. C's family then sues the hospital on behalf of his right to die. By this time, Mr. C has become comatose. The hospital is finally required by the court to comply with Mr. C's wishes.[5]

Three nurses discuss Mr. C's right to die versus the hospital's moral and legal duty to preserve life. Nurse A takes the position that Mr. C's right to die is his right and must be honored. Nurse B maintains that hospital staff members have no right to commit murder. Nurse C says that the physician ought to decide. Which nurse is right in this case, and on what moral grounds?

Case 7: Mrs. W., 50: Who Decides Not to Resuscitate? Mrs. W, a 50-year-old, is 50 percent burned. She has been alert, cheerful, happy, and positive. When Nurse A returned to her room after an hour, Mrs. W was not breathing. "I decided not to call a code. . . . I remembered the doctor saying 'Her spirits are good, but I still don't think she'll make it, but . . .' There would have been so much pain, and there was practically no chance that she would have survived the burns."[6] Nurse A told Dr. C and he decided not to resuscitate, because he did not know how much time had elapsed since Mrs. W. had stopped breathing.

Unlike Mr. C in the last case, Mrs. W had not expressed a wish to die. Would an additional lifesaving effort have been morally justified in this case? Nurse B believes so, but not Nurse A, who knew Mrs. W better and who found her not breathing. Who is right, and why?

Case 8: Ms. M, 52: Honoring the Patient's Wishes for a "Do Not Resuscitate" Directive. Ms. M is a 52-year-old woman who faces surgery for a possible malignancy of the brain. She asked not to be resuscitated. The order was written on her chart. When she suffered a cardiac arrest following surgery in which an inoperable cancer was found, the nurse resuscitated her. The result was that after three days, the kidneys she wished to donate were unusable.[7]

This case, unlike the case of Mr. C, could have resulted in a kidney transplant, which might have aided some other person. Was the nurse wrong to resuscitate the patient? On what grounds do you base your decision?

Case 9: Mr. W, 75: Paternalism versus Libertarianism. Mr. W, aged 75, was admitted to a community hospital with pneumonia, advanced pulmonary edema, urinary tract infection, and anemia. He did not respond well to treatment, but his wife asked that everything be done for him. On the 14th day, he stopped breathing. Nurse A, on finding him, reported that "vital signs were absent." She summoned Dr. B, who immediately gave a "Do Not Resuscitate" order. The cause of death was recorded as ventricular fibrillation. Mr. W had not been sent to the intensive care unit "due to a shortage of beds." Dr. B said afterwards, "I saw no sense calling Code Blue with a 75-year-old who has no future to look forward to. That's doing him a disservice with increasing hospital costs."[8] Nurse B disagrees with Nurse A and Dr. B.

In this case, should Nurse A have called Code Blue instead of calling Dr. B? Was Dr. B playing God or responding to medical reality? But then why did Dr. B make a gratuitous observation about Mr. W having no future? And why wasn't Mr. W put in intensive care, where he might have had a better chance to be resuscitated? What role is there for a nurse advocate in aiding Mr. W's best interests?

RELATED ETHICAL ISSUES

Trilogy of a Dying Patient's Rights

To respect a person consists in recognizing the dignity and inherent worth of that individual as being uncompromisable. Respect for persons is in some religiously oriented traditions defined as reverence for persons. Mother Theresa expresses this tradition when she says that her mission is to convert the lepers, the homeless, the poor and abandoned children, and the dying persons of Indian cities into angels. An example of respect is to treat patients in the order in which they arrive, on the principle of "first come, first served." This replaces preferential treatment or unfavorable treatment on the basis of prestige or social or economic standing. A patient's right to respect means that the patient is treated as an "end," not as a means only, in Kant's sense. In that sense, the patient's right to respect includes the right to know the truth and to be told the truth insofar as it is known. A conscious patient's right to respect implies importantly the right to informed consent prior to treatment or nontreatment. On the basis of a patient's right to respect, Carolyn in Case 4 has a right to know the truth about her diagnosis of leukemia and her imminent death. In another example, Mr. C. in Case 6 has a right to have his wish to die respected, as does Ms. M in Case 8, who does not wish to be resuscitated.

A second right, the right to receive treatment, means that a patient has the right to be given the best available treatment. The right to treatment flows out of the right to respect and is a special health care right. The patient's right to treatment means that the patient is not ignored or given custodial or palliative care if more aggressive measures are needed. For example, Mr. W's right to treatment includes the right to the intensive care unit, where he would in all likelihood have been resuscitated.

The patient's right to refuse and even to terminate all treatment is an especially important right of competent patients. Such a right assumes that hospital personnel are willing to take on the legal and moral responsibility associated with the death of patients who wish to discontinue treatment. This decision implies that health professionals will accept corresponding duties, such as providing competent, compassionate care while the patient is dying. The patient's right to terminate treatment also applies to Mr. C, the blind diabetic in Case 6. He too has the right to have his wishes honored. So does Ms. M, the woman with a brain tumor who refused resuscitation because she wanted to donate her kidneys. Finally, the trilogy of a dying patient's rights means a dying patient is treated with care and comfort and not left alone. For to show respect for a dying person is to provide maximum well-being for that person.

Quality versus Length of Life

Some of these cases illustrate the moral issue between the principle of saving all life versus the principle of preserving only a life of quality. Those who say all of life is a gift aim to protect all life, regardless of its quality. Others defend the idea that control of one's life and body are fundamental rights. These individuals are apt to evaluate the quality of life and would discontinue the respirator for the brain-dead in particular.

On the other hand, deciding who shall live or die can present a serious moral dilemma. The physician in the case of Mr. W arbitrarily decided that the patient's quality of life did not warrant his admission to an intensive care unit. Those who invoke a quality-of-life argument are, in effect, playing God. A safeguard, then, to a quality-of-life argument is to obtain freely given first-person consents for health professionals' interventions.

Relief of Individual Suffering versus the Principle of Double Effect

Another issue that concerns a dying patient is whether to relieve suffering in the presence of competing goals, expressed through the doctrine of *double effect.* This doctrine recommends doing the least of several evils when evil cannot be avoided. One example of double effect is that of giving a suffering terminal patient increasing doses of morphine, which relieves pain but which also inhibits respiration. Pope Pius XII addressed this topic specifically in 1957. He said, "If . . . the actual administration of drugs brings about two distinct effects, one the relief of pain and the other the shortening of life, the action is lawful."[9] According to the President's Commission for the Study of Ethical Problems, "health care professionals may provide treatment to relieve the symptoms of dying patients even when that treatment entails substantial risks of causing an earlier death."[10]

Ordinary versus Extraordinary

Treatment which at one time is extraordinary, scarce, and expensive later becomes ordinary. Antibiotics, dialysis, open-heart surgery, organ transplants, and cardiopulmonary resuscitation are examples of extraordinary treatments and procedures that have become ordinary. In an important papal statement of 1957, Pope Pius XII said, "One is held to use only ordinary means—according to circumstances of persons, places, times and culture—means that do not involve any grave burden for oneself or another."[11] The Pope's statement seems to say that deciding who lives and dies, especially among elderly patients, is relative to the degree of available technology in one's time and place.

In any event, the words "ordinary" and "extraordinary" are fraught with vagueness and ambiguity. The President's Commission identifies several, often confused and conflicting meanings of terms, such as "usualness," "complexity," "invasiveness," "artificiality," "expense," or "availability."[12] The Commission prefers "useful" and "burdensome to an individual patient" as having an important advantage over other distinctions, such as "common/usual."[13] A difficulty with the useful/burdensome distinction is that despite the reference "to an individual patient," this distinction overlooks other problems. What about the burden to the physician, nurses, family members, other hospital personnel, the patient, society in general? A further question is: Who decides whether a treatment or procedure is useful or burdensome to the patient if the patient cannot speak for himself or herself?

In one standard sense of the "ordinary" and "extraordinary" distinction, the extraordinary is associated with doing for a patient something exceptional, extra, heroic, supererogatory, or special. On this view, "ordinary" means applying conventional procedures and treatments, which are routine. However, to associate "ordinary" medicine with "useful" medicine and "extraordinary" with "burdensome to an individual" may do a disservice to the advancement of health care. The efforts made for Barney Clark, the recipient of the first artificial heart, shows that advances in health care depend occasionally on extraordinary rather than ordinary efforts. Unknown patients who selected burdensome, extraordinary means for themselves made it possible for caregivers to accumulate the experience that rendered those means ordinary. To give up the extraordinary flies in the face of the human spirit of struggling to improve the human condition. Moreover, a word like "useful" offers no great gain in clarification over "ordinary." For the minimum done for a patient might well be useless and call for the maximum to be done. For example, doing what was useful in the case of Mr. W might have involved putting him in intensive care, which would have been extraordinary. Since "useful" overlaps with "extraordinary," some of the same problems are apt to arise, namely, what to do for a given patient when all cannot be helped?

The ethically sensitive and intellectually critical nurse will in any event not be satisfied with any distinction that is not both effective and justifiable in considering what to do or refrain from doing for a given patient. One proposed usage is to drop the distinction altogether and do one's best in every situation. With reference to cardiopulmonary resuscitation, in particular, one tries to make it commonplace, as has occurred with so much in health care. This principle implies that Mr. W be transferred to an intensive care unit, where more resources for resuscitation are available. If he still has a life of quality, his hopes and expectations are unjustifiably ended by a physician who settles for the ordinary.

In the cases of Sandy, of Mr. C, or of Ms. M, these patients had no hope of recovery and treatment was refused. The appropriate thing to do is for nurses to help these people achieve a good death through compassionate, skilled nursing care. But in the case of the Johns Hopkins infant or with Mr. W, where something more could have been done to improve life chances, doing more would be the good thing to do. Also, some extraordinary efforts, like those of the "nut" who resuscitated Sandy or the nurse who resuscitated Ms. M, are not good. Moreover, countless ordinary, standard efforts are useful in helping patients.

Despite the difficulties, there are still advantages in using the ordinary/extraordinary distinction on occasion. Use of these terms sharpens one's awareness that the principle of what to do is decided on the basis of doing good and not harm.

THE ACTIVE/PASSIVE DISTINCTION IN EUTHANASIA

A moral issue that persists is the question whether letting die is morally equivalent to killing, or omission is equivalent to commission. The American Medical Association House of Delegates in 1973 adopted the following position on the distinction between active and passive euthanasia:

> The intentional termination of the life of one human being by another—mercy killing—is contrary to that for which the medical profession stands. . . . The cessation of . . . extraordinary means to prolong the life of the body when there is irrefutable evidence that biological death is imminent is the decision of the patient and/or his immediate family.[14]

Killing is wrong, but letting die in the sense of not exercising extraordinary efforts or discontinuing extraordinary efforts is morally permissible, according to the AMA.

Rachels has recently argued that the distinction between active and passive euthanasia is a distinction without a morally justifiable difference. Whether one drowns someone directly or does nothing to prevent a person from drowning, both the act and the omission are morally equivalent if the intent and result are the same. Rachels cites the example of the case of the Johns Hopkins Down's syndrome infant whose parents refused to give consent for surgical repair of a duodenal atresia.[15] The pediatrician mother defended her refusal to consent on the ground that omitting to help is not morally wrong, unlike outright killing. Rachels argues that not saving the infant is equivalent to murder if the intent and the result are the same. If killing a Down's infant is murder, so is letting it die by refusing to perform a minor piece of lifesaving surgery. Rachel compares two hypothetical cases involving the cousins of Smith and Jones. Smith stands to gain a large fortune by drowning his six year old cousin in the bathtub. Smith does so and covers his tracks. Jones, too, stands to gain a great deal if his cousin drowns. Jones' cousin slips and falls in the bathtub and drowns while Jones stands by passively. Rachels argues that there is no moral difference between them if the intentions and results are the same.[16]

One may present the counterargument that a patient died by himself or herself without assistance, and that the nurse or physician did not actively kill the patient. Rachels' active/passive equivalence may apply to those cases in which the active/passive distinction is used as a pretext for failure to save a life. But there are other types of cases in which there is a morally important difference between killing and letting die.

The case of Sandy, in irreversible and terminal coma, is an example of the nurse's deliberate shutting off the respirator to end the child's life. Had she not done so, the child's life would have continued for an indefinite time. Although, in this case, the prognosis was hopeless and irreversible, the saying, "Where there is life, there is hope," has its truth value. In some cases, killing is worse than not interfering with death. To not interfere with death, in contrast to active euthanasia, implies the possibility that a patient might recover, go into a remission, or survive long enough for a new and effective treatment to be discovered. Insulin, for example, saved the lives of diabetics. To not intefere with dying instead of practicing active euthanasia may "buy time" for a patient. That time may be spent in pointless suffering, or it may be a meaningful, enriching experience.

The flaw in Rachel's argument is that the intent and the consequences in either passive or active euthanasia are not always the same. In those cases, like the Johns Hopkins' infant with Down's syndrome, in which refusal to consent is used as a pretext for killing, killing and letting die are identical. Although many patients in cardiopulmonary intensive care units will probably die, such patients are better off whose dying is not interfered with rather than be killed outright. For not to interfere with dying instead of killing may effectively result in letting live. Without the active/passive distinction, one could argue that a dying patient might as well be killed, since not interfering with dying and killing are equivalent. With the case of Jack, the comatose football player, for example, if the nurse refuses to pull the plug, Jack might be back in school in another six months.

The case of Sandy presents a morally defensible case for preferring killing to not interfering with dying. But whether the nurse had the right to decide to remove Sandy from the respirator is an issue for further careful reflection. Without consulting the family and allied health professionals, such an act may be one of individual arrogance and arbitrariness. Decisions based on reflective dialogue are preferable to decisions made by individuals without consultation. In situations involving unbearable pain and futile prognosis, killing to shorten an unbearably painful dying process may be morally preferable to prolonging dying. Such a case was that of Charles Wertenberger.

> Mr. Wertenberger, upon learning that he was terminally ill, decided to bear the test of pain and live as full a life as possible as long as it was a meaningful one. In the end, he takes his own life in the company of, and assisted by his wife. . . .[17]

Nursing activities are aimed at effective intervention for improving both the quality and the length of life. The processes and goals show that not interfering with dying is, on the whole, morally preferable to killing.

Making omissions morally equivalent to commissions places too heavy a burden on health professionals, one that they cannot possibly fulfill. Not doing may have many reasons, such as avoiding the pain or expense of a useless procedure. The murderer, after all, is the cause of death and not the hopeless spectator.

Moreover, the use of words, such as "allow to die," or "permit to die," or "let die," is a dubious linguistic practice. Although these phrases are frequently heard, there is a difference between (a) a health professional who does not interfere with a patient's dying, and (b) a health professional who allows a patient to die by deciding for the patient when life supports are to be terminated. There is a distinction between decisions A and B. Choice of behavior A shows a health professional's recognition that a patient's life and death are the patient's ultimate right to decide and not a prerogative of health professionals. Choice of behavior B implies or suggests that the health professionals decide when a patient may die. If patients have any rights at all, they have rights to decide whether life support systems that are likely to be futile may be withdrawn. That decision belongs to the patient and not to the nurse and physician. The person who "allows" or "permits" decides. The person who allowed has a privilege but not a right. Therefore, dying patients alone have the right to decide to refuse or to terminate life-sustaining supports of all kinds. The patient does the allowing, or permitting, or letting, not the health profession-als. Thus, it is a linguistic mistake to characterize a health care deci-sion not to interfere with a patient's dying as being a case of allowing a patient to die.

VOLUNTARY AND INVOLUNTARY EUTHANASIA

A related issue to that of an active versus passive euthanasia or between killing and letting die is between voluntary and involuntary euthanasia. We all die, but when and under what circumstances is not always known. Some people die suddenly;[18] others die with time to prepare for their death within a finite time frame, ranging from a few days to a few years. In the case of Karen, a 16-year-old adolescent who refused further dialysis, her death involved her decision, consent, and wish. Tragic and terrible as death is for a 16-year-old, respect for her rationality and letting her decide shows that she died with informed consent, and thus illustrates voluntary euthanasia. One cannot apply voluntary euthanasia to a neonate or to a comatose person. One can, however, consider how they would like to be treated. For this purpose nearest of kin are given the power of proxy consent or what is called "substitute judgment."

The principle of voluntary euthanasia may be stated as follows: Whenever possible, consult the patient's wishes concerning the manner and procedures leading to that patient's death, including the with-drawal or withholding of life-sustaining treatment. Mr. C's wish to terminate treatment and die was ignored, thus violating the principle of voluntary euthanasia. The case of Jack leaves us with a dilemma. For the parent in this case wants a course of action taken that may not express the patient's preferences, and would thus violate the prin-ciple of voluntary euthanasia.

An advantage of applying the principle of voluntary euthanasia is that one treats a dying person as a rational being to be honored and respected as a person. Such treatment of a person exerts a moral barrier against other persons, such as family members, health profes-sionals, or officials who would decide who lives and dies and under what circumstances. In this connection, voluntary euthanasia is said to constitute a necessary condition of a good death.

In those cases in which patients have no opportunity to exercise voluntary euthanasia, one tries to do the next best thing, which is to consider what the patient in a rational frame of mind would want done.

Advance Directives
To offset the problem of health professionals not knowing their pat-ents' wishes regarding life-sustaining treatment, written and updated

advance directives are essential to the protection of patients' rights.

One model, the *Living Will Declaration* directs that such life-sustaining procedures as cardiopulmonary resuscitation and support, antibiotics, and artificially administered food and fluids be withheld or withdrawn in case of illness, disease, injury, or mental and physical deterioration that is without hope of recovery or of "regaining a meaningful quality of life."[19] Such *Living Wills* are now recognized by law in most states. Where still not legal, they provide significant evidence of a person's preference.

Durable power of attorney statutes exist in all 50 states. These statutes delegate the legal authority to act on the principal's behalf after the principal becomes incapacitated.[20] The power is designated primarily regarding property, but in some states the power may be extended to health care decisions.

Each of these advanced directives can be used legally to withdraw or withhold artificial feeding if not prohibited by state law. As these restrictions are challenged, there is an emerging consensus that artificial feeding is a life-sustaining treatment that may be refused like any other treatment in accordance with the patient's preference.[21]

Organ Transplants

A person's willingness to donate usable organs, as with the woman with the brain tumor who wished to donate her kidneys, shows how people can help one another. Views, however, differ on the moral permissibility of organ transplants or of the transfer of any bodily tissue. Jehovah's Witnesses, for example, object to the transfer of any bodily tissue, including blood transfusion, and consider such a transfer as a moral impurity.[22] Some religious and metaphysical views of the organism have held that all the organs naturally belong to a given organism, not to any other.[23] Others compare a person's body with machinery and find nothing wrong with replacing defective parts of bodies. Still others, out of respect for donors, impose restrictions on transplants. The patient's right to respect requires free and fully informed consent from the donor or nearest of kin, as with any other intrusion into the body.

A morally favorable attitude toward organ transplants may be found by appealing to Utilitarianism, which looks to the "greatest happiness of the greatest number." A positive attitude toward organ transplants also consists in appealing to the Christian love-based ethics as well as a metaphysical organicist's view, which holds that we are all part of the cosmic process and that nothing is impure. With appropriate safeguards of donors' and recipients' rights, more good than harm is served by favoring organ donations and transplants.

The nurse plays an important role in the altruistic donation of an organ of a brain-dead patient by communicating with appropriate authorities before the organs deteriorate. Moreover, the nurse can be supportive of the family by emphasizing the generosity of this contribution to others.

Suicide

Suicide is of particular concern to health professionals, who may be in a position to prevent it. Some cultures and individuals oppose suicide under all conditions. "Life is a gift," which no one has a right to take, is a summary of that position. In the cases before us, Tom, 26, in Case 5, is morally wrong to attempt suicide, because it is unnatural or contrary to the moral law or to the law of a religion. Suicide, they say, is evil. One practical argument against suicide is that if everyone who felt like committing suicide acted on such a feeling, there would be no human beings left.[24]

Some other cultures, such as the Japanese, and some individuals favor suicide over other negative values, such as dishonor. When Shakespeare's Brutus becomes aware that he will be marched through the streets of Rome in disgrace as a vanquished general, he prefers suicide. Cho-Cho-San in Puccini's *Madame Butterfly* prefers suicide to dishonor as a rejected and abandoned woman in 19th-century Japanese culture.

The topic of suicide holds out a fascination, partly morbid and partly concern with fundamental questions of being. Hamlet's "to be or not to be" affects everyone in this curiously morbid way. Hamlet, who at one time thinks he cannot right the wrong of his father's killing by his uncle, seriously considers suicide. Albert Camus, who thinks all of life is absurd without hope of a future, does not seem to object to suicide. Other thinkers, like William James, regard life as worthwhile. Prematurely "cashing in one's chips" is a "failure of nerve," a departure from the robust. Still other thinkers, like David Hume, Schopenhauer, and Mill, regard suicide as each person's private business, and immune from moral and legal censure. To Schopenhauer, to say suicide is wrong is "mere twaddle," for "no one has a greater right over anything in the world than over his own person and life."[25] Schopenhauer additionally thought it ridiculous to pass laws against suicide, since those who make a successful attempt can never be punished.

Some defenders of the right to commit suicide, however, seem to confuse suicide with self-sacrifice. The fireman who saves someone's life at the cost of his own does not thereby commit suicide. Yet R.B. Brandt says that

> suppose an army pilot's plane goes out of control over a heavily populated area; he has the choice of staying in the plane and bringing it down where it will do little damage but at the cost of certain death for himself, and of bailing out and letting the plane fall where it will very possibly kill many civilians.[26]

So we need a concept of suicide that does not confuse it with self-sacrifice.

Is suicide right or wrong? In some types of cases it is wrong. In other types of cases, in which it is regarded as the only alternative to prolonged futile suffering, as in Karen's case, it does not seem to be wrong. The case of Tom, the 26-year-old with AIDS, presents a dilemma, with good arguments on both sides of the suicide issue but with no conclusively right or wrong answer.

Suicide *per se* may not be wrong or right; it may be that other conditions accompanying suicide help us judge whether a given suicide is right or wrong. In this process, it helps to clarify the point that suicide is a self-regarding, self-inflicted death, which occasionally depends on assistance from others.

There are two analogies for a reflective nurse to consider in questions of suicidal patients. One analogy is that human beings are compared to property owners who may dispose of their bodies as they wish. On this view, suicide is morally permissible. More precisely, whether one commits suicide is neither moral nor immoral, but is amoral, being up to each person to decide. A second analogy is one in which human bodies are compared to property, only this time belonging to someone else. If life is either a gift or on loan in this sense, one may not do with one's body as one wishes. Instead, one depends on a higher benefactor to decide the time of death. Neither view seems free of difficulties. Surely, one cannot do just anything one pleases, even with one's life and body. Airplane hijackers who threaten to blow themselves up along with their hostages provide an example against the individual property view. Secondly, life for some people, like Karen, is no longer a gift, but rather a burden, which they do not wish to keep. Suicide, then, has not been shown to be morally right or wrong. It is an issue about which reasonable health professionals and patients may disagree.

Definitions of Death

Deciding what death is depends on one of two definitions: either irreversible cessation of respiration and circulation or "irreversible cessation of all functions of the brain."[27] A brain-death definition is appealed to for deciding vegetative cases, in which "cerebral silence" is a basis for donating organs for transplant. As Barney Clark's case illustrated, the heart can be kept beating indefinitely while other organ systems deteriorate and fail.

The concept of "death" masks an ambiguity between the heart and brain definitions. The brain-death definition affords more latitude for bodily experimentation and transplant uses than the heart-death definition. Since "there is no possibility that a person fitting" the brain-death criteria "will return to useful life,"[28] by identifying such beings as dead, one is then morally free to treat the remains as one treats other objects. If such a moral policy is generally adopted, it provides a ringing tribute to a 17th-century philosopher, René Descartes (1596–1650) who said that for a human being to exist is to think, and that for a human being not to think is not to exist.

A practical difficulty is that by ruling that if one organ is dead, the organism is dead, one is free to use the "dead" as means for other ends, on the assumption that cerebral activity defines the person. The question is: Can one be a nonthinking person? If the answer is: "No," then the brain-death definition is morally acceptable, with all of its social and economic consequences, including Elitism. If, however, the answer is "Yes," then the world will soon be overpopulated with mindless or brainless beings who may morally not be tampered with because they are not yet regarded as dead. However, they must be cared for by others and receive the benefit of resources.

The growing appeal of the brain-death definition is not only a tribute to Descartes. It is also a way of showing the role of the mind-body problem in relation to health care ethics. Although people now speak of the brain in place of the mind, the two are equivalent, at least on the identity theory, which holds that the mind is nothing more than a brain state. Secondly, the mind-body problem of showing how the body and the brain or mind are related is also a basic presupposition of teaching right from wrong and of doing health care ethics. For if our brains and bodies were different, our ethics would be also. If we had the brains of bats, we might have no ethics. We could expect either more or less responsibility from one another if we had either greater or fewer mental capacities. We are defined by our minds.

Personhood

To be a person, as distinct from being human, derives from the Latin *persona,* meaning a mask from which an actor spoke.[29] In subsequent Roman law, a person was identified as a bearer of rights and responsibilities. A person is a human being who is in a position to perform social roles, like being a nurse, physician, engineer, teacher, waiter, husband, wife, mother, or child. Human characteristics, such as laughing, crying, eating, drinking, eliminating, being hungry, thirsty, and afraid, are biological features. These answer the question: What is a human being? To have social roles and acquire recognition as a member of a community means one can write and read, work, take a vacation, vote, treat patients, reconcile conflicts, develop friendships, and show sympathy for others, for example. To be able to do so is to live not only as a human being, but as a person. As humanhood is biological, personhood is biographical. Personhood calls for respect and recognition of individual rights. Such rights provide individuals with freedoms, powers, entitlements, responsibilities, and boundaries which others may not trespass without a rightholder's permission.

Pivotal to a person as a rightholder is the right to informed consent, a point well made by Paul Ramsey. According to Ramsey, "a human being or person is more than a patient or experimental subject, he is a personal subject. . . ."[30] Consent establishes and sustains a relation of fidelity between persons, according to Ramsey. One writer endorses the *Oxford English Dictionary* definition of a person as "a self-conscious or rational being."[31] Although J. Fletcher refers to humans, the criteria he uses aptly identify persons. Fletcher's criteria of personhood include neocortical activity, an effective I.Q. (operationally at least 20-40), exemplified in a sense of the past and future, self-awareness, consciousness of others, the capacity to communicate with others, and the ability to form and sustain significant human relationships with others.[32] One who has hopes, plans, projects, a past, the sense of the present, joys, frustration, the capacity to regret, and a sense of a future with expectations and prospects, all of which presuppose consciousness—such a being is said to have a life[33] as a person. If one can plan a vacation, drive a car, play a musical instrument, or have some similar project, then one is living a biographical life and is said to be a person. To live as a person is more than just breathing and eliminating.

A reason for distinguishing a human from a person is that additional restrictions can be agreed upon and imposed on who qualifies as worthy of receiving scarce health care resources. This distinction facilitates ethical decision making in regard to those who have priority for being helped to live and those who are valued as being less important.

A related reason is that one invests scarce health care resources and medical attention on persons, treating them as ends, never as means only, in accordance with Kant's substantive ethical principle. One form this principle takes is the right to informed consent and respect for a person as a rightholder, one who has some control of what happens in and to his or her life and body. This is sometimes referred to as the right to self-determination. As a rightholder, a person has a veto power, a moral barrier over what others may morally do to him or her.

A further reason for distinguishing a human from a person is to restrict the attribute of being a person to beings who meet the personhood criteria. Becoming human happens over time. Potentiality is a term that applies to biological processes rather than social roles. One does not attribute potentiality to persons. To speak of a potential or unborn person or child is a contradiction. Personhood is a conferred role depending on social role achievements.

A disadvantage in distinguishing humans from persons is that one is apt to decide quite arbitrarily who counts as a person and consequently rule out those one dislikes or deems unworthy. The application of flat deductive rules, like deciding who lives or dies on the grounds of personhood, without reference to a case-by-case approach, commits an ethnocentric fallacy of simply preferring one's own kind. This practice leaves the resolution of who lives or dies to those with the most power. Making "person" synonymous with being a member of an elite club is an obvious misuse of language.

There are nevertheless advantages in distinguishing humans from persons, as long as such a distinction is not excessively restrictive. For one needs some criteria for deciding who lives or dies. Those with severe mental, social, or emotional incompetence may not qualify as persons. When there is only so much room at the table, hard choices have to be made. The softest of these is a reasonably restrictive set of criteria for personhood, such as a minumum I.Q. and the capacity to form and sustain interpersonal relationships.

Applying Personhood to "Do Not Resuscitate" Orders: Tracing and Examining Arguments for Appropriate Metaphors and Models

A philosophical move, which may be helpful in deciding what nurses are to do about DNR orders, is to consider a viewpoint and trace it to some acknowledged metaphor, analogy, or comparison on which defense of that viewpoint depends. One may compare a comatose person either to a "vegetable" or to a spiritual object, such as an angel. One may compare a bedridden man of 75 to a piece of useless "deadwood" or to a wise ruler. Thirdly, one examines the metaphor to determine how it applies or breaks down in practice and in practical discourse. So if one is a "vegetable," he or she cannot be a person. A comatose individual who after being "on a respirator for eight months is now back in school,"[34] to cite a case against "pulling the plug," shows that such an individual is not necessarily or always a vegetable. Such a case refutes the metaphor of a given person being a vegetable, and provides a counterexample to the advisability of "pulling the plug," as Jack's mother wanted the nurse to do in Case 3. Thus, one tests an analogy to see if it applies in practical discourse. Questions of truth or falsity arise here. One may consider, fourthly, whether supplementary or alternative metaphors or analogies aid in defense of a given viewpoint.

In regard to a comatose or dying patient, one may ask the question, "Does patient X own his or her body?" If X owns her or his body, then X has the right to control what happens in and to her or his body, including, importantly, the right to refuse all treatment, including the right to forgo resuscitation. To own property is to be the boss over what one owns. If individuals do not own their bodies and lives, and if life is to be taken only by the "one who gives life," then health professionals are obligated not to cause death.

The point is that each metaphor may be examined for its illumination and practical applicability as well as for its implied difficulties.

Life, for example, is not always a gift, as the cases of Sandy or Mr. C amply show. Yet, life was regarded as a gift by Mr. W's wife, who spoke on his behalf; and life is regarded for most of us most of the times as a gift, which reveals Aquinas's insight. However, one can also see how Aquinas's metaphor of life as a gift breaks down when it comes up against some hard cases, such as some of those cited here.

On the other hand, human life is not quite like someone's property or factory, on which one can do anything one wishes. A person with a contagious disease can be quarantined, for example. One can see dangers in both extremes. Trying to save everyone has counterproductive consequences. Too many malfunctioning or nonfunctioning beings cannot support the growing demands of sustaining life now or in the future. On the other hand, playing God by deciding who has the required quality of life and who therefore lives or dies also reveals a serious moral pitfall of arbitrarily abridging the equal rights of individuals to decide whether to live or die. Persons' rights to informed consent are crucial to their "rational life plans," whatever else they may want, to cite J. Rawls.

Let's take a closer look, however, at Ms. M, the patient in Case 8. The patient asks the nurse not to resuscitate her under certain circumstances. To comply with this patient's right to die requires the nurse—on one view, that all life is a gift—to commit murder. But is it murder? It is not, if that life is no longer a gift to that person.[35] In hopelessly terminal cases, if we consult the patients' most fundamental interests as friends, in Aristotle's sense, we might then recognize that since their life prospects are hopeless, were we in our friends' place, we would not consider life a gift. To be a friend in that type of hopeless case is to help, even if it means ending our friend's life, as Freud's physician was willing to do. If a nurse does not resuscitate a terminal patient who has asked not to be resuscitated, we would not think it wrong.[36] The appeal of such rights is not to the older view of option rights, which says, "Don't interfere," but the newer view of rights, which says, "Help me, care for me." A view of rights that addresses a patient's or nurse's vital, rational interests seems the more adequate at certain key moments in one's life. These deeper rights to live well are associated with a good life and provide the conditions for effectively exercising one's freedom. But if it is not already evident, a defense of such rights comes down on the side of a life of quality, but not without the constraints one finds with well-considered rights, such as the test of other people's retrospective judgments.

To have rights is to have a form of moral standing. With rights, like one's right to a paycheck, one knows where one stands. In health care, a resulting trilogy of patients' rights includes the right to be treated with respect, to receive treatment, and to refuse treatment. These rights are vitally important to one's moral standing as a person, regardless of whether one is a dying patient refusing resuscitation, a nurse, or a physician. Beyond that, rights break down, in the recognition that tragedy and stalemate, too, are aspects of the ethical life of persons, which no formalization or objectivity can overcome.

RELIGIOUS ASPECTS OF THE NURSING CARE OF THE DYING

Religious beliefs are for some people ultimate values that guide and justify the believer's moral conduct in important matters of living and dying. Firmly held religious beliefs influence perceptions of human relationships, religious duties and obligations, and notions of immortality following death. For those patients and families it is essential that all prescribed religious practices are fulfilled. In contrast, some patients have been inactive in religious matters, but when death is imminent, they confront and reevaluate religious beliefs learned as children. As a consequence, some will request the comfort of appropriate religious ritual. The nurse respects these values regardless of the nurse's own beliefs of deism, agnosticism, or atheism. The nurse offers to contact the appropriate clergy or religious representative and follows through until the patient's religious desires are fulfilled.

Since religions and individuals who identify themselves with a particular sect vary widely in their beliefs and practices, each patient's desires regarding religious rites and rituals need to be considered. On admission, the patient is usually asked to state a religious preference. As part of the assessment process the nurse has the opportunity to elicit the patient's wishes for religious involvement. If the answer is affirmative, then a hospital chaplain of that faith is reached. If the patient's response is negative toward religious involvement, the nurse respects that point of view as well. This view provides the nurse with the singular opportunity to offer expressions of concern and caring as the last human contact while alive. The dying person's need for human presence emphasizes the concept of personhood until the last breath is drawn.

Some of the major religions have particular rituals and rites for the dying, which should be observed. Other religions do not have specific rites for the dying. Instead, these nonritualistic religions emphasize human attachments, care, and concern throughout life up to the moment of death. These groups have leaders, visitors, or simply members who visit the dying and provide support. Whatever the patient's or nurse's constellation of religious beliefs or nonbeliefs, the nurse has the opportunity to coordinate human support, care, and concern for the dying person in the effort to soften the impersonal, technical, and sometimes disrespectful means of prolonging dying. The nurse accepts the reality of a patient's belief system, whether religion is or is not an important value, as deeply rooted in that person's personality and way of life. The values of an individual facing death are an expression of personal choice and an extension of the person's right to freedom of thought and of speech.

Health Care, Society, Literature, Nursing, and Religion

The role of religious beliefs is to give dying patients reassurance that the lives they led were good rather than useless or evil. Religion, thus conceived, is designed to help overcome the sense of alienation of the individual dying patient in the face of modern societal demands for youth, productivity, and pleasure. Religion increasingly finds a pastoral and therapeutic role, with a message of love, communion, and emotional support. Religions help strengthen family and community life, keep families from falling apart, counsel suicidal persons, alcoholics, the jobless, the undervalued, and the diseased, and offer them reassurance of their essential worth. Religion means a bringing together. In the fragmented state of society, religion has the role of uniting people through love and wisdom in human relationships. It aims to give individuals reassurance that their lives are meaningful.

It is no accident that Robert Veatch's three models of patient-health professional relationships include the "priestly model" along with the engineering and collegial models. People seek trust, love, compassion, character, goodness, and individual security, and they find it by appealing to priestly relationships with health professionals.

The force of religion is also expressed through literary works, like Tolstoy's *The Death of Ivan Ilich*. In this novel, the dying man who is rejected by his family is accepted to the end by his servant, who nurses his cancer wounds and cares for him with religious love. Although religions differ in the form of their expression, they seek to unite the true, the good, the faithful, and the beautiful.

A therapeutic perception may be that even though most religions believe in or seek God, what they also believe in and seek is some idea of the good in human relations and experience. God for the nonbeliever may be spelled with two o's as another way of interpreting religious experience.[37] Finally, a religious belief or "blik," as R.M. Hare has put it, orients and guides one's moral beliefs. We may reason out what is good or bad for the dying patient, but religion helps us to put our hearts into it.

THE ROLE OF THE NURSE IN THE CARE OF THE DYING PATIENT

Helping an indidvidual to die well is to support that person's sense of self-respect, dignity, and choice until the last moment of life. Achievement of this goal requires skilled and compassionate nursing care to minimize suffering and maximize comfort. The nurse provides calm, sensitive, individualized care to each person so that this final human experience is as free from pain and anxiety as possible.[38]

Patients differ enormously in their attitudes toward death. The term "attitude" has affective, cognitive, and behavioral dimensions. These attitudes, along with ethical and religious or humanistic principles, are integral parts of how individuals think and feel about death, and ultimately how they behave when faced with death.[39] Some patients want to know all of the truth as their condition deteriorates. Other patients steadfastly find benign reasons for their symptoms of failing health. The individual's personality, maturity, cultural and ethnic orientations, education, religious belief or its absence, age, role, social status, and family relationships are but some of the variables that influence the patient's response to imminent death.

One widely recognized work on the attitudes of the dying stresses stage approaches. Elisabeth Kübler-Ross describes five stages through which dying persons move. The first stage is one of denial and isolation, in which the evidence of impending death is rejected and ignored or regarded as false. "No, not me," "It's not true," or "It's just arthritis (not cancer)," are typical denials. In the second stage, outrage, and bitter anger and resentment are expressed toward death as unjust and unfair. "Why me?" is a typical response to this stage. The third stage is characterized as a bargaining phase in which the individual promises to reform or to make amends to postpone death until the marriage or birth of a grandchild, for example. "Yes, but after . . ." is a remark typical of this stage. In view of the advancement of the disease process, however the dying person recognizes the bargaining to be futile and becomes depressed. The fourth stage, depression, is a reaction to the anticipated loss of life and of loved ones. "Yes, I am slipping" is acknowledgment of impending death. The fifth stage is one in which the inevitability of death is accepted. "I have done my best" is one expression of acceptance and resignation.[40]

Kübler-Ross views these stages as normal and adaptive for the individual's progression toward acceptance of death. She views the stage of acceptance of death as the culmination of the necessary work of grieving to be done by the patient. Kübler-Ross sees the role of the health care provider or counselor to facilitate the dying patient's movement through these stages with "minimal regression . . . to denial or anger" after a more advanced stage has been reached.[41] Yet she concedes that patients move back and forth between stages and may hold two stages simultaneously.

Kalish points to the possibility that the stages are so familiar that there is danger of their "becoming a self-fulfilling prophecy. . . . It is difficult to ascertain whether the stages are universal, modal, culture-bound, or even adaptive, since no consistent research findings have been reported, and medical clinicians themselves are in disagreement."[42] Kalish identifies the ethical issue as one that questions the practice of intervening with dying persons to help them pass through the five stages, given the lack of research.[43]

Other investigations with different questions and different methods have produced other insights. One study by Hinton, who conducted interviews with the dying, demonstrated that dying persons want to understand their prognosis and are aware, especially those with children and with discomfort, of their condition, even without being given an official medical diagnosis.[44] Another investigation conducted with the dying adds another category to their awareness of their condition. Weisman calls this "middle knowledge," which lies between open acknowledgment of death and its denial. He warns against trying to set firm categories, since patients appear to know and want to know their conditions, yet talk as if they did not want to be reminded of information received.[45] The nursing implication is, "Wait until the patient is ready to discuss his or her condition and to focus the discussion on those questions and issues with which the patient is presently able to cope."

In several studies reported by Kalish, the coping ability of dying patients is enhanced by "good marital relationships, having good interpersonal relationships in general, expressing greater life satisfaction, and maintaining open communication about dying."[46] Competent and sensitive nurses support the coping abilities of dying patients as they struggle to maintain control and equanimity in the face of declining powers.

Another investigation shows that patients who live longer than predicted are likely to have good human relations and maintain intimacy until death. They have the capacity to ask for and receive support in relation to medical care and emotional relationships. They accept the fact of a serious illness, but not the inevitability of death. They are able to express resentment about their illness and treatment, but are seldom deeply depressed.[47]

Thus, another function of the nurse is to regard the anger and resentment of a dying patient as the natural expression of powerlessness without personal animosity. The anger serves the purpose of ventilating negative emotions.

Nursing Interventions

A useful assumption is that fear of death is natural and present in everyone and that attempts at control, attaining power, and relating to the transcendent are ways of reducing that fear. Thus, an important goal of nursing practice is to enhance the patient's right to autonomy as a manifestation of power over self and limits on the interventions of care providers. One way of accomplishing this goal is through involving the individual in the planning and implementation of care as the prime decision maker.[48] If, for example, the dying patient decides that a visit with loved ones is more important than a dressing change or treating a bowel obstruction, that is a priority to be respected. This is a way of lessening the fear of abandonment by significant others and to bolster the sense of control by "making available those experiences that the patient values."[49]

Symptom control is important to the self-esteem of persons in fear of losing control and to those who find pain frightening and burdensome. The prospect of uncontrolled pain is a specter that haunts most patients. Mental dysfunctions, nausea, constipation, diarrhea, infections, bedsores, and respiratory problems may be equally distressing. Most can be controlled through well-known measures and the remainder through aggressive therapies. Each patient's situation is best considered individually as an effort to control present and anticipated symptoms. Staff and resource shortages, as in the case of Mr. W, who was not put in intensive care, can result in loss of control of symptoms with resulting death.

Pain can almost always be controlled. Causes of pain are expected to be identified and followed by specific interventions, such as prophylactic nailing of pathological fractures and radiation or chemotherapy for relieving symptoms.[50] The choice of drugs and combinations of drugs to relieve pain, apprehension, and depression are increasing and improving constantly. The recommended administration of narcotics, such as morphine, in small, frequent doses is recommended for the rapid control of pain for patients not previously taking narcotics.[51] Effective control of pain can be maintained, along with alertness, through continual experimentation. For some patients who are close to death, the patient or family may agree to sedation in order to avoid pain. The President's Commission recommends that the administration of narcotics be regularly scheduled so that each new dose takes effect as the last one wanes. Sometimes increased frequency is more effective than increased dosage. Orders written as PRN enable the nurse caring for the patient to adjust the dose to prevent pain without excessive sedation. However, respiratory depression and oversedation can be reversed by use of naloxone (Narcan) in prescribed amounts and intervals.[52] The concerns of nurses and other caregivers regarding the "dying patients becoming addicted to narcotics are both mistaken and, in any case, irrelevant. Few patients develop problems because of physical dependence. . . . Furthermore, physical and psychological addiction, when it occurs, is not particularly troubling to a patient who is dying, nor should be to caregivers."[53] This statement is a direct application of Kantian ethics, which treats humans as ends rather than as means only. This statement applies the principle to every dying patient for control of pain and of symptoms that otherwise dehumanize the dying patient.

The nurse can effectively utilize nursing observations of the patient's responses to medications as the basis for recommending changes in drugs, in dosage, or in frequency. From systematic nursing assessments of patients' responses to the illness and to the therapeutic regimens, the nurse evaluates the effectiveness of current therapies and raises the issue of change when indicated. Competent nursing care is essential to control of pain and other symptoms, enabling the patient to live as fully as possible for as long as possible. A nurse who promises control of a patient's pain and who demonstrates the truth of that statement eases the patient's fear of and attention to pain. The patient is more able to trust the staff on other matters and is usually more cooperative as a consequence.

The trust that a dying patient is able to invest in skilled and compassionate nursing staff may contribute directly to reducing the patient's fears of abandonment and of losing control of the situation. The family's trust in the competence and concern of the nurse may reduce the family's fears that the patient will be neglected in their absence. Trust among patient, family, and care providers is significant when mental dysfunctions appear as a consequence of the disease or of treatment. Anxiety and depression are expected expressions of behavior in dying patients. Consistently given sympathy and support by the nurse along with pain and symptom control, comfort measures, mild psychotropic drugs, and attention to the environment can give relief.

Whatever the symptoms of the dying patient—and some, such as dyspnea, can be quite agonizing—there are relieving measures that can be used. These measures cover a wide range of specific nursing techniques such as bathing, positioning, suctioning, skin care, care of bedsores, bowel and urinary control, providing an esthetic environment free from noxious smells, and administering analgesics on time and without unnecessary discomfort. The nurse's opportunities to implement the Kantian principle of treating persons as ends are varied and plentiful. The nurse caring for the dying has multiple chances and ways to help make this experience deep and meaningful for patient, family, and self.

The central principle is that the nurse as advocate of the dying person seeks to protect the basic human values of dignity, respect, and autonomy while providing the highest standards of care possible. The nurse's competence and compassion will largely determine how well this last human experience comes to an end. The nurse's concern can be extended to the family through kindnesses and courtesies, which show respect for them as well as to the dying person. Family members can be guided in offering nourishment, in wiping the brow, or in holding the patient's hand and lending their presence. In this last phase of relationship, unfinished projects and unresolved tensions can be put aside as family members and significant others, with the help and support of nurses, conduct this last human experience with the sensitivity and consideration that the finality of death warrants.

The Hospice Concept

The hospice movement provides compassionate, skilled care for the dying adult and child that is consistent with the Kantian imperative of treating humans as ends. The term *hospice* is defined as a "lodging for travelers, young persons, or the underprivileged."[54] The term "hospitable," which follows the word "hospice" in the dictionary, is defined as "given to generous and cordial reception of guests."[55] These terms were translated into care of the dying by the founder of the modern hospice movement, Dr. Cicely Saunders, a physician and former nurse, now director of St. Christopher's Hospital in London. Saunders' conception of the hospice is to provide the dying with a comfortable, cheerful environment with the amenities of a home in which family members, friends, children, and pets are welcomed and given hospitality. Pain and other symptoms are controlled so that the dying process will be a meaningful, enriched, final separation from life and one's loved ones. The patient is cared for skillfully and compassionately until the last breath. Patients feel secure in the skill and concern of their nurses and care providers. Thus, there is less suffering and less anxiety about the control of pain and symptoms and more serenity about imminent death. The topic of dying and death is openly discussed. Emotional support is consistently given by everyone, including patients to one another, since the concept of a sharing, caring community pervades the hospital. At St. Christopher's and elsewhere in England, "Brompton's cocktail," which contains heroin as one of its ingredients, is given orally as often as necessary to keep the patient free from pain and from the anticipation of pain. The patient need never suffer while waiting for the next dose of medication to come due. Addiction does not necessarily happen, but if it does, priority is given to freedom from pain and to helping the patient achieve a "good" death.

In the United States, the hospice concept has undergone variations. Some hospice programs, such as that in New Haven, Connecticut, began as a home care program with community health nurses and progressed to include full-time hospice care. At St. Luke's Hospital in New York City, the hospice team, which includes nurses, assumes responsibility for the supervision of the care of dying patients in units throughout the hospital. The team gives care, advocates for the patient's best interests and wishes to the unit staff, counsels the family and staff concerning their feelings about death, and works toward providing a caring environment for the dying patient. Another hospice program in Summit, New Jersey, involves the family, community, and hospital staff in providing care at home and in the hospital if needed. Hospice staff are on call 24 hours of every day so that no one need feel abandoned.

These and many other programs in the United States not discussed are consistent with the hospice concept. The dying patient is identified and supported as a self-determining human being worthy of respect, care, and affection until the very last moment of life. The traditional isolation of the dying is transformed into inclusion of the individual as a member of the community of the living, fully participating in all of life's joys. The physical suffering of the dying is controlled. The patient need not fear pain. The patient need not fear abandonment. Death is treated as an inevitable and acceptable part of life that comes to everyone.

CONCLUSION

Death is a tragedy to each individual. Death to each person is, as L. Wittgenstein remarked, "not an event of life. Death is not lived through."[56] Some physicists say that in billions of years, the universe will be a "black hole," which means that nothing will be left. That is how some people believe it is for the individual who dies. To those who continue to live, the griefs and satisfactions of life continue. For them, the death of others is an event lived through.

The nurse at a dying patient's bedside can give succor and support to that patient, helping the patient through the stages of dying, sharing the patient's grief with compassion, support, and understanding. The nurse with ethical sensitivity, oriented by a love-based ethics at a dying patient's last hours, gives as one person to another in the recognition that they have this life and this fate in common. The nurse who can share as a person is aware that she or he, too, will die, and that how one ends life, whether well or badly, depends partly on the wisdom and love or lack of it shown by relevant others at this time.

Discussion Questions

1. How is the distinction between *ordinary* and *extraordinary* useful in deciding whether to treat a patient who tests HIV positive?
2. What moral reasons are there to support or oppose Rachels' argument concerning the moral equivalence of active and passive euthanasia?
3. What, if anything, is morally wrong with "allowing" rather than "enabling" someone to die?
4. What strength or difficulty do you find in Schopenhauer's argument against prohibiting suicide?

REFERENCES

1. President's Commission for the Study of Ethical Problems in Medicine and Biomedical and Behavioral Research. Deciding to Forego Life-Sustaining Treatment. Washington, DC: U.S. Government Printing Office; 1983: 17–18.
2. Heifetz MD. with Mangel C. *The right to die*. New York: Berkley; 1975: 59–60.
3. Muyskens J. *Moral problems in nursing*. Totowa, NJ: Littlefield, Adams; 1983: 92–93.
4. Davis AJ, Aroskar MA. *Ethical dilemmas and nursing practice*. 2nd ed. Norwalk, CT: Appleton-Century-Crofts; 1983: 223.
5. Cross J. Whose life is it anyway? Empire State Report, March 1983, 25.
6. Muyskens. *Moral problems in nursing*. 92.
7. Levine M. Nursing ethics and the ethical nurse. J Nursing. 1977. 77(5):843.
8. Carson R, Siegler M. Does "doing everything" include CPR? Hasting Center Report. 1982. 12(5):27.
9. Pope Pius XII. Symposium on anesthesiology. In: Hayes EJ, Hayes PJ, Kelly DE. *Moral principles of nursing*. New York: Macmillan; 1964: 131.
10. President's Commission. *Deciding to forego life-sustaining treatment*. 90.
11. Ibid.; 85.
12. Ibid.; 62.
13. Ibid.; 85.
14. Rachels J. Active and passive euthanasia. N Engl J Med. 1975. 292(2):78.
15. Ibid.
16. Ibid.
17. Kohl M. Karen Quinlan: Human rights and wrongful killing. In: Bandman EL, Bandman B. (eds). *Bioethics and Human Rights: A Reader for Health Professionals*. Lanham, Md., University Press of America, 1986; 125.
18. President's Commission. *Deciding to forego life-sustaining treatment*. 16.
19. Society for the Right to Die. *Living will delcaration*. New York: Author; 1985.
20. Society for the Right to Die. *The physician and the hopelessly ill patient*. New York: Author; 1985: 26.
21. Ibid.; 32.
22. Machlin R. Consent, coercion and conflicts of rights. In: Arras J, Hunt R. (eds). *Ethical Issues in Modern Medicine*. 2nd ed. Palo Alto, CA: Mayfield; 1983: 231–238.
23. McCormick R. Organ transplants: Ethical principles. In: Reich W. (ed). *Encyclopedia of Bioethics*. New York: The Free Press; 1978: 1169–1172.
24. Kant I. *Fundamental principles of the metaphysics of morals*. Indianapolis: Bobbs-Merrill; 1949: 39.
25. Schopenhauer A. On Suicide. In: Beck R, Orr J. (eds). *Ethical Choice*. New York: Free Press; 1970: 78.
26. Brandt RB. The morality and rationality of suicide. In: Beauchamp T, Perlin S. (eds). *Ethical Issues in Death and Dying*. Englewood Cliffs, NJ: Prentice-Hall; 1978: 125.

27. Guidelines for the Determination of Death. In: *Legal and Ethical Aspects of Treatment for Critically and Terminally Ill Patients.* New York: American Society for Law and Medicine and Concern for Dying; 1981: 54–63.
28. Black P. Definitions of brain death. In: *Ethical Issues in Death and Dying.* 9.
29. Downie RS. *Roles and values.* London: Methuen; 1971: 131.
30. Ramsey P. *The patient as person.* New Haven: Yale University Press; 1970: 5.
31. Singer P. Value of life. In: *Encyclopedia of Bioethics.* Vol. 2: 823.
32. Fletcher J. *Four indicators of humanhood: The enquiry matures.* Hastings Center Report. 1974. 4(6):51.
33. Ruddick W. Parents, children and medical decisions. In: *Bioethics and Human Rights: A Reader for Health Professionals.* 165–170.
34. Davis and Aroskar. *Ethical dilemmas and nursing practice.* 223.
35. Bandman B, Bandman E. The nurse's role in an interest-based view of patient's rights. In: Spicker S, Gadow S. (eds). *Nursing Image and Ideals.* New York: Springer; 1980: 135–136.
36. Ibid.
37. Hare RM. Religion and morals. In: Mitchell B. (ed). *Faith and Logic.* London: Allen & Unwin; 1957: 192.
38. American Nurses' Association. *Code for nurses.* 6.
39. Kalish RA. Death, attitudes toward. In: *Encyclopedia of Bioethics.* Vol. 1: 286.
40. Kübler-Ross E. *On death and dying.* New York: Macmillian; 1969.
41. Kalish. *Death, attitudes toward.* 287.
42. Kalish. *Death, attitudes toward.* 287.
43. Ibid.
44. Ibid.
45. Ibid.
46. Ibid.; 288.
47. Ibid.
48. American Nurses' Association. *Code for nurses.* 4.
49. *President's Commission. Deciding to forego life-sustaining treatment.* 276.
50. Ibid.; 278.
51. Ibid.; 279.
52. Ibid.; 283.
53. Ibid.; 284
54. *Webster's New Collegiate Dictionary.* Springfield, MA: Merriam; 1974: 553.
55. Ibid.
56. Wittgenstein L. *Tractatus logicus philosophicus.* New York: Humanities Press; 1951: 185.

Appendix

American Nurses' Association Code for Nurses*

Preamble

A code of ethics makes explicit the primary goals and values of the profession. When individuals become nurses, they make a moral commitment to uphold the values and special moral obligations expressed in their code. The *Code for Nurses* is based on belief about the nature of individuals, nursing, health, and society. Nursing encompasses the protection, promotion and restoration of health; the prevention of illness, and the alleviation of suffering in the care of clients, including individuals, families groups, and communities. In the context of these functions, nursing is defined as the diagnosis and treatment of human responses to actual or potential health problems.

Since clients themselves are the primary decision making matters concerning their own health, treatment, and well-being, the goal of nursing actions is to support and enhance the client's responsibility and self-determination to the greatest extent possible. In this context, health is not necessarily an end in itself, but rather a means to a life that is meaningful from the client's perspective.

When making clinical judgments, nurses base their decisions on consideration of consequences and of universal moral principles, both of which prescribe and justify nursing actions. The most fundamental of these principles is respect for persons. Other principles stemming from this basic principle are autonomy (self-determination), beneficience (doing good), nonmaleficence (avoiding harm), veracity (truthtelling), confidentiality (respecting privileged information), fidelity (keeping promises), and justice (treating people fairly).

In brief, then, the statements of the code and their interpretation provide guidance for conduct and relationships in carrying out nursing responsibilities consistent with the ethical obligations of the profession and with high quality in nursing care.

Introduction

A code of ethics indicates a profession's acceptance of the responsibility and trust with which it has been invested by society. Under the terms

---

*Adopted by the American Nurses Association, 1976, 1985 and reprinted by permission.]

of the implicit contract between society and the nursing profession, society grants the profession considerable autonomy and authority to function in the conduct of its affairs. The development of a code of ethics is an essential activity of a profession and provides one means for the exercise of professional self-regulation.

Upon entering the profession, each nurse inherits a measure of both the responsibility and the trust that have accrued to nursing over the years, as well as the corresponding obligation to adhere to the profession's code of conduct and relationships for ethical practice. The *Code for Nurses with Interpretive Statements* is thus more a collective expression of nursing conscience and philosophy than a set of external rules imposed upon an individual practitioner of nursing. Personal and professional integrity can be assured only if an individual is committed to the profession's code of conduct.

A code of ethical conduct offers general principles to guide and evaluate nursing actions. It does not assure the virtues required for professional practice within the character of each nurse. In particular situations, the justification of behavior as ethical must satisfy not only the individual nurse acting as a moral agent but also the standards for professional peer review.

The *Code for Nurses* was adopted by the American Nurses' Association in 1950 and has been revised periodically. It serves to inform both the nurse and society of the profession's expectations and requirements in ethical matters. The code and the interpretive statements together provide a framework within which nurses can make ethical decisions and discharge their responsibilities to the public, to other members of the health team, and to the profession.

Although a particular situation by its nature may determine the use of specific moral principles, the basic philosophical values, directives, and suggestions provided here are widely applicable to situations encountered in clinical practice. The *Code for Nurses* is not open to negotiation in employment settings, nor is it permissible for individuals or groups of nurses to adapt or change the language of this code.

The requirements of the code may often exceed those of the law. Violations of the law may subject the nurse to civil or criminal liability. The state nurses' associations, in fulfilling the profession's duty to society, may discipline their members for violations of the code. Loss of the respect and confidence of society and of one's colleagues is a serious sanction resulting from violation of the code. In addition, every nurse has a personal obligation to uphold and adhere to the code and to ensure that nursing colleagues do likewise.

Guidance and assistance in applying the code to local situations may be obtained from the American Nurses' Association and the constituent state nurses' associations.

Code for Nurses

1. The nurse provides services with respect for human dignity and the uniqueness of the client, unrestricted by considerations of social or economic status, personal attributes, or the nature of health problems.
2. The nurse safeguards the client's right to privacy by judiciously protecting information of a confidential nature.
3. The nurse acts to safeguard the client and the public when health care and safety are affected by the incompetent, unethical, or illegal practice of any person.
4. The nurse assumes responsibility and accountability for individual nursing judgments and actions.
5. The nurse maintains competence in nursing.
6. The nurse exercises informed judgment and uses individual competence and qualifications as criteria in seeking consultation, accepting responsibilities, and delegating nursing activities to others.
7. The nurse participates in activities that contribute to the ongoing development of the profession's body of knowledge.
8. The nurse participates in the profession's efforts to implement and improve standards of nursing.
9. The nurse participates in the profession's effort to establish and maintain conditions of employment conducive to high quality nursing care.
10. The nurse participates in the profession's effort to protect the public from misinformation and misrepresentation and to maintain the integrity of nursing.
11. The nurse collaborates with members of the health professions and other citizens in promoting community and national efforts to meet the health needs of the public.

International Council of Nurses
Code for Nurses: Ethical Concepts
Applied to Nursing*

- The fundamental responsibility of the nurse is fourfold: to promote health, to prevent illness, to restore health and alleviate suffering.

*Adopted by the International Council of Nurses, May 1973 and reprinted by permission.

- The need for nursing is universal. Inherent in nursing is respect for life, dignity and rights of man. It is unrestricted by considerations of nationality, race, creed, color, age, sex, politics or social status.
- Nurses render health services to the individual, the family and the community and coordinate their services with those of related groups.

Nurses and People

- The nurse's primary responsibility is to those people who require nursing care.
- The nurse, in providing care, promotes an environment in which the values, customs, and spiritual beliefs of the individual are respected.
- The nurse holds in confidence personal information and uses judgment in sharing this information.

Nurses and Practice

- The nurse carries personal responsibility for nursing practice and for maintaining competence by continual learning.
- The nurse maintains the highest standards of nursing care possible within the reality of a specific situation.
- The nurse uses judgment in relation to individual competence when accepting and delegating responsibilities.
- The nurse when acting in a professional capacity should at all times maintain standards of personal conduct which reflect credit upon the profession.

Nurses and Society

- The nurse shares with other citizens the responsibility for initiating and supporting action to meet the health and social needs of the public.

Nurses and Co-Workers

- The nurse sustains a cooperative relationship with co-workers in nursing and other fields.
- The nurse takes appropriate action to safeguard the individual when his care is endangered by a co-worker or any other person.

Nurses and the Profession

- The nurse plays the major role in determining and implementing desirable standards of nursing practice and nursing education.

- The nurse is active in developing a core of professional knowledge.
- The nurse, acting through the professional organization, participates in establishing and maintaining equitable social and economic working conditions in nursing.

The World Medical Association Declaration of Geneva*

Physician's Oath

At the time of being admitted as a member of the medical profession: I solemnly pledge myself to consecrate my life to the service of humanity; I will give to my teachers the respect and gratitude which is their due; I will practice my profession with conscience and dignity; the health of my patient will be my first consideration; I will maintain by all the means in my power, the honor and the noble traditions of the medical profession; my colleagues will be my brothers; I will not permit considerations of religion, nationality, race, party politics or social standing to intervene between my duty and my patient; I will maintain the utmost respect of human life from the time of conception, even under threat, I will not use my medical knowledge contrary to the laws of humanity; I make these promises solemnly, freely, and upon my honor.

*Adopted by the General Assembly of the World Medical Association, Geneva, Switzerland, September 1948 and amended by the 22nd World Medical Assembly, Sydney, Australia, August 1968. Reprinted by permission.

American Medical Association Principles of Medical Ethics*

Preamble

The medical profession has long subscribed to a body of ethical statements developed primarily for the benefit of the patient. As a member

*Adopted by the American Medical Association in 1980 and reprinted with permission.

of this profession, a physician must recognize responsibility not only to patients, but also to society, to other health professionals, and to self. The following Principles adopted by the American Medical Association are not laws, but standards of conduct which define the essentials of honorable behavior for the physician.

1. A physician shall be dedicated to providing competent medical service with compassion and respect for human dignity.
2. A physician shall deal honestly with patients and colleagues, and strive to expose those physicians deficient in character or competence, or who engage in fraud or deception.
3. A physician shall respect the law and also recognize a responsibility to seek changes in those requirements which are contrary to the best interests of the patient.
4. A physician shall respect the rights of patients, of colleagues, and of other health professionals, and shall safeguard patient confidences within the constraints of the law.
5. A physician shall continue to study, apply, and advance scientific knowledge, make relevant information available to patients, colleagues, and the public, obtain consultation, and use the talents of other health professionals when indicated.
6. A physician shall, in the provision of appropriate patient care, except in emergencies, be free to choose whom to serve, with whom to associate, and the environment in which to provide medical services.
7. A physician shall recognize a responsibility to participate in activities contributing to an improved community.

American Hospital Association
A Patient's Bill of Rights*

The American Hospital Association presents a Patient's Bill of Rights with the expectation that observance of these rights will contribute to more effective patient care and greater satisfaction for the patient, the physician, and the hospital organization. Further, the Association presents these rights in the expectation that they will be supported by the hospital on behalf of its patients, as an integral part of the healing process. It is recognized that a personal relationship between the phy-

*Approved by the American Hospital Association House of Delegates, February 6, 1973, and reprinted by permission of the American Hospital Association, c 1975.

sician and the patient is essential for the provision of proper medical care. The traditional physician-patient relationship takes on a new dimension when care is rendered within an organizational structure. Legal precedent has established that the institution itself also has a responsibility to the patient. It is in recognition of these factors that these rights are affirmed.

1. The patient has the right to considerate and respectful care.
2. The patient has the right to obtain from his physician complete current information concerning his diagnosis, treatment, and prognosis in terms the patient can be reasonably expected to understand. When it is not medically advisable to give such information to the patient, the information should be made available to an appropriate person in his behalf. He has the right to know, by name, the physician responsible for coordinating his care.
3. The patient has the right to receive from his physician information necessary to give informed consent prior to the start of any procedure and/or treatment. Except in emergencies, such information for informed consent should include but not necessarily be limited to the specific procedure and/or treatment, the medically significant risks involved, and the probable duration of incapacitation. Where medically significant alternatives for care or treatment exist, or when the patient requests information concerning medical alternatives, the patient has the right to such information. The patient also has the right to know the name of the person responsible for the procedures and/or treatment.
4. The patient has the right to refuse treatment to the extent permitted by law and to be informed of the medical consequences of his action.
5. The patient has the right to every consideration of his privacy concerning his own medical care program. Case discussion, consultation, examination, and treatment are confidential and should be conducted discreetly. Those not directly involved in his care must have the permission of the patient to be present.
6. The patient has the right to expect that all communications and records pertaining to his care should be treated as confidential.
7. The patient has the right to expect that within its capacity a hospital must make reasonable response to the request of a patient for services. The hospital must provide evaluation, service, and/or referral as indicated by the urgency of the case. When medically permissible, the patient may be transferred to another facility only after he has received complete information and explanation concerning the needs for and alternatives

for such a transfer. The institution to which the patient is to be transferred must first have accepted the patient for transfer.

8. The patient has the right to obtain information as to any relationship of his hospital to other health care and educational institutions insofar as his care is concerned. The patient has the right to obtain information as to the existence of any professional relationships among individuals, by name, who are treating him.

9. The patient has the right to be advised if the hospital proposes to engage in or perform human experimentation affecting his care or treatment. The patient has the right to refuse to participate in such research projects.

10. The patient has the right to expect reasonable continuity of care. He has the right to know in advance what appointment times and physicians are available and where. The patient has the right to expect that the hospital will provide a mechanism whereby he is informed by his physician or a delegate of the physician of the patient's continuing health care requirements following discharge.

11. The patient has the right to examine and receive an explanation of his bill regardless of source of payment.

12. The patient has the right to know what hospital rules and regulations apply to his conduct as a patient.

No catalog of rights can guarantee for the patient the kind of treatment he has a right to expect. A hospital has many functions to perform, including the prevention and treatment of disease, the education of both health professionals and patient, and the conduct of clinical research. All these activities must be conducted with an overriding concern for the patient, and, above all, the recognition of his dignity as a human being. Success in achieving this recognition assures success in the defense of the rights of the patient.

The Nuremberg Code*

The great weight of the evidence before us is to the effect that certain types of medical experiments on human beings, when kept within

*Reprinted from *Trials of War Criminals before the Nuernberg Military Tribunals under Control Council Law No. 10,* vol. 2 (Washington, D.C.: U.S. Government Printing Office, 1949), pp. 181-82.

reasonably well-defined bounds, conform to the ethics of the medical profession generally. The protagonists of the practice of human experimentation justify their views on the basis that such experiments yield results for the good of society that are unprocurable by other methods or means of study. All agree, however, that certain basic principles must be observed in order to satisfy moral, ethical, and legal concepts:

1. The voluntary consent of the human subject is absolutely essential. This means that the person involved should have legal capacity to give consent; should be so situated as to be able to exercise free power of choice, without the intervention of any element of force, fraud, deceit, duress, overreaching, or other ulterior form of constraint or coercion; and should have sufficient knowledge and comprehension of the elements of the subject matter involved as to enable him to make an understanding and enlightened decision. This latter element requires that before the acceptance of an affirmative decision by the experimental subject there should be made known to him the nature, duration, and purpose of the experiment; the method and means by which it is to be conducted; all inconveniences and hazards reasonably to be expected; and the effects upon his health or person which may possibly come from his participation in the experiment.

   The duty and responsibility for ascertaining the quality of the consent rests upon each individual who initiates, directs or engages in the experiment. It is a personal duty and responsibility which may not be delegated to another with impunity.
2. The experiment should be such as to yield fruitful results for the good of society, unprocurable by other methods or means of study, and not random and unnecessary in nature.
3. The experiment should be so designed and based on the results of animal experimentation and a knowledge of the natural history of the disease or other problem under study that the anticipated results will justify the performance of the experiment.
4. The experiment should be so conducted as to avoid all unnecessary physical and mental suffering and injury.
5. No experiment should be conducted where there is an *a priori* reason to believe that death or disabling injury will occur; except, perhaps, in those experiments where the experimental physicians also serve as subjects.
6. The degree of risk to be taken should never exceed that determined by the humanitarian importance of the problem to be solved by the experiment.
7. Proper preparations should be made and adequate facilities

provided to protect the experimental subject against even remote possibilities of injury, disability, or death.

8. The experiment should be conducted only by scientifically qualified persons. The highest degree of skill and care should be required through all stages of the experiment of those who conduct or engage in the experiment.

9. During the course of the experiment the human subject should be at liberty to bring the experiment to an end if he has reached the physical or mental state where continuation of the experiment seems to him to be impossible.

10. During the course of the experiment the scientist in charge must be prepared to terminate the experiment at any stage, if he has probable cause to believe, in the exercise of the good faith, superior skill and careful judgment required of him that a continuation of the experiment is likely to result in injury, disability, or death to the experimental subject.

A LIVING WILL
And Appointment of a
Surrogate Decision Maker

To My Family, My Physician,
My Lawyer, and All Others
Whom it May Concern

Death is as much a reality as birth, growth, and aging—it is the one certainty of life. In anticipation of decisions that may have to be made about my own dying and as an expression of my right to refuse treatment, I _____

(print name)

being of sound mind, make this statement of my wishes and instructions concerning treatment.

By means of this document, which I intend to be legally binding, I direct my physician and other care providers, my family, and any surrogate designated by me or appointed by a court, to carry out my wishes. If I become unable, by reason of physical or mental incapacity, to make decisions about my medical care, let this document provide the guidance and authority needed to make any and all such decisions.

If I am permanently unconscious or there is no reasonable expectation of my recovery from a seriously incapacitating or lethal illness or condition, I do not wish to be kept alive by artificial means. I request that I be given all care necessary to keep me comfortable and free of pain, even if pain-relieving medications may hasten my death, and I direct that no life-sustaining treatment be provided except as I or my surrogate specifically authorize.

This request may appear to place a heavy responsibility upon you, but by making this decision according to my strong convictions, I intend to ease that burden. I am acting after careful consideration and with understanding of the consequences of your carrying out my wishes. *List optional specific provisions in this space below. (See other side)*

Reprinted by permission.

Durable Power of Attorney for Health Care Decisions (Cross out if you do not wish to use this section)

To effect my wishes, I designate _____ , residing at _____ (Phone #) _____ , (or if he or she shall for any reason fail to act, _____ (Phone #) _____ , residing at_____) as my health care surrogate— that is, my attorney-in-fact regarding any and all health care decisions to be made for me, including the decision to refuse life-sustaining treatment—if I am unable to make such decisions myself. This power shall remain effective during and not be affected by my subsequent illness, disability or incapacity. My surrogate shall have authority to interpret my Living Will, and shall make decisions about my health care as specified in my instructions or, when my wishes are not clear, as the surrogate believes to be in my best interests. I release and agree to hold harmless my health care surrogate from any and all claims whatsoever arising from decisions made in good faith in the exercise of this power.

I sign this document knowingly, voluntarily, and after careful deliberation, this_____ day of_____ , 19_____ .

_____
(signature)

Address _____

_____

I do hereby certify that the within document was executed and acknowledged before me by the principal this _____ day of _____ , 19 _____ .

_____

_____
Notary Public

Witness_____

Printed Name _____

Address _____

_____

Witness_____

Printed Name_____

Address_____

_____

Copies of this document have been given to:

(Optional) My Living Will is registered with Concern for Dying (No. _____)
Distributed by Concern for Dying, 250 West 57th Street, New York, NY 10107 (212) 246-6962

How to Use Your Living Will

The Living Will should clearly state your preferences about life-sustaining treatment. You may wish to add specific statements to the Living Will in the space provided for that purpose. Such statements might concern:

- Cardiopulmonary resuscitation
- Artifical or invasive measures for providing nutrition and hydration
- Kidney dialysis
- Mechanical or artifical respiration
- Blood transfusion
- Surgery (such as amputation)
- Antibiotics

You may also wish to indicate any preferences you may have about such matters as dying at home.

The Durable Power of Attorney for Health Care

This optional feature permits you to name a surrogate decision maker (also known as a proxy, health agent or attorney-in-fact), someone to make health care decisions on your behalf if you lose that ability. As this person should act according to your preferences and in your best interests, you should select this person with care and make certain that he or she knows what your wishes are and about your Living Will.

You should not name someone who is a witness to your Living Will. You may want to name an alternate agent in case the first person you select is unable or unwilling to serve. If you do name a surrogate decision maker, the form must be notarized. (It is a good idea to notarize the document in any case.)

Important Points to Remember

- Sign and date your Living Will.
- Your two witnesses should not be blood relatives, your spouse, potential beneficiaries of your estate or your health care proxy.
- Discuss your Living Will with your doctors; and give them copies of your Living Will for inclusion in your medical file, so they will know whom to contact in the event something happens to you.

- Make photo copies of your Living Will and give them to anyone who may be making decisions for you if you are unable to make them yourself.
- Place the original in a safe, accessible place, so that it can be located if needed—not in a safe deposit box.
- Look over your Living Will periodically (at least every five years), initial and redate it so that it will be clear that your wishes have not changed.

Index